LUPUS

Edited by **Wahid Ali Khan**

Lupus
http://dx.doi.org/10.5772/65819
Edited by Wahid Ali Khan

Contributors

Konstantinos Tselios, Alexandros Sarantopoulos, Ioannis Gkougkourellas, Panagiota Boura, Andrei Stepanovich Trofimenko, Antoni Hrycek, Eugeniusz Hrycek, Iwona Banasiewicz – Szkrobka, Pawel Buszman, Aleksander Zurakowski1, Xin Luo, Qinghui Mu, Michael Edwards, S. Ahmed, Christopher Reilly, Takeshi Kuroda, HIroe Sato, Georgy Nevinsky, Wahid Ali Khan, Gaffar Sarwar Zaman

Published by InTech
Janeza Trdine 9, 51000 Rijeka, Croatia

Publishing Process Manager Maja Bozicevic
Technical Editor SPi Global
Cover InTech Design team

First published May, 2017
Printed in Croatia
Legal deposit, Croatia: National and University Library in Zagreb

Additional hard copies can be obtained from orders@intechopen.com

Lupus, Edited by Wahid Ali Khan
p. cm.
Print ISBN 978-953-51-3179-3
Online ISBN 978-953-51-3180-9

For EU product safety concerns:
IN TECH d.o.o., Prolaz Marije Krucifikse Kozulić 3, 51000 Rijeka, Croatia,
info@intechopen.com or visit our website at intechopen.com.

Meet the editor

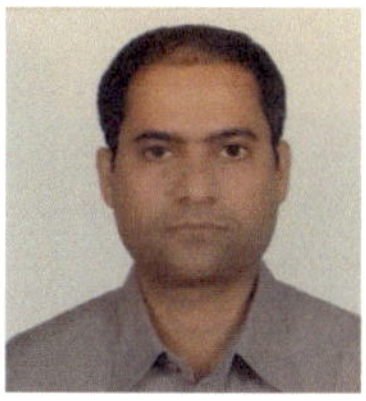

Dr. Wahid Ali Khan is an Assistant Professor in the Department of Clinical Biochemistry, College of Medicine, King Khalid University, Abha, KSA. Dr. Khan has served as a member of the editorial board of more than six international journals and guest editor for two journals. His research interest includes the role of estrogen and its metabolites in various autoimmune diseases including lupus. He is also interested in cloning of interferon alpha 2b and finding out its role in the pathogenesis of lupus. Dr. Khan has published more than 25 articles, 4 reviews, and 2 book chapters. He is also the editor of three books, which had been well recognized and documented by international research community.

Contents

Preface

It gives me great pleasure to present the book *Lupus* that highlights the important updates regarding this subject. This book *Lupus* is one of its own kinds that consist of four major sections: "Introduction to Lupus," "Antibodies and Lymphocytes in Lupus," "Additional Complications in Lupus," and "Diet and Microbes in Lupus." The first section includes two chapters that mainly deal with introduction and physiology of lupus. The first chapter in this section discusses generally about lupus and main factors predisposing to this disease. The second chapter deals with the introduction of lupus, historical perspectives and physiology, epidemiology, and relationship of SLE with heredity and genes.

SLE is an autoimmune disease that is known for the production of autoantibodies against various types of autoantigens. Although the presence of these autoantibodies has been well established among SLE patients, we still don't know much about their mechanism of action and how they act against different antigens. SLE is also characterized by a number of immune system aberrations involving deficiencies in both innate and adaptive immune mechanism including intercommunication between T and B lymphocytes and other antigen-presenting cells. Tregs represent a subpopulation of the CD4+ T lymphocytes depleted from the periphery of active lupus SLE patients and highly associated with decreased activity that might be used as possible marker for this disease. The second section, i.e., "Antibodies and Lymphocytes in Lupus," addresses all these issues and consists of three chapters with two chapters explaining autoantibody issues in lupus and one on T lymphocytes.

The third section of the book, i.e., "Additional Complications in Lupus," explains different types of complications that arise either due to the SLE itself such as atherosclerosis or due to the therapy used to treat this disease such as idiopathic osteonecrosis and atypical femoral fracture. SLE is also a disease that can affect various tissues and organ systems including the heart. Patients with SLE are at higher risk of developing atherosclerosis, and some adipocytokines/adipokines are known to play an important role for this process in SLE patients. Glucocorticoid is the first line of treatment for SLE patients, and because of its serious adverse effects, it is responsible for idiopathic osteonecrosis and atypical femoral fracture in SLE patients.

The fourth section, i.e., "Diet and Microbes in Lupus," consists of one chapter only that delineates the role of diet and microbes in the pathogenesis of SLE. I believe that this book would serve as an important resource for all students/scientists who seek knowledge from various aspects of lupus. I am very much confident that this book would be of great use for all those who want to know the latest update on lupus.

Wahid Ali Khan
Department of Clinical Biochemistry
College of Medicine, King Khalid University
Abha, Kingdom of Saudi Arabia

Section 1

Introduction to Lupus

Chapter 1

Introductory Chapter: Systemic Lupus Erythematosus - Different Predisposing Factors

Wahid Ali Khan

Additional information is available at the end of the chapter

http://dx.doi.org/10.5772/intechopen.69277

1. Introduction

Systemic lupus erythematosus (SLE) is a complex, multisystem autoimmune disease characterized by impaired immune tolerance resulting in the production of pathogenic autoantibodies and immune complexes [1]. Prevalence of SLE ranges between 20 and 150/100,000 and its incidence ranges between 1 and 10/100,000 [2]. American College of Rheumatology revised their criteria for the classification of SLE [3]. Their incidence is moat common in some ethnic group such as Asians, Australian Aborigines, African Americans, and Hispanics. Incidence rate has been raised in recent years that may probably due to better detection techniques for the disease. In the past few decades, the prognosis for SLE patients has been improved, and it was found that about 90% of the cases have 10-year survival rate [4]. This might be due to the fact that a combination of diagnosis of earlier disease and of milder disease and partially due to the development of various serological test used for SLE and combined used of steroids and various immunosuppressive drugs and availability of the techniques such as renal dialysis and transplantation [5]. Although, the exact cause of SLE remains elusive, but there is a consensus that it might be due to the combination various factors such as immunological, genetic and environmental. All these factors may somehow responsible for the chronic course of the disease. It is found that autoreactive T cells hold responsible for the activation of B cells that might be stimulated to produce antibodies by high levels of cytokines (pro-inflammatory) such as interleukin 10, interleukin 6, tumor necrosis factor-α and interferon γ in different SLE patients [6]. In addition, production of antibody might be elevated further by B and T cells through interaction via co-stimulatory molecules that inhibit apoptosis. Autoantibodies produce from these cells are very likely responsible for the pathogenic effect on tissues in different SLE patients [7]. In addition, impaired production of IL-10 and IL-12 causing B cell activation and inhibition in the normal function of T cells [8]. Interleukin 12 responsible for the down-regulation of interleukin 10 and lower level somehow correlate with elevated activity and nephritis [9]. More recently, it has been assumed that the stimulus of autoantibodies production is the inability to depose apoptotic cells from the body [10].

2. Different factors predisposing to SLE

SLE is an autoimmune disease which involves multisystem disorder whose etiology is unknown but supposes to be multifactorial in origin. Different epidemiological data showed that there are many factors that might trigger SLE. These include gender, age, racial, hormonal, genetic, and environmental factors.

2.1. Hormonal factors

The incidence and prevalence of SLE varies considerably worldwide [11]. In addition, gender discrepancies are also observed in SLE burden, with a higher number of cases was found in women as compared to men. It has been observed that this disease has been affected to about 80–90% women of all the reported cases [12]. Prevalence of SLE is far more in women in comparison to men [13]. In addition, if we compare female to male ratio during childhood, it was found to about 12:1 [14]. These data showed that hormone plays an important role in etiology of SLE [15]. Hormones such as estrogen have both anti-inflammatory and pro-inflammatory properties depending upon different influencing factors [16]. There are various studies that can explain the role of estrogen and its metabolites in SLE [15, 17]. The 2-hydroxyestrogens was found to be 10 times lower in patients with SLE than the control subjects, and the ratio of 16-hydroxyestrone/2-hydroxyestrogen was found to be 20 times higher in these SLE patients [18]. Previous studies also showed that SLE patients have increased the concentration of serum 16-hydroxyestrone. α-Hydroxylation of estrogen was found to increased in SLE patients, producing more estrogen metabolites that were reported to elevate B cell differentiation and activation of T cells [19]. Another important mechanism through which estrogen plays a role in SLE etiopathogenesis is the involvement of quinone-semiquinone redox cycling of estrogen to produce free radicals that can damage DNA. This would probably alter its antigenicity leading to the induction and increased level of SLE autoantibodies that somehow cross-reacting with native DNA [20].

Estrogens are known to have higher immune reactivity in females and are also contribute to triggering autoimmune diseases including SLE [14]. Various conditions (physiological, therapeutic, and pathological) such as menstrual cycle, inflammatory cytokines, chronic stress, treatment with a corticosteroid, oral contraceptives, and steroid hormone replacement might cause variation in serum estrogen concentration and this variation in concentration contribute to SLE in different groups of the population [21].

2.2. Genetic factors

The difference (polymorphism) in various types of genes may also enhance the risk for the development of SLE, and in most of the cases, different genetic factors are thought to contribute to the pathogenesis of this disease. In most of the cases, SLE is caused by a mutation in multiple genes and rarely seen by a mutation in the single gene. Multiple genes, that are causing SLE, are linked to the function of the immune system and difference in this most likely effect proper controls and targeting of the immune system. Genetic factors along with environmental factors play an important role in the determination of SLE susceptibility [22]. It is suggested that genetic factors play an important role not only in disease susceptibility but also in the development of SLE phenotype [22]. The genes that can increase SLE susceptibility are the genes included in the interferon pathway, also containing IRF5, IF1H1, and STAT4 [23]. The biggest genetic risk for SLE is confirmed by deficiencies of complement pathway proteins such as C1q, B and C4A, and C2. Mutation in TREX1 gene causing the accumulation of DNA that encodes for 3'repair endonuclease activity. The defect in these genes is although rare but susceptibility in most patients arises from a combination of normal variation in different genes. High-density SNP screening of the major histocompatibility complex in SLE showed strong evidence for independent susceptibility regions including HLADR2, HLADR3, and HLA-DRB1 [24]. There are other types of genes that can regulate the immune system, are also implicated in SLE. These genes include those that can influence the function or survival of T and B lymphocytes (BANK-1, PTPN22, OX4OL, BLK, LYN, PD-1) or those involved in the clearance of immune complex including FcγRIIa, ITGAM, and complement proteins. The class II alleles HLA-DR2 and HLA-DR3 were found to be the most prominent genetic risk factors for SLE in some group (Caucasian group) and these alleles showed twofold to threefold increased the risk for this disease [25]. There are two alleles namely HLA-DQ and –DR, which interestingly showed a close association with SLE autoantibodies [26]. The signal transducer and activator of transcription (STAT4) genes were first identified in rheumatoid arthritis and later on, it shows strong association with SLE [27]. Careful analyses of this gene revealed that there is a strong association of this gene not only with SLE nephritis but also with double-stranded DNA, autoantibodies and younger age of onset [28]. The difference in the promoter of certain genes (pentraxin C-reactive protein, CRP) has been linked with SLE or SLE nephritis in some ethnic group [29]. CRP is an important candidate for SLE susceptibility. This protein is found to be an effective innate immune modulator that brings out the clearance of cell debris and apoptotic bodies and we know that any defect in the clearance of apoptotic waste is belief to be an important process that mainly responsible for the promotion and development of autoantibodies in SLE patients [29]. From all these studies, it is observed that genetic factors play an important role in SLE pathogenesis. These evidence suggest that these factors play a role not only in disease susceptibility but also in the development of disease phenotype.

2.3. Environmental factors

Although hormonal and genetic factors predispose towards SLE but the initiation of the disease may trigger from various environmental and exogenous factors. Different environmental toxicants and agents, such as alcohol, smoking, various chemical, ultraviolet light, various infectious agents, hormone, and therapeutic agents, have been involving in inducing SLE. All these environmental agents along with other types of factors have been associated with the occurrence of SLE [30]. Infectious agents may disturb immune regulation and stimulate various immune response through molecular mimicry; food influence the production of inflammatory mediators; drug or toxin alter cellular responsiveness and antigenicity of self-antigen;

and different chemical and physical agents like ultraviolet light, alcohol, etc. induce inflammation, causes cellular apoptosis, and also damage tissue and DNA. Various types of drugs like procainamide and hydralazine (aromatic amines or hydrazines) induce lupus-like symptoms in those individuals who are ingested or in contact with these agents [31, 32]. In addition, more use of hair dyes, which consists of aromatic amines, have been associated with the development of SLE [33]. Sunlight exposure is one of the main environmental factors associated with the induction and exacerbation of SLE. Exposure of ultraviolet light is found to be an important factor that may trigger SLE in many patients. This exposure of skin with ultraviolet light alter the position and structure of DNA as well as Ro and nRNP antigen and somehow increase its immunogenicity [34]. Several dietary factors along with various infectious agents are involved in the pathogenesis of SLE. There are the reports that showed that ingestion of alfalfa sprouts that consists of L-canavanine, might involved in the development of lupus-like syndrome [35]. The use of environmental estrogen had been increasing over the years and they are present in the human body from the consumption of meat and milk product from lives stock that is given synthetic estrogen [36]. Moreover, these estrogens have also been used by postmenopausal women and for contraceptive purposes. Hormone replace therapy as well as oral contraceptives has been shown to be a risk factor in the development of SLE [37]. The environmental estrogen with another endocrine hormone may act as an important agent to trigger autoimmunity in susceptible individuals. The development of SLE may depend on several factors such as genetic background, dose, sex, age, a period of exposure, and status of the immune system at the time of contact of these environmental agents.

Author details

Wahid Ali Khan

Address all correspondence to: wahidalikhan@rediffmail.com

Department of Clinical Biochemistry, College of Medicine, King Khalid University, Abha, Kingdom of Saudi Arabia

References

[1] Oon S, Wilson NJ, Wicks I. Targeted therapeutics in SLE: Emerging strategies to modulate the interferon pathway. Clinical and Translational Immunology. 2016;**5**:e79

[2] Squatrito D, Emmi D, Silvestri E, et al. Pathogenesis and potential therapeutic targets in systemic lupus erythematosus from bench to bedside. Autoimmune Highlights. 2014;**5**:33–45

[3] Hochberg MC. Updating the American College of rheumatology revised criteria for the classification of systemic lupus erythematosus. Arthritis & Rheumatology. 1997;**40**:1725

[4] Peschken CA, Esdaile JM. Systemic lupus erythematosus in North Americans Indians: A population base study. The Journal of Rheumatology. 2000;**27**:1884–1891

[5] Goldblatt F, Isenberg DA. New therapies for systemic lupus erythematosus. Clinical & Experimental Immunology. 2005;**140**:205–212

[6] Davas EM, Tsirogianni A, Kappou I, et al. Serum IL-6, TNFα, p55 srTNFα, p75 srTNFα, sr II-2α levels and disease activity in systemic lupus erythematosus. Clinical Rheumatology. 1999;**18**:17–22

[7] Hagelberg S, Lee Y, Bergman I, et al. Long term follow up of childhood lupus nephritis. The Journal of Rheumatology. 2002;**29**:2635–2642

[8] Emilie D, Mariette X. Interleukin 10: A new therapeutic target in systemic lupus erythematosus? Joint Bone Spine. 2001;**68**:1–5

[9] Min DJ, Cho ML, Cho CS, et al. Decreased production of interleukin-12 and interferon-gamma is associated with renal involvement is systemic lupus erythematosus. Scandinavian Journal of Rheumatology. 2001;**30**:159–163

[10] Taylor PR, Carugati A, Fadok VA, et al. A hierarchical role for classical pathway complement proteins in the clearance of apoptotic cell in vivo. The Journal of Experimental Medicine. 2000;**192**:359–366

[11] Danchenko N, Satia JA, Anthony MS, Epidemiology of systemic lupus erythematosus: A comparison of worldwide disease burden. Lupus. 2006;**15**:308–318

[12] Siegel M, Lee SL. The epidemiology of systemic lupus erythematosus. Seminars in Arthritis and Rheumatism. 1973;**3**:1–54

[13] Jacobson DL, Gange SJ, Rose NR, Graham NMH. Epidemiology an estimated population burden of selected autoimmune disease in the United States. Clinical Immunology and Immunopathology. 1997;**84**:223–243

[14] Ramsey-Goldman R, Manzi S. Systemic lupus erythematosus. Women and Health. Academic Press. 2000:704

[15] Khan WA, Habib S, Khan WA, et al. Enhanced binding of circulating SLE autoantibodies to catecholestrogen-copper-modified DNA. Molecular and Cellular Biochemistry. 2008;**315**:143–150

[16] Straub RH. The complex role estrogen in inflammation. Endocrine Reviews. 2007;**28**: 521–574

[17] Cohen-Solal JF, Jeganathan V, Grimaldi CM, et al. Sex hormone and SLE: Influencing the fate of autoreactive B cells. Current Topics in Microbiology and Immunology. 2006;**305**:67–88

[18] Weidler C, Harle P, Schedel J, et al. Patients with rheumatoid arthritis and systemic lupus erythematosus have increased renal excretion of mitogenic estrogen in relation to andogenous antiestrogen. The Journal of Rheumatology. 2004;**31**:489–494

[19] Lahita RG. The connective tissue diseases and the overall influence of gender. International journal of fertility and menopausal studies. 1996;**41**:156–160

[20] Khan WA, Moinuddin, Khan MWA, Chabbra HS. Catecholestrogen: Possible role in systemic lupus erythematosus. Rheumatology. 2009;**48**:1345–1351

[21] Cutolo M, Sulli A, Capellino S, et al. Sex hormone influence on the immune system: Basic and clinical agents in autoimmunity. Lupus. 2004;**13**:635–638

[22] Ceciarelli F, Perricone C, Borgiani P, et al. Genetic factors in systemic lupus erythematosus: Contribution in disease phenotypes. Journal of Immunology Research. 2015;**745647**: 1–11

[23] Hagberg N, Ronnblom S. Sytemic lupus erythematosus – A disease with a dysregulated type I interferon system. Scandinavian Journal of Immunology. 2015;**82**:199–207

[24] Barcellos LF, May SL, Ramsay PP, et al. High-density SNP screening of the major histocompatibily complex in systemic lupus erythematosus demonstrate strong evidence for independent susceptibility genes. PLoS Genetics. 2009;**5**:e1000696

[25] Tsao BP, Wu H. The genetics of human lupus. In: Wallace DJ, Hahn BH, editors. Dubois Lupus Erythematosus. 7th ed. Philadelphia: Lippincott Williams & Wilkins; 2007. pp. 54–81

[26] Fernando MM, Stevens CR, Sabeti PC, et al. Identification of two independent risk factors for lupus within the MHC in United Kingdom families. PLoS Genetics. 2007;**3**:e192

[27] Remmers EF, Plenge RM, Lee AT, et al. STAT4 and the risk of rheumatoid arthritis and systemic lupus erythematosus. The New England Journal of Medicine. 2007;**357**:977–986

[28] Taylor KE, Remmers EF, Lee AT, et al. Specificity of the STAT4 genetic association for severe disease manifestation of systemic lupus erythematosus. PLOS Genetics. 2008;**4**:e1000084

[29] Edberg JC, Wu J, Langefeld CD, et al. Genetic variation in the CRP promoters: Association with systemic lupus erythematosus. Human Molecular Genetics. 2008;**17**:1147–1155

[30] Mak A, Tay SH. Environmental factors, toxicants and systemic lupus erythematosus. International Journal of Molecular Sciences. 2014;**15**:16043–16056

[31] Adoms LE, Mongey AB. Role genetic factors in drug-related autoimmunity. Lupus. 1994;**3**:443–447

[32] Reidenberg MM, Drayer DE, Lorenzo B, et al. Acetylation phenotypes and environmental chemical exposure of people with idiopathic systemic lupus erythematosus. Arthritis & Rheumatology. 1993;**36**:971–973

[33] Freui-Titulaer LW, Kelley DB, Grow AG, et al. Connective tissues decrease in southern Georgia: A case–control study of etiology factors. American Journal of Epidemiology. 1989;**130**:404–409

[34] Furukawa F, Kashihara-Sawami M, Lyons MB, et al. Binding of antibodies to the extractable nuclear antigens SS-A/Ro and SSB/La is induce on the surface of human keratinocytes by ultraviolet lights (UVL): Implications for the pathogenesis of photosensitive cutaneous lupus. Journal of Investigative Dermatology. 1990;**94**:77–85

[35] Prete PE. The mechanism of action of L-canavanine in inducing autoimmune phenomena. Arthritis & Rheumatology. 1985;**28**:1198–1200

[36] Ahmed SA, Hissong BD, Verthelyi D, et al. Gender and risk of autoimmune disease: Possible role of estrogenic compound. Environmental Health Perspectives. 1999;**107**: 681–686

[37] Sanchez-Guerrero J, Liaug MH, Karlson EW, et al. Postmenopausal estrogen therapy and the risk for developing systemic lupus erythematosus. Annals of Internal Medicine. 1995;**122**:430–433

Chapter 2

Introduction and Physiology of Lupus

Gaffar Sarwar Zaman

Additional information is available at the end of the chapter

http://dx.doi.org/10.5772/intechopen.68635

Abstract

Lupus is an autoimmune disease, which means that the immune system erroneously acts against its own healthy tissues. It usually follows a chronic course and hence can also be termed as a chronic disease. It may involve only a single organ, but in its due course, it usually involves multiple organs of the body. There are various types of rashes in systemic lupus erythematosus (SLE), the butterfly-like rash being the most famous. Up to now, many classifications of lupus have been given, but the classification into the discoid lupus and the disseminated lupus is being most widely accepted. From the time of Hippocrates, it was assumed to be present, and after many research studies, it is still a dreaded disease. Females are more affected than males by this disease. In the past, the survival rate of SLE was very poor. Now the survival rate has increased, thanks to the newer drugs and other strategies taken against this disease. The main causes of death from SLE were renal disease, neoplasm, CVD, cerebrovascular disease, respiratory disease and infection. It has been found that various genes cause the disease. In a small fraction of patients, the disease may be attributed to a single gene. But majority of the patients with this disease have multiple genes.

Keywords: chronic disease, autoimmune, autoantibodies, immune system, multiple organs

1. Introduction

1.1. Definition of lupus

Systemic lupus erythematosus (SLE), which is simply known as lupus, is an autoimmune disease in which the immune system of the body erroneously onslaughts tissues in various parts of the body which are healthy [1, 2]. It may show only single organ sign or multiple system sign at the onset. It can affect the brain, skin, joints and other parts of the body. It is an autoimmune problem that has a wide-ranging clinical presentation, encircling various parts of the body (**Figures 1** and **2**).

1.2. Varieties of lupus skin reactions

Varieties of lupus skin eruptions:

(1) Acute cutaneous lupus (also called as the butterfly lupus rash or malar rash).

(2) The subacute cutaneous lupus: There are two types: (a) the first one is very sensitive to exposure to the sun and depicts red coloured pimples as the skin eruptions development begins. (b) The second variety begins as flat lesions and get larger as they enlarge to the exterior.

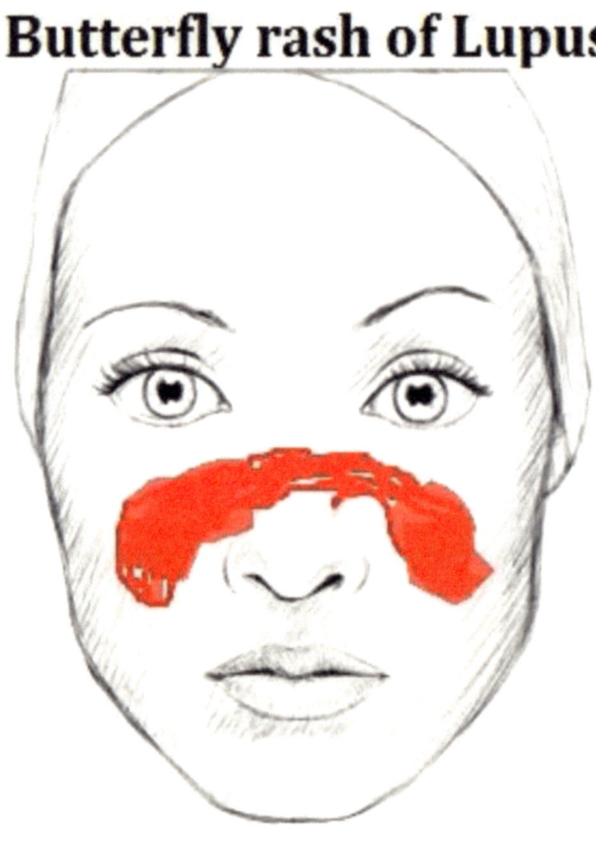

Figure 1. The butterfly rash of lupus. It is a type of condition of the skin, which is denoted by the appearance of spots/ skin eruptions over the cheekbones and also over the bridge of the nose.

http://dx.doi.org/10.5772/intechopen.68635

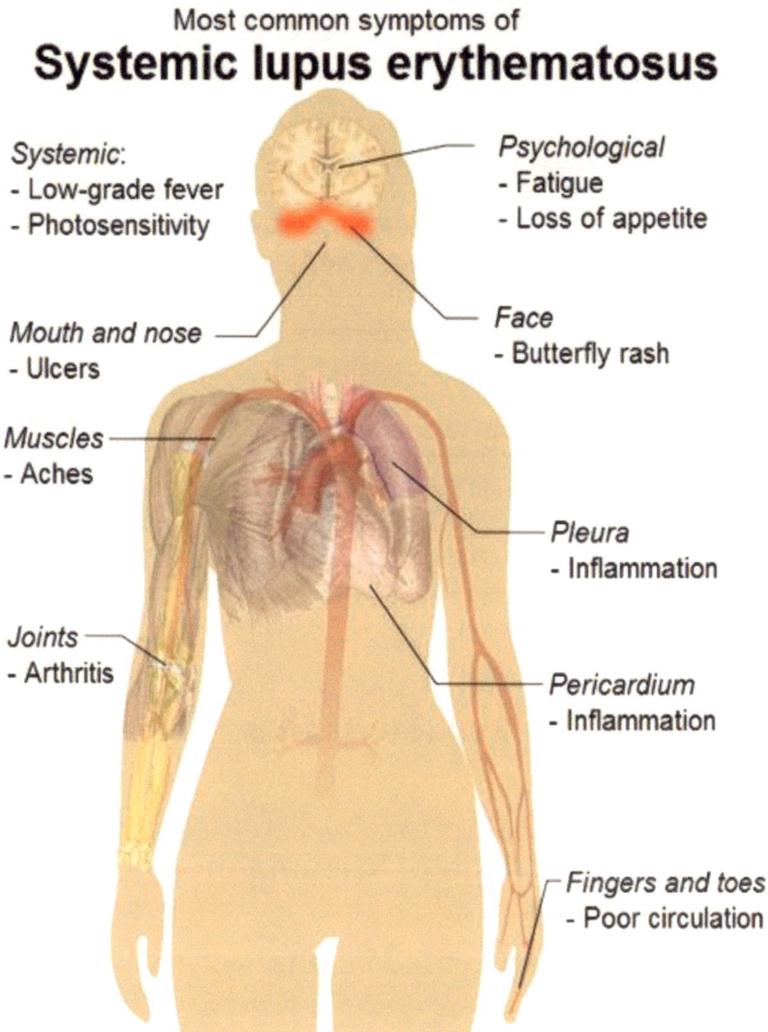

Figure 2. The most usual systemic effects of systemic lupus erythematosus, which affects various organs as shown [131].

(3) Chronic cutaneous lupus (also called discoid lupus erythematosus—DLE): these skin eruptions are found in a very few of SLE patients.

The disease SLE can attack people of all ages, races and both males and females, but it has been observed that more than 90% of new patients having SLE are women in their conceiving years. The prevalence of SLE, which has been reported recently, is 20–150 per 100,000. Data from metropolitan areas in the United States stipulated the prevalence to be 104–170 per 100,000 women [3]. The lowest incidence rates are observed in Caucasian populations [4].

1.3. Classification

Up to now, it has been divided into two parts: the discoid lupus and the disseminated lupus.

In 1971, classification criteria for SLE originated for the first time; they were subsequently revised in 1982 [5], and formally accepted by the American College of Rheumatology (ACR) in the year 1997 [6]. Whilst they have been accepted as 'classification yardstick', ACR (**Figure 3**) has been vastly used as diagnostic criteria for SLE. To diagnose a patient with SLE, the patient must have at least 4 of 11 ACR classification (**Table 1**) yardsticks. In 2012, the Systemic Lupus International Collaborating Clinics (SLICC) foundation re-evaluated and made it valid [6, 7], and now according to them, the SLE patient must have at least 4 of 17 SLICC yardsticks, which should include at least one immunologic and one clinical criterion.

One of the most important scales to assess disease activity in SLE is the systemic lupus erythematosus disease activity index (SLEDAI) [8–10]. One of the famous modified indexes is known as the safety of estrogens in lupus erythematosus national assessment (SELENA) trial also called SELENA-SLEDAI system [11].

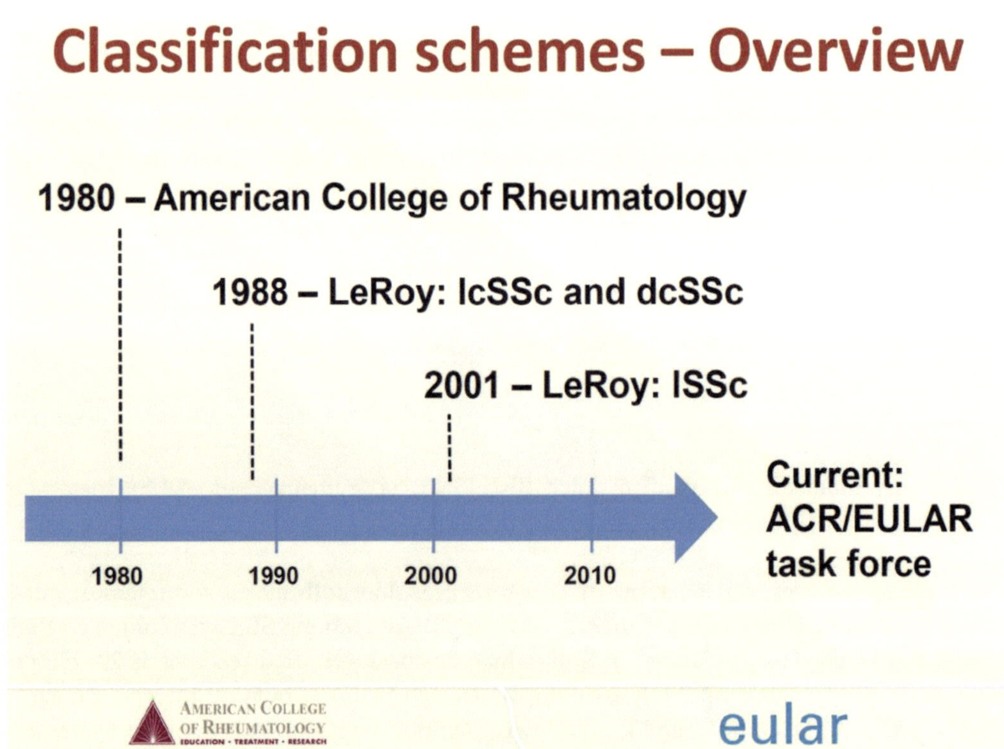

Figure 3. Classification schemes for lupus [ACR-endorsed Criteria for Rheumatic Diseases: http://www.rheumatology.org/Practice-Quality/Clinical-Support/Criteria/ACR-Endorsed-Criteria].

Criterion	Definition
1. Malar rash	Fixed erythema, flat or raised, over the malar eminences, tending to spare the nasolabial folds
2. Discoid rash	Erythematous raised patches with adherent keratotic scaling and follicular plugging; atrophic scarring may occur in older lesions
3. Photosensitivity	Skin rash as a result of unusual reaction to sunlight, by patient history or physician observation
4. Oral ulcers	Oral or nasopharyngeal ulceration, usually painless, observed by physician
5. Nonerosive arthritis	Involving two or more peripheral joints, characterized by tenderness, swelling, or effusion
6. Pleuritis or pericarditis	1. Pleuritis-convincing history of pleuritic pain or rubbing heard by a physician or evidence of pleural effusion 1. *OR* 2. Pericarditis-documented by electrocardigram or rub or evidence of pericardial effusion
7. Renal disorder	1. Persistent proteinuria > 0.5 g/d or > than 3+ if quantitation not performed 1. *OR* 2. Cellular casts—may be red cell, hemoglobin, granular, tubular, or mixed
8. Neurologic disorder	1. Seizures—in the absence of offending drugs or known metabolic derangements; e.g., uremia, ketoacidosis, or electrolyte imbalance 1. *OR* 2. Psychosis—in the absence of offending drugs or known metabolic derangements, e.g., uremia, ketoacidosis, or electrolyte imbalance
9. Hematologic disorder	1. Hemolytic anemia—with reticulocytosis 1. *OR* 2. Leukopenia—<4000/mm^3 on > 2 occasions 1. *OR* 3. Lyphopenia—< 1500/mm^3 on > 2 occasions 1. *OR* 4. Thrombocytopenia—<100,000/mm^3 in the absence of offending drugs
10. Immunologic disorder	1. Anti-DNA: antibody to native DNA in abnormal titer 1. *OR* 2. Anti-Sm: presence of antibody to Sm nuclear antigen 1. *OR* 3. Positive finding of antiphospholipid antibodies on: 1. An abnormal serum level of IgG or IgM anticardiolipin antibodies, 2. A positive test result for lupus anticoagulant using a standard method, or 3. A false-positive test result for at least 6 months confirmed by Treponema pallidum immobilization or fluorescent treponemal antibody absorption test

Criterion	Definition
11. Positive antinuclear antibody	An abnormal titer of antinuclear antibody by immunofluorescence or an equivalent assay at any point in time and in the absence of drugs

Reference: ACR-endorsed criteria for rheumatic diseases: http://www.rheumatology.org/Practice-Quality/Clinical-Support/Criteria/ACR-Endorsed-Criteria

Table 1. 1997 update of the 1982 American College of Rheumatology revised criteria for classification of systemic lupus Eeythematosus.

2. Historical perspective and physiology

Now, the origin of this disease is understandable clearly. It is conjectured that hormonal, environmental, genes, genetic variation and heredity play a significant role in its development [12]. It has been seen that if one member of a twin is affected the chances that the other twin may also be affected is 24%.

Documented proof of lupus can be tracked down to the time of the ancient Greek physician Hippocrates. In the year 400 BC, he wrote about herpes esthiomenos [13], which is conjectured to be lupus only. It has been seen that Hippocrates (**Figure 4**) mentioned about red, circumscribed inflammatory and often suppurating lesion on the skin or an internal mucous surface resulting in necrosis of tissue, which may depict present day lupus.

It has also been documented that there was a saint named Lupus, who lived in the sixth century A.D. [14].

The history can be traced back into three parts as follows:

(1) The traditional or classical phase during which the skin disarray was narrated.

(2) The conventional period during which the entire body symptoms and signs of lupus were found out after careful searching unearthed and organised in a systematic way.

(3) The contemporary period or modern phase which was portended by the unearthing of the LE cell in 1948 and is differentiated by other related discoveries in the field of science.

2.1. Traditional or classical phase

In the biography of St. Martin, for first time, we get an evidence of the word 'lupus' being used [15].

The word 'lupus' (which in Latin means 'wolf') is officially recognized to be coined by the Rogerius Grugardi, a physician who lived in the thirteenth century. He is accredited with coining 'noli me tangere', which means 'do not touch me'. He gave the term to the lesions and ulcers of the face associated with this disease. As time passed, the term underwent changes as the position of the disease changed. But the term 'lupus' remained. He used this term to

http://dx.doi.org/10.5772/intechopen.68635

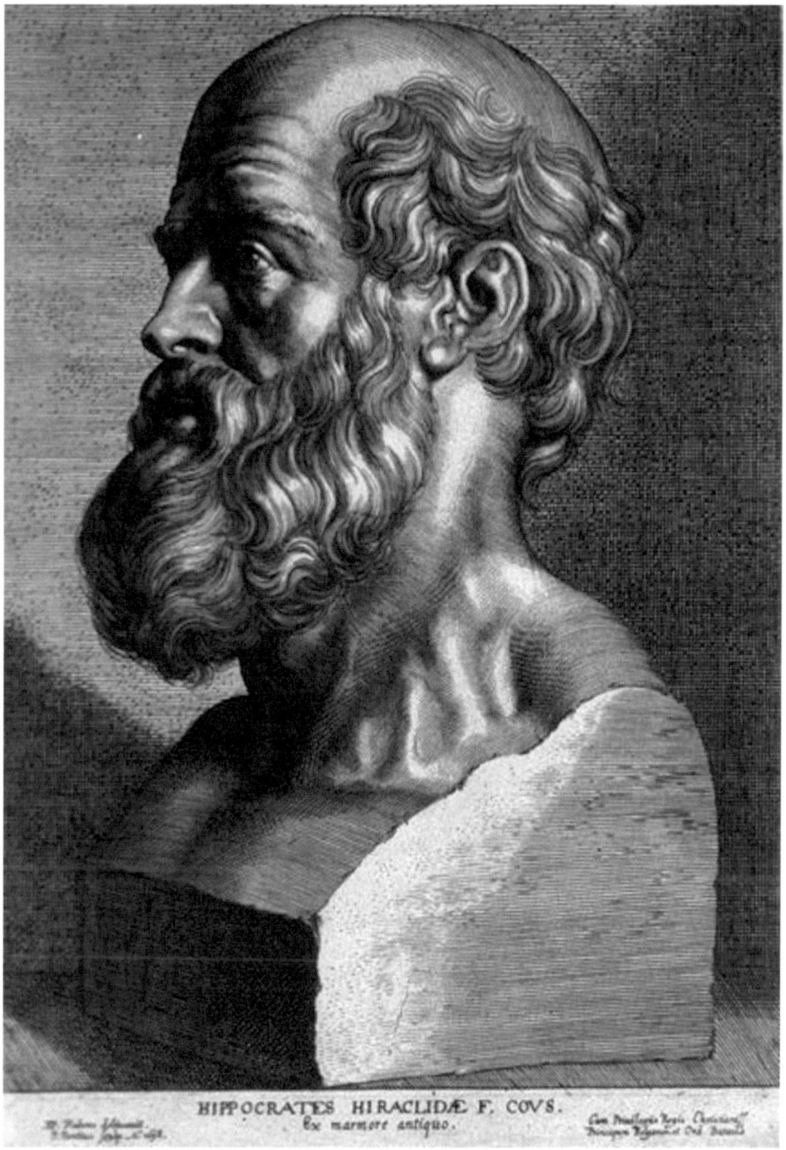

Figure 4. Hippocrates, engraving by Peter Paul Rubens, 1638 [Courtesy of the National Library of Medicine [http://laphamsquarterly.org/contributors/hippocrates].

delineate vicious lacerations of the face, which could be compared to the bite of a wolf. It was told that the characteristic butterfly rash analogous with lupus have a similarity with the teeth marks of a wolf's onslaught. The other hypothesis remarks that the terrifying impression on the face of a person resembled the impressions on the face of the wolf. The petrifying impression of people afflicted with lupus brings to the mind the terrifying tale of werewolves (**Figure 5**). These were mythologically described as humans who had magical power to meta-

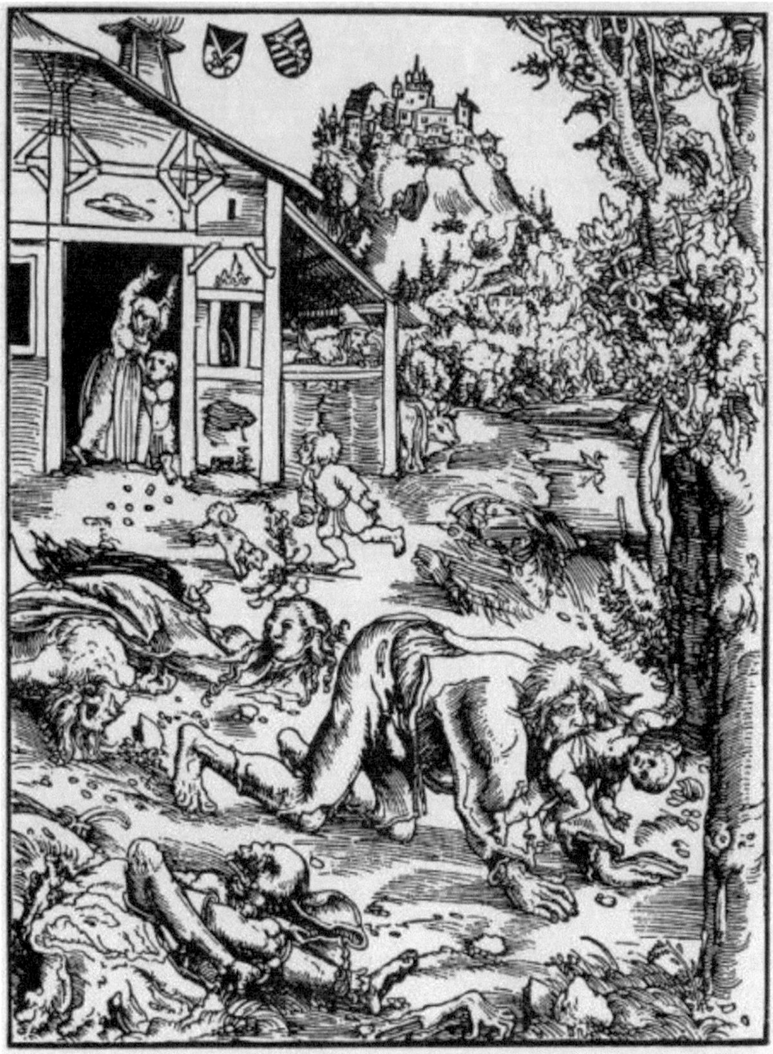

Figure 5. Werewolf attack—Woodcut of the sixteenth century by Lucas Cranach the Elder, 1512 [132].

morphose into animals. It was, therefore, the superstitious belief of the middle ages that the impressions on people faces afflicted with lupus resembled were wolves [16, 17].

2.2. Conventional or neoclassical phase

A student of Grugardi, Roland of Parma, wrote more about this disease. He also gave a detailed account of its different stages, which are not in use nowadays [18]. Erasmus Wilson (1809–1884) confused lupus with tuberculosis and syphilis [19] (**Figures 6** and **7**).

Robert Willan (1757–1812) was the one who first classified lupus based on clinical observations. Before him, the classification of lupus was mainly done according to symptomatology.

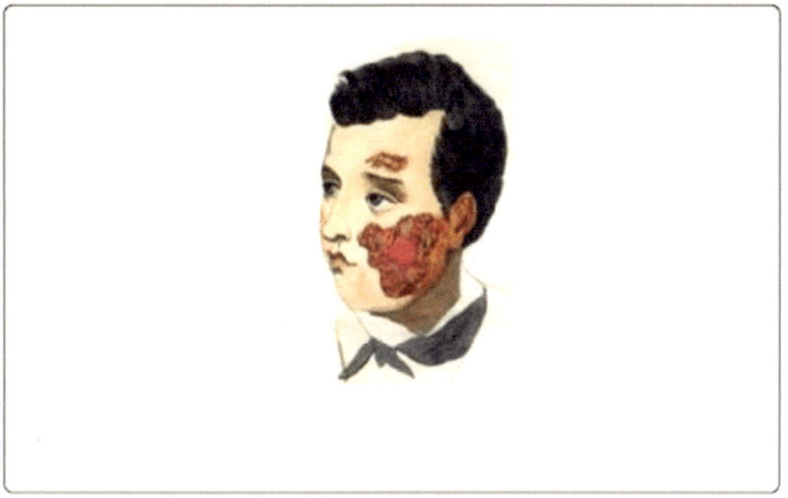

Figure 6. Lupus Vulgaris picture taken from Cazenave and Schedel's book [133].

Willan (**Figure 8**) segregated his findings into three parts: (i) lupus that extirpates the uppermost layer, (ii) lupus that extirpates the surface up to the bottom and (iii) lupus that is associated with overgrowth and dysplasia [20]. His student Thomas Bateman (1778–1821) helped him in publishing a book regarding lupus [21, 22].

Established and conventional elucidations of the variegated skin manifestations were made by Thomas Bateman.

It was in 1612 that the St. Louis Hospital was built by Biet (a pupil of Bateman) and Alibert. In the beginning, its main purpose was to help victims of plague. From1800, it started treating skin disorders. Laurent Theodore Biett (1781–1840) and Cazenave (1802–1877), who are renowned in the work of lupus, came from this school. Henri Schedel and Cazenave wrote book Abrege Pratique Des Maladies De La Peau in the year 1828.

Notable contributions were also made by Cazenave (**Figures 6** and **7**), who is credited with formulating the phrase lupus érythémateux (lupus erythematosus) in the mid-nineteenth century (**Figure 9**); creditable contributions were also made by Moriz Kaposi (1837–1902) in the late nineteenth century (**Figure 10**).

The contusions now alluded to as discoid lupus was described in 1833 by Cazenave who gave a characteristic account of the contusions; the typical distribution of the butterfly rash in the face was written by Ferdinand von Hebra in 1846.

The photosensitivity of the lesions of lupus was first described by Jonathon Hutchinson (1828–1913).

The beginning of the conventional period of lupus is accredited to the year 1872 in which Kaposi, a Viennese physician, at first delineated the whole body affecting character of lupus. It was first suggested by Kaposi about the two distinct varieties of lupus erythematosus: the

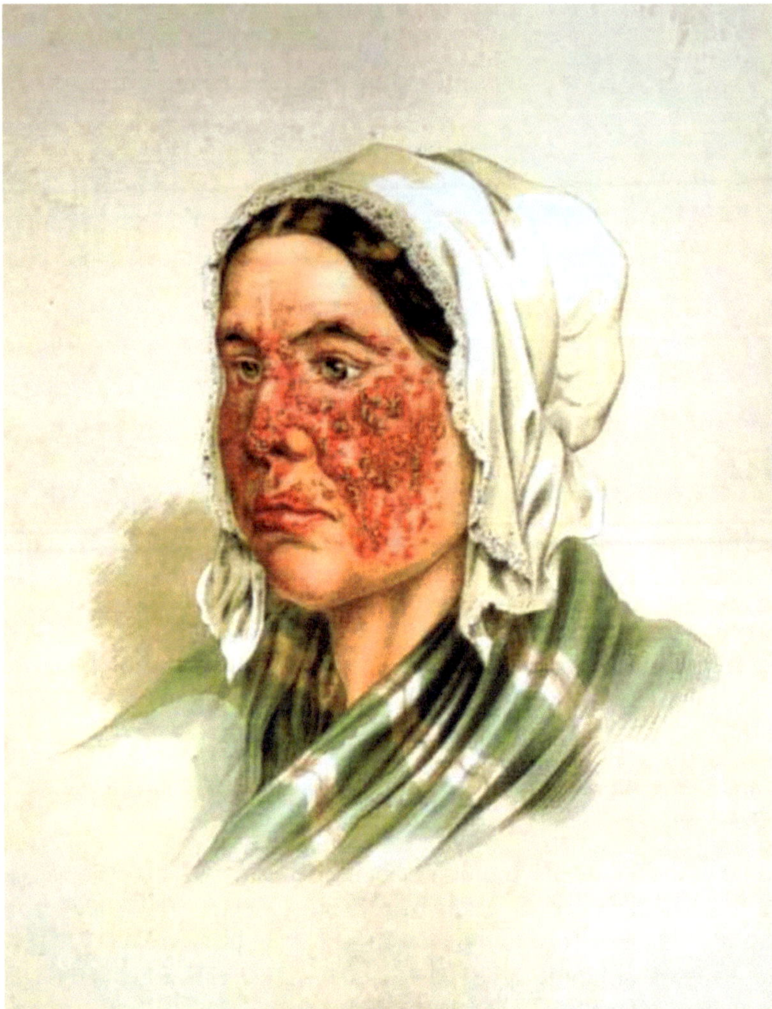

Figure 7. Drawing of lupus—1856 [Lupus erythematosus. Atlas der Hautkrankheiten. Farblithographie von Anton Elfinger. Heft I, Tafel 6, 59 × 45 cm (1856)].

discoid conformation and a disseminated conformation. In addition, he quantified the systemic manifestations of the disseminated form, which included lymphadenopathy, subcutaneous nodules, fever, arthritis with synovial hypertrophy of both small and large joints, anaemia, weight loss and involvement of the central nervous system [23]. Sir William Osler (**Figure 11**) also contributed much to the SLE concept. It was the works of this founding father of John Hopkins Hospital and Jadassohn (**Figure 12**) that the disseminated or systemic form of lupus was firmly confirmed [24, 25].

Over the following 30 years, disease studies registered the actuality of wire-loop lesions in individuals with glomerulonephritis and nonbacterial verrucous endocarditis (Libman-Sacks

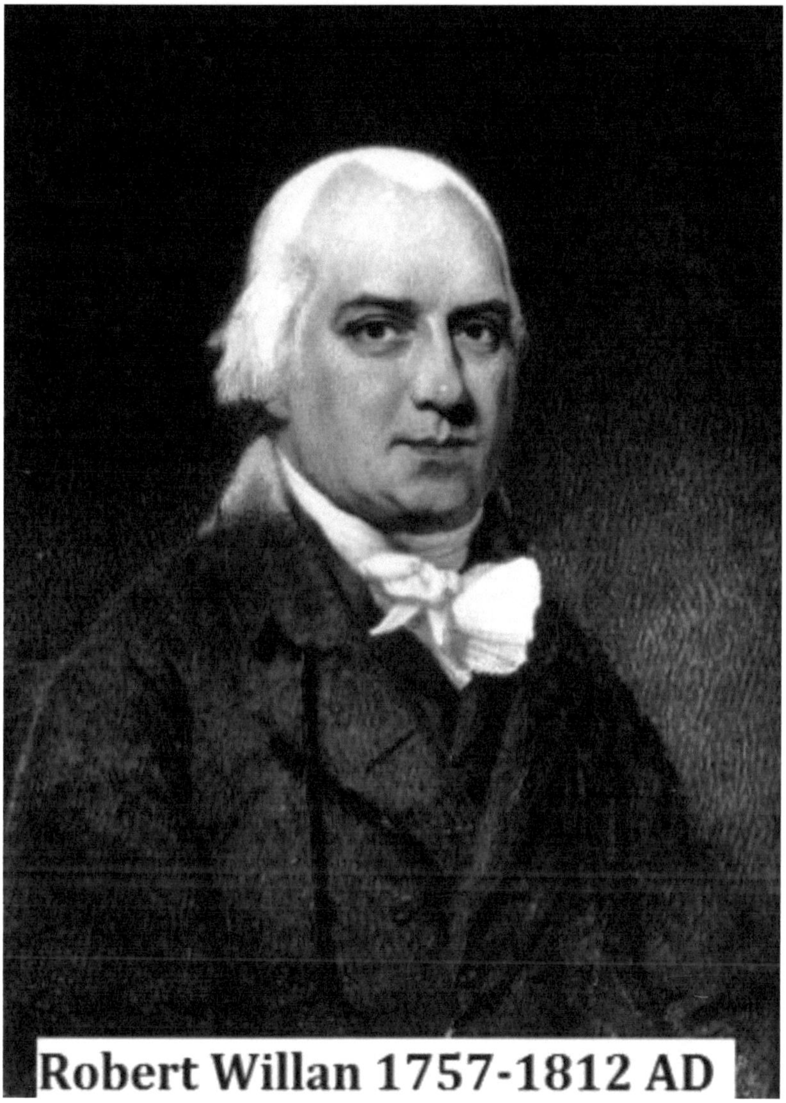

Figure 8. A painting of Robert Willan (1757–1812) [Painting by unknown, Photographed by A. C. Cooper. http://catalogue.wellcome.ac.uk/record=b1162089].

disease), discovered and named by Emanuel Libman and Benjamin Sacks [26, 27]; it was these reviews at the autopsy table that led to the fabrication of collagen disease, which was suggested by Kemperer and colleagues in the 1940s [28]. Major advancements in the field of lupus occurred during 1920–1930 by the pathologists working at Mt. Sinai Hospital in New York.

The first use of sulphonamides for the treatment of lupus occurred in 1938. Although it was unable to cure the disease, it brought some relief to the patients from the symptoms [29]. For centuries, two principles were being accepted and they were not considered wrong. Giovanni

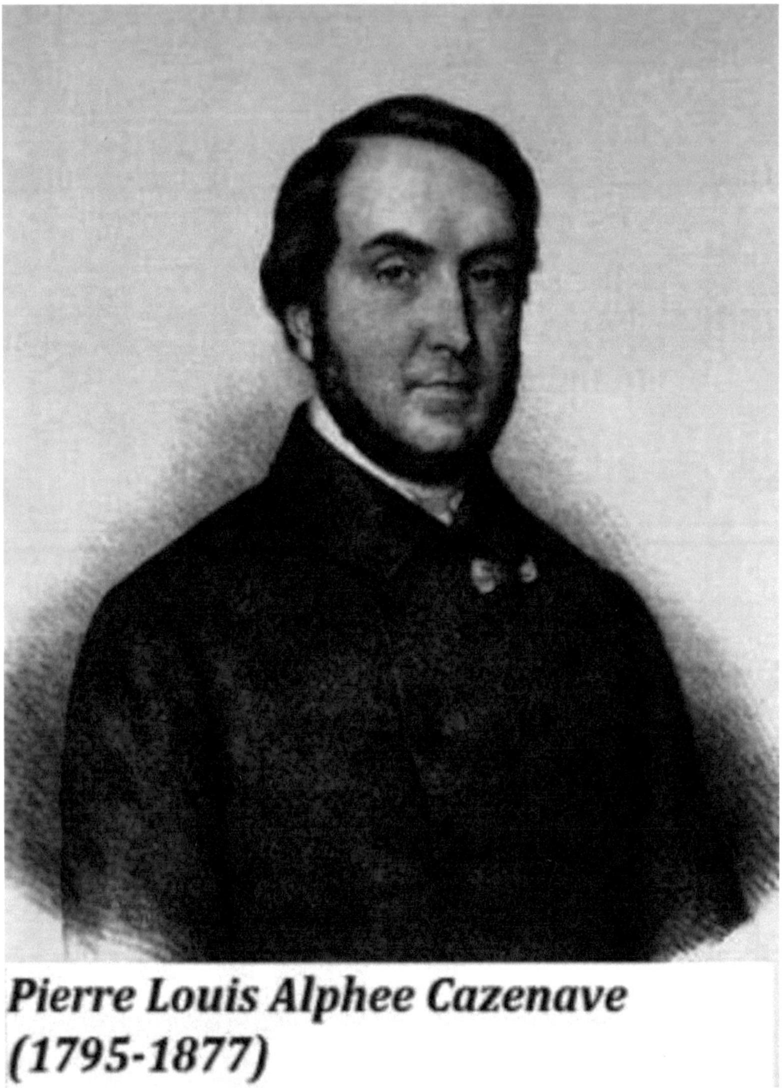

Figure 9. Pierre Louis Alphee Cazenave (1795–1877) [https://upload.wikimedia.org/wikipedia/commons/5/5d/Cazenave%2C_P.-L._Alph%C3%A9e.jpg] | Author=unknown/anonymous | Date=before 1877 |].

B. Morgagni (1682–1771) stated that a particular organ is affected by each different variety of lupus. Paul Ehrlich (1854–1915) stated the second principle in which he said that autoimmune destruction in lupus is false [30]. A German pathologist, Fritz Klinge (1892–1974), refused to accept the first principle. His study of rheumatic fever and rheumatoid arthritis showed that lupus affects connective tissue in addition to the heart [30].

Wilheim Generich, a German dermatologist, studied extensively and proved that parts of our own body can attack its own [31].

http://dx.doi.org/10.5772/intechopen.68635

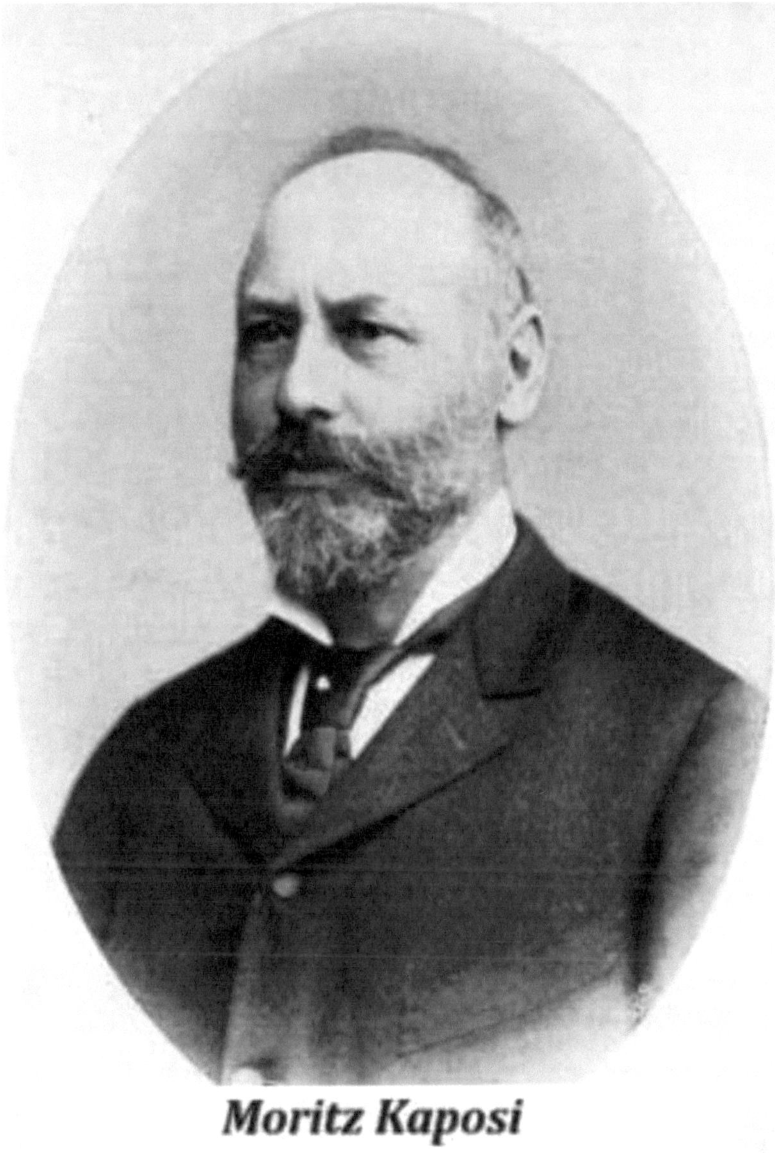

Figure 10. Moritz Kaposi (23 October 1837–6 March 1902) [From the images from the History of Medicine (NLM), US National Library of Medicine (NLM). The NLM considers this item to be in public domain. https://es.wikipedia.org/wiki/Moritz_Kaposi#/media/File:Moriz_Kaposi.jpg].

2.3. The modern phase

In 1948, the unanticipated event in a healthcare in the mid-1900s which announced the modern era was the finding of the LE cell by Hargraves et al. [32]. These findings set the scene for the present period of the utilization of immunology for studying lupus erythematosus;

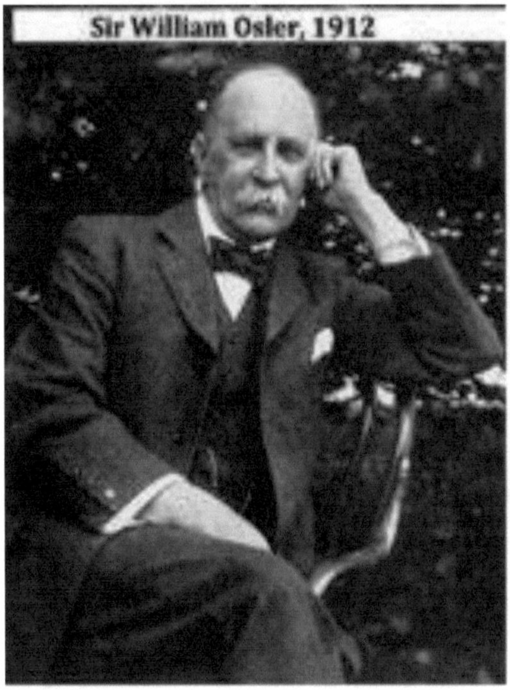

Figure 11. Sir William Osler (12 July 1849–29 December 1919) [This file is licensed under the Creative Commons Attribution 4.0 International license].

immunology also facilitated the recognition of people with much lighter forms of the disease. This, along with the use of cortisone for the treatment of this disease made life much easier for mankind [33].

In the 1950s, two new tests as being associated with lupus: the biologic false-positive test for syphilis [34] and the immunofluorescent test for antinuclear antibodies [35].

In 1957, Friou utilized the method of indirect immunofluorescence to show that antinuclear antibodies were present in the blood of people having systemic lupus [35]. After sometime, antibodies to deoxyribonucleic acid (DNA) [36] and antibodies to extractable nuclear antigens (nuclear ribonucleoprotein (nRNP), Sm, Ro, La), etc. were discovered.

Two notable advances in this age have been the invention of animal models of lupus and the discovery of the role of genetic predisposition with lupus occurrence.

The hereditary materialization of systemic lupus was first discovered by Leonhardt in 1954 and later confirmed by various observations by Arnett and Shulman [37]. Eventually, lupus having familial aggregation, the concurrence of lupus in monozygotic twin pairs and the relation of genetic markers with lupus have been delineated and reported over the last 20 years [38].

http://dx.doi.org/10.5772/intechopen.68635

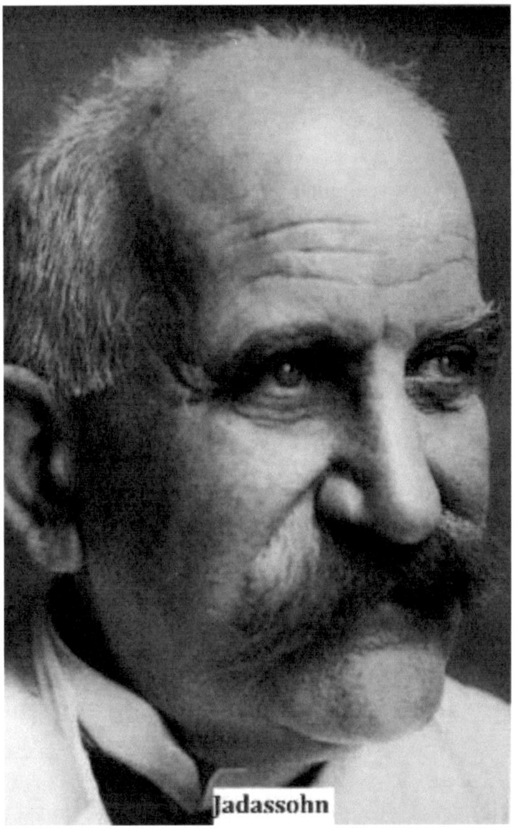

Figure 12. Joseph Jadassohn (10 September 1863–24 March 1936) [British Journal of Dermatology, vol. XLVIII (1937)].

3. Epidemiology of lupus

3.1. Incidence and prevalence of SLE

It can be said with evidence from many studies that lupus mainly affects young women, having a peak during the ages of 15–40 years. However, the onset age can be taken from infancy and the last age will be the old age [39].

Most of the studies on SLE have reported incidence of 1–10 per 100,000 person-years.

It has been found that the incidence and prevalence of SLE in blacks almost twice or thrice the rate found in whites [40–63]. SLE has been found in all the six continents of the world ((North America, Europe, South America, Australia, Africa and Asia) [64–69]. According to a large study done in Michigan, it was seen that according to the American College of Rheumatology definition, incidence rates were five and a half per 1 lakh population-years, 95% confidence interval being 5–6.1. It was found that female populations had a comparatively higher incidence (the

95% confidence interval being almost nine) and the male population had a lesser 95% confidence limit (in between one and two). It was observed that blacks had a higher incidence rate than whites. Black females also had a higher incidence rate than white females. It was seen that the age-standardised prevalence was more almost six times more in blacks than in whites [70]. Another study, which was done in a predominantly white population in the United States, showed that the incidence rate was almost 3%. It was also seen that the incidence in women was much more (almost nine times more in women than in men) than that in men [71].

Many studies (epidemiological) have found that Caucasians have a twofold to threefold lower incidence and prevalence rates than Asians [72–79]. Moreover, it was found in many studies that Asians had more severe symptoms and signs of the disease, more aggressive kidney involvements, and the autoantibody positivity was also higher in Asians than in non-Asians [76, 79–83].

3.2. Progression of the disease

It has been seen that kidney involvement is more common in males than in females—males also had kidney damages earlier in the course of their disease than females, who got the disease late in their disease course [84].

Regardless of age/other factors involved, it has been found that American, Hispanic, Asian and African SLE patients tend to have more renal serosal, hematological and neurological manifestations [69, 85–90]. It may be possible that differences seen in the different ethnic groups may be due to genetic causes, or, possibly due to socio-economic conditions which have been prevalent from ages [91–93].

There is a lupus also known as pediatric lupus it usually presents before 16 years of age. In this disease, major organ systems are involved and the patient presents with neuropsychiatric complications [88, 94–99].

When lupus occurs late in life, it usually has a more gradual onset. They have less organ systems involved, and the disease is mild in them, but the progress and natural course, for some unknown reasons, is bad [100–108].

3.3. What is the mortality rate in these patients?

In the past, the survival rate of SLE was very poor. Now the survival rate has increased, thanks to the newer drugs and other strategies taken against this disease. Also, the detection of the milder forms of this disease or detection of the disease in the earlier stages has also made it possible to increase the survival rate. Improved survival rate has been noted in studies from patients in Sweden, Taiwan, Canada, Minnesota and California [41, 109–112].

Up to now, according to many surveys, the risk of death for SLE patients is still two times that of normal patients. The 95% CI is 2.3–3.8 approximately [113].

http://dx.doi.org/10.5772/intechopen.68635

3.4. Causes of death in patients with SLE

In 2014, Thomas et al. reported that the main causes of death from SLE were renal disease, neoplasm, cardiovascular disease (CVD), cerebrovascular disease, respiratory disease and infection [114]. This data was also supported by a Canadian study [115].

It was seen in many other studies that treatment of infection with prednisone and other immunosuppressive agents was related to the death of SLE patients [116, 117]. In addition, acute confusional states, seizures were reported to cause a higher proportion of deaths in SLE [118–123].

4. Relationship of SLE with heredity and genes

SLE is a long-standing disease of variable stringency, sometimes becoming more severe and sometimes becoming less severe, with courses that can be fatal—if not treated early. The preclinical phase of the disease is denoted by autoantibodies which can be found in other systemic autoimmune diseases and results in a noticeable autoimmune phase.

The finding of SLE in identical twins, first-degree relatives having increased rate of SLE, and the sons and daughters of SLE patients having more risk of developing the disease contemplate an inheritance determined by polygenes. It has been found that various genes cause the disease. In a small fraction of patients (<5%), the disease may be attributed to a single gene. For instance, patients having homozygous deficiencies of some parts of complement have a danger of evolving SLE or a lupus-like disease [124]. But majority of the patients require multiple genes. Researches have proved that it is estimated that at least four sensitive genes are required for the formation of the disease [125, 126]. In addition, many other types of genes, especially polymorphic non-MHC genes have been reported to occur in SLE, especially genes that encode mannose-binding protein (MBP), tumour necrosis factor a, the T cell receptor, interleukin 6 (IL-6), CR1, immunoglobulin Gm and Km allotypes, FcgRIIA and FcgRIIIA (both IgG Fc receptors), and heat shock protein 70 [127, 128].

SLE patients have imperfect removal of immune complexes by phagocytic cells [129]. This is due to the decreased numbers of CR1 receptors for complement and defective receptors on cell surfaces [32, 33]. It has also been found from a recent study that non-inflammatory swallowing up of apoptotic cells is damaged in patients with SLE [130].

Author details

Gaffar Sarwar Zaman

Address all correspondence to: gffrzaman@gmail.com

King Khalid University, Abha, KSA, Saudi Arabia

References

[1] Handout on Health: Systemic Lupus Erythematosus. 2015. Available from: http://www.niams.nih.gov [Accessed: 12 June 2016]

[2] Shankar S, Behera V. Advances in management of systemic lupus erythematosus. Journal of Mahatma Gandhi Institute of Medical Sciences. 2014;**19**:28-36

[3] Jacobson DL, Gange SJ, Rose NR, Graham NM. Epidemiology and estimated population burden of selected autoimmune diseases in the United States. Clinical Immunology and Immunopathology. 1997;**84**(3):223-243

[4] Danchenko N, Satia JA, Anthony MS. Epidemiology of systemic lupus erythematosus: A comparison of worldwide disease burden. Lupus. 2006;**15**(5):308-318

[5] Tan EM, Cohen AS, Fries JF, Masi AT, McShane DJ, Rothfield NF, et al. The 1982 revised criteria for the classification of systemic lupus erythematosus. Arthritis & Rheumatology. 1982;**25**:1271-1277. DOI: 10.1002/art.1780251101. [PubMed] [Cross Ref]

[6] Hochberg MC. Updating the American College of Rheumatology revised for the classification of systemic lupus erythematosus. Arthritis Rheumatology. 1997;**40**:1725. DOI: 10.1002/art.1780400928. [PubMed] [Cross Ref]

[7] Petri M, Orbai AM, Alarcón GS, Gordon C, Merrill JT, Fortin PR, et al. Derivation and validation of the Systemic Lupus International Collaborating Clinics classification criteria for systemic lupus erythematosus. Arthritis Rheumatology. 2012;**64**:2677-2686. DOI: 10.1002/art.34473. [PMC free article] [PubMed] [Cross Ref]

[8] Lam GKV, Petri M. Assessment of systemic lupus erythematosus. Clinical and Experimental Rheumatology. 2005;**23**:S120-S132. [PubMed]

[9] Urowitz MB, Gladman DD. Measures of disease activity and damage in SLE. Baillieres Clinical Rheumatology. 1998;**12**:405-413. DOI: 10.1016/S0950-3579(98)80027-7. [PubMed] [Cross Ref]

[10] Petri M, Genovese M, Engle E, Hochberg M. Definition, incidence and clinical description of flare in systemic lupus erythematosus. Arthritis Rheumatology. 1991;**34**:937-944. DOI: 10.1002/art.1780340802. [PubMed] [Cross Ref]

[11] Smith CD1, Cyr M. The history of lupus erythematosus. From Hippocrates to Osler. Rheumatic Disease Clinics of North America. 1988;**14**:1-14

[12] Petri M, Kim MY, Kalunian KC, Grossman J, Hahn BH, Sammaritano LR, et al. Combined oral contraceptives in women with systemic lupus erythematosus. The New England Journal of Medicine. 2005;**353**:2550-2558. DOI: 10.1056/NEJMoa051135. [PubMed] [Cross Ref]

[13] Adams F. The Genuine Works of Hippocrates. Baltimore, USA: Williams & Wilkins CD; 1939. pp. 300-330

[14] de voragnine J, Ryan G, Ripperger H. The Golden Legend of Jacobus de Voragine. In: Ryan G, Ripperger H, trans. New York: Arno Press; 1969. pp. 515–516

[15] Lisnevskaia L, Murphy G, Isenberg D. Systemic lupus erythematosus. Lancet (London, England). 2014;**384**(9957):1878-1888. DOI:10.1016/s0140-6736(14)60128-8. PMID 24881804

[16] Bateman T. A Practical Synopsis of Cutaneous Diseases. 4th ed. Philadelphia, London: Collins & Croft: 1818. p. 305

[17] Wilson E. On Disease of the Skin. 5th ed. Philadelphia, London: Blanchard & Lea; 1863. p. 315

[18] Holubar K. Terminology and iconography of lupus erythematosus. A historical vignette. The American Journal of Dermatopathology. 1980;**2**:239-242

[19] Bateman T. A Practical Synopsis of Cutaneous Diseases, According to the Arrangements of Dr. Willan. 8th ed. London: Longman, Rees, Orme, Brown, Green and Longman; 1936

[20] Wallace D, Dubois HB. Lupus Erythematosus. 5th ed. USA: Williams & Wilkins; 1997. p. 3-16

[21] Lahita RG. Introduction. In: Lahita RG, editor. Systemic Lupus Erythematosus. New York: John Wiley and Sons; 1987. pp. 1-3 (fifth edition published 2010)

[22] Boltzer JW. Systemic lupus erythematosus. I. Historical aspects. Maryland State Medical Journal. 1983;**37**:439

[23] Kaposi MH. Neue Beitrage zur Keantiss des lupus erythematosus. Archives of Dermatological Research. 1872;**4**:36

[24] Osler W. On the visceral manifestations of the erythema group of skin diseases (third paper). The American Journal of the Medical Sciences. 1904;**127**:1

[25] Jadassohn J. Lupus erythematodes. In: Mracek F, editor. Handbach der Hautkrakheiten. Wien: Alfred Holder; 1904. pp. 298-404

[26] Libmann E. Sacks B. A hitherto undescribed form of volvular and mural endocarditis. Archives of Internal Medicine Journal. 1924;**33**:701

[27] Hoffman BJ. Sensitivity to sulfadiazine resembling acute disseminated lupus erythematosus. Archives of Dermatological Research. 1945;**51**:190-192

[28] Klemperer P, Pollack AD, Baehr G. Landmark article May 23, 1942: Diffuse collagen disease. Acute disseminated lupus erythematosus and diffuse scleroderma. The Journal of the American Medical Association. 1984;**251**:1593-1594

[29] Rich AR. Hypersensitivity in disease, with special reference to periarteritisnodosa, rheumatic fever, disseminated lupus erythematosus and rheumatoid arthritis. Harvey Lectures. 1947;**42**:106-147

[30] Baehr G, Klemperer P, Schifrin A. A diffuse disease of the peripheral circulation usually associated with lupus erythematosus and endocarditis. Transactions of the Association of American Physicians Journal. 1935;**50**:139

[31] Klemperer P. Pollack AD, Baehr G. Pathology of disseminated lupus erythematosus. Archives of Pathology (Chicago). 1941;**32**:569

[32] Hargraves MM, Richmond H, Morton R. Presentation of two bone marrow elements: The tart cell and the LE cell. Proceedings of the Staff Meetings Mayo Clinic. 1948;**23**:25

[33] Hench PS. Introduction: Cortisone and ACTH in clinical medicine. Proceedings of the Staff Meetings Mayo Clinic. 1950;**25**:474-476

[34] Moore JE, Lutz WB. The natural history of systemic lupus erythematosus: An approach to its study through chronic biological false positive reactions. Journal of Chronic Diseases. 1955;**2**:297

[35] Friou GJ. Clinical application of lupus serum nucleoprotein reaction using fluorescent antibody technique. Journal of Clinical Investigation. 1957;**36**:890

[36] Deicher HR, Holman HR, Kunkel HG. The precipitin reaction between DNA and a serum factor in SLE. Journal of Experimental Medicine. 1959;**109**:97

[37] Arnett FC, Shulman LE. Studies in familial systemic lupus erythematosus. Medicine 1976;**55**:313

[38] Hochberg MC. The application of genetic epidemiology to systemic lupus erythematosus. Journal of Rheumatology. 1987;**14**:867-869

[39] Ward MM, Pyun E. Studenski S. Long-term survival in systemic lupus erythematosus. Patient characteristics associated with poorer outcomes. Arthritis & Rheumatology. 1995;**38**:274-283

[40] Uramoto KM, Michet Jr. CJ, Thumboo J, Sunku J, O'Fallon WM, Gabriel SE. Trends in the incidence and mortality of systemic lupus erythematosus, 1950-1992. Arthritis & Rheumatology. 1999;**42**:46-50. [PubMed: 9920013]

[41] Naleway AL, Davis ME, Greenlee RT, Wilson DA, McCarty DJ. Epidemiology of systemic lupus erythematosus in rural Wisconsin. Lupus. 2005;**14**:862-866. [PubMed: 16302684] Pons-Estel et al. Page 7 Semin Arthritis Rheum. Author manuscript; available in PMC 2010 February 1. NIH-PA Author Manuscript NIH-PA Author Manuscript NIH-PA Author Manuscript

[42] Peschken CA, Esdaile JM. Systemic lupus erythematosus in North American Indians: A population based study. Journal of Rheumatology. 2000;**27**:1884-1891. [PubMed: 10955328]

[43] Nossent JC. Systemic lupus erythematosus on the Caribbean island of Curacao: An epidemiological investigation. Annals of the Rheumatic Diseases. 1992;**51**:1197-1201. [PubMed: 1466595]

[44] Vilar MJ, Sato EI. Estimating the incidence of systemic lupus erythematosus in a tropical region (Natal, Brazil). Lupus. 2002;**11**:528-532. [PubMed: 12220107]

[45] Stahl-Hallengren C, Jonsen A, Nived O, Sturfelt G. Incidence studies of systemic lupus erythematosus in Southern Sweden: Increasing age, decreasing frequency of renal manifestations and good prognosis. Journal of Rheumatology. 2000;**27**:685-691. [PubMed: 10743809]

[46] Jonsson H, Nived O, Sturfelt G, Silman A. Estimating the incidence of systemic lupus erythematosus in a defined population using multiple sources of retrieval. British Journal of Rheumatology. 1990;**29**:185-188. [PubMed: 2357500]

[47] Voss A, Green A, Junker P. Systemic lupus erythematosus in Denmark: Clinical and epidemiological characterization of a county-based cohort. Scandinavian Journal of Rheumatology. 1998;**27**:98-105. [PubMed: 9572634]

[48] Nossent HC. Systemic lupus erythematosus in the Arctic region of Norway. Journal of Rheumatology. 2001;**28**:539-546. [PubMed: 11296955]

[49] Hopkinson ND, Doherty M, Powell RJ. Clinical features and race-specific incidence/prevalence rates of systemic lupus erythematosus in a geographically complete cohort of patients. Annals of the Rheumatic Diseases. 1994;**53**:675-680. [PubMed: 7979581]

[50] Nightingale AL, Farmer RD, de Vries CS. Incidence of clinically diagnosed systemic lupus erythematosus 1992-1998 using the UK General Practice Research Database. Pharmacoepidemiology and Drug Safety. 2006;**15**:656-661. [PubMed: 16389657]

[51] Somers EC, Thomas SL, Smeeth L, Schoonen WM, Hall AJ. Incidence of systemic lupus erythematosus in the United Kingdom, 1990-1999. Arthritis Rheumatology. 2007;**57**:612-618. [PubMed: 17471530]

[52] Gudmundsson S, Steinsson K. Systemic lupus erythematosus in Iceland 1975 through 1984. A nationwide epidemiological study in an unselected population. Journal of Rheumatology. 1990;**17**:11621167. [PubMed: 2290155]

[53] Lopez P, Mozo L, Gutierrez C, Suarez A. Epidemiology of systemic lupus erythematosus in a northern Spanish population: Gender and age influence on immunological features. Lupus. 2003;**12**:860-865. [PubMed: 14667105]

[54] Alamanos Y, Voulgari PV, Siozos C, Katsimpri P, Tsintzos S, Dimou G, et al. Epidemiology of systemic lupus erythematosus in northwest Greece 1982-2001. Journal of Rheumatology. 2003;**30**:731-735. [PubMed: 12672191]

[55] Maskarinec G, Katz AR. Prevalence of systemic lupus erythematosus in Hawaii: Is there a difference between ethnic groups? Hawaii Medical Journal. 1995;**54**:406-409. [PubMed: 7737852]

[56] Boyer GS, Templin DW, Lanier AP. Rheumatic diseases in Alaskan Indians of the southeast coast: High prevalence of rheumatoid arthritis and systemic lupus erythematosus. Journal of Rheumatology. 1991;**18**:1477-1484. [PubMed: 1765971]

[57] Hochberg MC. Prevalence of systemic lupus erythematosus in England and Wales, 1981-2. Annals of the Rheumatic Diseases. 1987;**46**:664-666. [PubMed: 3499873]

[58] Molokhia M, McKeigue P. Risk for rheumatic disease in relation to ethnicity and admixture. Arthritis & Rheumatology. 2000;**2**:115-125. [PubMed: 11094421]

[59] Gourley IS, Patterson CC, Bell AL. The prevalence of systemic lupus erythematosus in Northern Ireland. Lupus. 1997;**6**:399-403. [PubMed: 9175027]

[60] Al-Arfaj AS, Al-Balla SR, Al-Dalaan AN, Al-Saleh SS, Bahabri SA, Mousa MM, et al. Prevalence of systemic lupus erythematosus in central Saudi Arabia. Saudi Medical Journal. 2002;**23**:87-89. [PubMed: 11938371]

[61] Bossingham D. Systemic lupus erythematosus in the far north of Queensland. Lupus. 2003;**12**:327-331. [PubMed: 12729060]

[62] Segasothy M, Phillips PA. Systemic lupus erythematosus in Aborigines and Caucasians in central Australia: A comparative study. Lupus. 2001;**10**:439-444. [PubMed: 11434580]

[63] Hart HH, Grigor RR, Caughey DE. Ethnic difference in the prevalence of systemic lupus erythematosus. Annals of the Rheumatic Diseases. 1983;**42**:529-532. [PubMed: 6625702]

[64] McCarty DJ, Manzi S, Medsger Jr. TA, Ramsey-Goldman R, LaPorte RE, Kwoh CK. Incidence of systemic lupus erythematosus. Race and gender differences. Arthritis & Rheumatology. 1995;**38**:1260-1270. [PubMed: 7575721]

[65] Johnson AE, Gordon C, Palmer RG, Bacon PA. The prevalence and incidence of systemic lupus erythematosus in Birmingham, England. Relationship to ethnicity and country of birth. Arthritis & Rheumatology. 1995;**38**:551-558. [PubMed: 7718010]

[66] Hopkinson ND, Doherty M, Powell RJ. The prevalence and incidence of systemic lupus erythematosus in Nottingham, UK, 1989-1990. British Journal of Rheumatology. 1993;**32**:110-115. [PubMed: 8428221]

[67] Chakravarty EF, Bush TM, Manzi S, Clarke AE, Ward MM. Prevalence of adult systemic lupus erythematosus in California and Pennsylvania in 2000: Estimates obtained using hospitalization data. Arthritis & Rheumatology. 2007;**56**:2092-2094. [PubMed: 17530651]

[68] Samanta A, Feehally J, Roy S, Nichol FE, Sheldon PJ, Walls J. High prevalence of systemic disease and mortality in Asian subjects with systemic lupus erythematosus. Annals of the Rheumatic Diseases. 1991;**50**:490-492. [PubMed: 1877855]

[69] Hochberg MC. The incidence of systemic lupus erythematosus in Baltimore, Maryland, 1970-1977. Arthritis and Rheumatism. 1985;**28**:80-86. [PubMed: 3966940]

[70] Somers EC, et al. Population-based incidence and prevalence of systemic lupus erythematosus: The Michigan lupus epidemiology and surveillance program. Arthritis Rheumatology 2014;**66**(2):369-378. DOI: 10.1002/art.38238

[71] Jarukitsopa S, et al. Epidemiology of systemic lupus erythematosus and cutaneous lupus in a predominantly white population in the United States. Arthritis Care & Research (Hoboken). 2015;**67**(6):817-828. DOI: 10.1002/acr.22502

[72] Ferucci ED, Johnston JM, Gaddy JR, et al. Prevalence and incidence of systemic lupus erythematosus in a population-based registry of American Indian and Alaska Native people, 2007-2009. Arthritis & Rheumatology. 2014;**66**:2494-2502

[73] Lim SS, Bayakly AR, Helmick CG, et al. The incidence and prevalence of systemic lupus erythematosus, 2002-2004: The Georgia Lupus Registry. Arthritis & Rheumatology. 2014;**66**:357-368

[74] See L, Kuo C, Chou I, et al. Sex- and age-specific incidence of autoimmune rheumatic diseases in the Chinese population: A Taiwan population-based study. Seminars in Arthritis and Rheumatism. 2013;**43**:381-386

[75] Jakes RW, Bae S, Louthrenoo W, et al. Systematic review of the epidemiology of systemic lupus erythematosus in the Asia-Pacific region: Prevalence, incidence, clinical features, and mortality. Arthritis Care & Research. 2012;**64**:159-168

[76] Flower C, Hennis AJM, Hambleton IR, et al. Systemic lupus erythematosus in an Afro-Caribbean population: Incidence, clinical manifestations and survival in the Barbados national lupus registry. Arthritis Care & Research. 2012;**64**:1151-1158

[77] Pons-Estel GJ, Alarco'n GS, Scofield L, et al. Understanding the epidemiology and progression of systemic lupus erythematosus. Seminars in Arthritis and Rheumatism. 2010;**39**:257-268

[78] Mok CC, To CH, Hod LY, et al. Incidence and mortality of systemic lupus erythematosus in a southern Chinese population, 2000-2006. Journal of Rheumatology. 2008;**35**:1978-1982

[79] Mok C. Epidemiology and survival of systemic lupus erythematosus in Hong Kong Chinese. Lupus. 2011;**20**:767-771

[80] Golder V, Connelly K, Staples M, et al. Association of Asian ethnicity with disease activity in SLE: An observational study from the Monash Lupus Clinic. Lupus. 2013;**22**:1425-1430

[81] Connelly K, Morand EF, Hoi AY. Asian ethnicity in systemic lupus erythematosus: An Australian perspective. Internal Medicine Journal. 2013;**43**:618-624

[82] Ong C, Nicholls K, Becker G. Ethnicity and lupus nephritis: An Australian single centre study. Internal Medicine Journal. 2011;**41**:270-278

[83] Cervera R, Khamashta MA, Font J, et al. Systemic lupus erythematosus: Clinical and immunologic patterns of disease expression in a cohort of 1000 patients. The European Working Party on Systemic Lupus Erythematosus. Medicine (Baltimore). 1993;**72**:113-124

[84] Pons-Estel GJ. Understanding the epidemiology and progression of systemic lupus erythematosus. Seminars in Arthritis and Rheumatism. 2010;**39**(4):257. DOI: 10.1016/j.semarthrit.2008.10.007

[85] Alarcon GS, Friedman AW, Straaton KV, Moulds JM, Lisse J, Bastian HM, et al. Systemic lupus erythematosus in three ethnic groups: III. A comparison of characteristics early in the natural history of the LUMINA cohort. LUpus in MInority populations: Nature vs Nurture. Lupus. 1999;**8**:197-209

[86] Pons-Estel BA, Catoggio LJ, Cardiel MH, Soriano ER, Gentiletti S, Villa AR, et al. The GLADEL multinational Latin American prospective inception cohort of 1,214 patients with systemic lupus erythematosus: Ethnic and disease heterogeneity among "Hispanics". Medicine (Baltimore). 2004;**83**:1-17. [PubMed: 14747764]

[87] Cooper GS, Parks CG, Treadwell EL, St Clair EW, Gilkeson GS, Cohen PL, et al. Differences by race, sex and age in the clinical and immunologic features of recently diagnosed systemic lupus erythematosus patients in the southeastern United States. Lupus. 2002;**11**:161-167. [PubMed: 11999880]

[88] Ward MM, Studenski S. Clinical manifestations of systemic lupus erythematosus. Identification of racial and socioeconomic influences. Archives of Internal Medicine. 1990;**150**:849-853. [PubMed: 2327845]

[89] Alarcón GS, McGwin Jr. G, Petri M, Reveille JD, Ramsey-Goldman R, Kimberly RP. Baseline characteristics of a multiethnic lupus cohort: PROFILE. Lupus. 2002;**11**:95-101. [PubMed: 11958584]

[90] Bastian HM, Roseman JM, McGwin Jr. G, Alarcón GS, Friedman AW, Fessler BJ, et al. Systemic lupus erythematosus in three ethnic groups. XII. Risk factors for lupus nephritis after diagnosis. Lupus. 2002;**11**:152-160. [PubMed: 12004788]

[91] Alarcón GS, McGwin Jr. G, Bartolucci AA, Roseman J, Lisse J, Fessler BJ, et al. Systemic lupus erythematosus in three ethnic groups. IX. Differences in damage accrual. Arthritis & Rheumatology. 2001;**44**:2797-2806. [PubMed: 11762940]

[92] Rivest C, Lew RA, Welsing PM, Sangha O, Wright EA, Roberts WN, et al. Association between clinical factors, socioeconomic status, and organ damage in recent onset systemic lupus erythematosus. Journal of Rheumatology. 2000;**27**:680-684. [PubMed: 10743808]

[93] Cooper GS, Treadwell EL, St Clair EW, Gilkeson GS, Dooley MA. Sociodemographic associations with early disease damage in patients with systemic lupus erythematosus. Arthritis & Rheumatology. 2007;**57**:993-999. [PubMed: 17665464]

[94] Font J, Cervera R, Espinosa G, Pallares L, Ramos-Casals M, Jimenez S, et al. Systemic lupus erythematosus (SLE) in childhood: analysis of clinical and immunological findings in 34 patients and comparison with SLE characteristics in adults. Annals of the Rheumatic Diseases. 1998;**57**:456-449. [PubMed:9797549]

[95] Bakr A. Epidemiology treatment and outcome of childhood systemic lupus erythematosus in Egypt. Pediatric Nephrology. 2005;**20**:1081-1086. [PubMed: 15940546]

[96] Lehman TJ, McCurdy DK, Bernstein BH, King KK, Hanson V. Systemic lupus erythematosus in the first decade of life. Pediatrics. 1989;**83**:235-239. [PubMed: 2913553]

[97] Carreno L, Lopez-Longo FJ, Monteagudo I, Rodriguez-Mahou M, Bascones M, Gonzalez CM, et al. Immunological and clinical differences between juvenile and adult onset of systemic lupus erythematosus. Lupus. 1999;**8**:287-292. [PubMed: 10413207]

[98] Sibbitt Jr. WL, Brandt JR, Johnson CR, Maldonado ME, Patel SR, Ford CC, et al. The incidence and prevalence of neuropsychiatric syndromes in pediatric onset systemic lupus erythematosus. Journal of Rheumatology. 2002;**29**:1536-1542. [PubMed: 12136916]

[99] Quintero-Del-Rio AI, Van M. Neurologic symptoms in children with systemic lupus erythematosus. Journal of Child Neurology. 2000;**15**:803-807. [PubMed: 11198495]

[100] Mak SK, Lam EK, Wong AK. Clinical profile of patients with late-onset SLE: Not a benign subgroup. Lupus. 1998;**7**:23-28. [PubMed: 9493145]

[101] Pu SJ, Luo SF, Wu YJ, Cheng HS, Ho HH. The clinical features and prognosis of lupus with disease onset at age 65 and older. Lupus. 2000;**9**:96-100. [PubMed: 10787005]

[102] Ho CT, Mok CC, Lau CS, Wong RW. Late onset systemic lupus erythematosus in southern Chinese. Annals of the Rheumatic Diseases. 1998;**57**:437-440. [PubMed: 9797573]

[103] Formiga F, Moga I, Pac M, Mitjavila F, Rivera A, Pujol R. Mild presentation of systemic lupus erythematosus in elderly patients assessed by SLEDAI. SLE Disease Activity Index. Lupus. 1999;**8**:462-465. [PubMed: 10483015]

[104] Ward MM, Polisson RP. A meta-analysis of the clinical manifestations of older-onset systemic lupus erythematosus. Annals of the Rheumatic Diseases. 1989;**32**:1226-1232. [PubMed: 2803325]

[105] Maddison P, Farewell V, Isenberg D, Aranow C, Bae SC, Barr S, et al. The rate and pattern of organ damage in late onset systemic lupus erythematosus. Journal of Rheumatology. 2002;**29**:913-917. [PubMed:12022349]

[106] Costallat LT, Coimbra AM. Systemic lupus erythematosus: Clinical and laboratory aspects related to age at disease onset. Clinical and Experimental Rheumatology. 1994;**12**:603-607. [PubMed: 7895393]

[107] Boddaert J, Huong DL, Amoura Z, Wechsler B, Godeau P, Piette JC. Late-onset systemic lupus erythematosus: A personal series of 47 patients and pooled analysis of 714 cases in the literature. Medicine (Baltimore). 2004;**83**:348-359. [PubMed: 15525847]

[108] Bertoli AM, Alarcón GS, Calvo-Alen J, Fernandez M, Vila LM, Reveille JD. Systemic lupus erythematosus in a multiethnic US cohort. XXXIII. Clinical [corrected] features, course, and outcome in patients with late-onset disease. Arthritis & Rheumatology. 2006;**54**:1580-1587. [PubMed: 16645994]

[109] Urowitz MB, Gladman DD, Abu-Shakra M, Farewell VT. Mortality studies in systemic lupus erythematosus. Results from a single center. III. Improved survival over 24 years. Journal of Rheumatology. 1997;**24**:1061-1065. [PubMed: 9195509]

[110] Pistiner M, Wallace DJ, Nessim S, Metzger AL, Klinenberg JR. Lupus erythematosus in the 1980s: A survey of 570 patients. Seminars in Arthritis and Rheumatism. 1991;**21**:55-64. [PubMed: 1948102]

[111] Bjornadal L, Yin L, Granath F, Klareskog L, Ekbom A. Cardiovascular disease a hazard despite improved prognosis in patients with systemic lupus erythematosus: Results from a Swedish population based study 1964-95. Journal of Rheumatology. 2004;**31**:713-719. [PubMed: 15088296]

[112] Wang LC, Yang YH, Lu MY, Chiang BL. Retrospective analysis of mortality and morbidity of pediatric systemic lupus erythematosus in the past two decades. Journal of Microbiology, Immunology and Infection. 2003;**36**:203-208. [PubMed: 14582566]

[113] Yurkovich M, Vostretsova K, Chen W, et al. Overall and cause specific mortality in patients with systemic lupus erythematosus: A meta-analysis of observational studies. Arthritis Care & Research. 2014;**66**:608-616

[114] Thomas G, Mancini J, Jourde-Chiche N, et al. Mortality associated with systemic lupus erythematosus in France assessed by multiplecause-of-death analysis. Arthritis & Rheumatology. 2014;**66**:2503-2511

[115] Bernatsky S, Boivin JF, Joseph L, et al. Mortality in systemic lupus erythematosus. Arthritis & Rheumatology. 2006;**54**:2550-2557

[116] Xu G, Liu M, Yu K. A prospective study of nosocomial infection in patients with systemic lupus erythematosus. Chinese Journal of Rheumatology. 2003;**7**:216-219

[117] Danza A, Ruiz-Irastorza G. Infection risk in systemic lupus erythematosus patients: Susceptibility factors and preventive strategies. Lupus. 2013;**22**:1286-1294

[118] Zhou H, Zhang F, Tian X, et al. Clinical features and outcome of neuropsychiatric lupus in Chinese: Analysis of 240 hospitalized patients. Lupus. 2008;**17**:93-99

[119] Li M, Zhang W, Leng X, et al. Chinese SLE treatment and Research group (CSTAR) registry: I. Major clinical characteristics of Chinese patients with systemic lupus erythematosus. Lupus. 2013;**22**:1192-1199

[120] Hanly JG, McCurdy G, Fougere L, et al. Neuropsychiatric events in systemic lupus erythematosus: Attribution and clinical significance. Journal of Rheumatology. 2004;**31**:2156-2162

[121] Sanna G, Bertolaccini ML, Cuadrado MJ, et al. Neuropsychiatric manifestations in systemic lupus erythematosus: Prevalence and association with antiphospholipid antibodies. Journal of Rheumatology. 2003;**30**:985-992

[122] Mok CC, Lau CS, Wong RW. Neuropsychiatric manifestations and their clinical associations in southern Chinese patients with systemic lupus erythematosus. Journal of Rheumatology. 2001;**28**:766-771

[123] Kasitanon N, Louthrenoo W, Piyasirisilp S, et al. Neuropsychiatric manifestations in Thai patients with systemic lupus erythematosus. Asian Pacific Journal of Allergy and Immunology. 2002;**20**:179-185

[124] Walport MJ, Davies KA, Botto M. C1q and systemic lupus erythematosus. Immunobiology. 1998;**199**:265-285

[125] Schur PH. Genetics of systemic lupus erythematosus. Lupus. 1995;**4**:425-437

[126] Sullivan KE. Genetics of systemic lupus erythematosus. Clinical implications. Rheumatic Disease Clinics of North America. 2000;**26**:229-256

[127] Salmon JE, Millard S, Schachter LA, et al. Fc gamma RIIA alleles are heritable risk factors for lupus nephritis in African Americans. The Journal of Clinical Investigation. 1996;**97**:1348-1354

[128] Mir A, Porteu F, Levy M, et al. C3b receptor (CR1) on phagocytic cells from SLE patients: Analysis of the defect and familial study. Clinical & Experimental Immunology. 1988;**73**:461-466

[129] Kiss E, Csipo I, Cohen JH, et al. CR1 density polymorphism and expression on erythrocytes of patients with systemic lupus erythematosus. Autoimmunity. 1996;**25**:53-58.

[130] Herrmann M, Voll RE, Zoller OM, et al. Impaired phagocytosis of apoptotic cell material by monocyte-derived macrophages from patients with systemic lupus erythematosus. Arthritis & Rheumatology. 1998;**41**:1241-1250

[131] Haggstrom, M. Medical gallery of Mikael Häggström 2014. Wiki Journal of Medicine. 2014;**1**(2). DOI: 10.15347/wjm/2014.008. ISSN 2002-4436. Public domain

[132] The Jack and Belle Linsky Collection in the Metropolitan Museum of Art. New York, NY: Metropolitan Museum of Art; 1984. p. 101. ISBN 978-0-87099370-1

[133] Cazenave PLA, Schedel HE. Abrege Pratique des maladies de la peau. 3rd ed. Paris: Bechet jeune; 1838. p. 11

Section 2

Antibodies and Lymphocytes in Lupus

Chapter 3

Catalytic Antibodies in Norm and Systemic Lupus Erythematosus

Georgy A. Nevinsky

Additional information is available at the end of the chapter

http://dx.doi.org/10.5772/67790

Abstract

Systemic lupus erythematosus (SLE) is known as a systemic polyethiologic diffuse autoimmune disease characterized by connective tissue disorganization and the paramount damage of skin and visceral capillaries. Usually, SLE symptoms include high fever, hair loss, mouth ulcers, chest pain, swollen lymph nodes, painful and swollen joints, increased fatigue, and appearance of red rash more often on the face. The exact reason of SLE appearance is not really clear. Detection of catalytic Abs (abzymes) was shown to be the earliest indicator of different AI disease development. Some abzymes are cytotoxic and can play a dangerous negative role in the pathogenesis of AI diseases. SLE is characterized by the appearance of abzymes with several different catalytic functions including hydrolysis of peptides and proteins, DNA, RNA, and oligosaccharides. In addition, monoclonal SLE abzymes are characterized by extraordinary diversity in the affinity to the substrates, physicochemical and catalytic characteristics, optimal conditions of catalysis, cytotoxicity, etc. Production of abzymes in SLE mice is associated with changes in the differentiation of hematopoietic stem cells of bone marrow, increase in lymphocyte proliferation, and significant suppression of cell apoptosis in different organs. In this chapter, abzymes with different catalytic activities in SLE are described.

Keywords: systemic lupus erythematosus, catalytic antibodies, hydrolysis of RNA, DNA myelin basic protein, and oligosaccharides, apoptosis, cytotoxicity, diversity of monoclonal antibodies

1. Introduction

According to classical conception, antibodies (Abs) are specific proteins produced by the immune systems with exclusive function of antigen binding. Antibodies can act similarly to specific enzymes, but in contrast to enzymes, they cannot catalyze chemical conversions of their ligands. For most part of antibodies, this observation is correct. At the same time during the last 30 years, it was shown that Abs against chemically stable analogues modeling the transition states of chemical reaction can catalyze many different reactions [1–8]. Such artificial catalytic antibodies were called abzymes (derived from antibody enzymes). Abzymes (Abzs) can catalyze more than 200 different chemical reactions and are new biological catalysts attracting great interest during recent years and are well described (for review see [1–8] and refs therein).

First, natural Abzs were found in patients with bronchial asthma; they hydrolyze vasoactive intestinal peptide [9]. Then IgGs hydrolyzing DNA were revealed in the blood of patients with systemic lupus erythematosus (SLE) [10]. The third natural Abzs were SLE IgGs with RNase activity [11]. To date, many catalytic Abs (IgGs and/or IgAs, IgMs) catalyzing hydrolysis of different RNA, DNA, nucleotides, oligopeptides, proteins, lipids, and oligosaccharides were revealed in the sera of patients with various autoimmune and viral diseases (for review, see Refs. [8, 12–22] and refs therein).

Some idiotypic Abzs against foreign antigens and auto-Abzs to self-antigens having different catalytic activities may be spontaneously induced by primary antigens simulating in varying degrees the transition states of chemical reactions [8, 12–22]. At the same time, some antiidiotypic Abs against active centers of many enzymes are also catalytically active [8, 12–22, 23–28]. Healthy humans do more often not demonstrate catalytic Abs or their activities are extremely low. It was shown that detection of Abzs is the earliest indicator of different autoimmune diseases (ADs) development [8, 12–22]. At the outset and early stages of ADs analyzed, the repertoire of abzymes is more often relatively narrow, but it is expanding very much with the progress of AI diseases; the generation of diverse Abzs with many various activities and functions may be observed [8, 12–22]. Some abzymes are cytotoxic and dangerous for people; they can play a very important negative role in the different AD pathogenesis [8, 12–22]. However, specific positive roles have been also proposed for several abzymes. Increase in Abzs activities is associated with a specific reorganization of the immune system including change in differentiation profile and level of proliferation of hematopoietic stem cells of bone marrow as well as lymphocyte proliferation in different organs of SLE and experimental autoimmune encephalomyelitis (EAE) in mice [29–32]. Different mechanisms of abzymes production were revealed in healthy animals after external immunization and in autoimmune mice during their spontaneous or antigen-induced development of autoimmune processes [29–32].

Catalysis of different reactions by abzymes is potentially important for many different fields; specific reaction for a synthesis of new drugs, which may be useful for therapy, estimation of abzyme's possible role in innate and adaptive immunity, as well as for understanding of destructive responses and self-tolerance in ADs [33–37].

In this chapter, Abzs with various catalytic activities in SLE are described and compared with abzymes in case of other autoimmune pathologies. In addition, a possible role of different defects of immune systems resulting in changes of differentiation profile of hematopoietic stem cells (HSCs) of mice bone marrow as well as an increase in lymphocyte proliferation in thymus, bone marrow, spleen, and a significant suppression in these organs of cell apoptosis associated with the abzymes production is discussed.

2. Features of the immune status of patients with systemic lupus erythematosus

As mentioned above, SLE is systemic polyethiologic diffuse autoimmune disease, symptoms of which for different patients vary significantly and may be from mild to severe. The exact reason and mechanisms of SLE development till yet is not clear [38]. Genetic, environmental, hormonal, and immune factors may play an important role for the development of SLE. Many different autoimmune diseases (ADs) including SLE are characterized by spontaneous generation of primary antibodies to nucleotides, nucleic acids and their complexes, proteins, polypeptides, polysaccharides, etc. [8, 16–22, 36, 38–42]. Anti-DNA auto-Abs without catalytic activities are detectable even in the sera of healthy humans and their relative titres vary from individual to individual significantly [43, 44].

SLE is usually considered to be associated with autoimmunization of patients with DNA, since sera of such patients usually contain anti-DNA Abs and DNA in increased concentrations comparing with that for healthy volunteers [38]. However, comparing to healthy donors, anti-DNA antibody concentrations are higher not only in patients with SLE (36% of patients) [43, 45], but also in Hashimoto's thyroiditis (23%) [43], multiple sclerosis (17–18%) [43, 46, 47], rheumatoid arthritis (7%), myasthenia gravis (6%), and Sjogren's syndrome (18%) [43]. In addition, from the cloning of the IgG repertoire from directly active plaques and periplaque regions of brain and from B-cells of the cerebrospinal fluid of MS patient, new keys to the understanding of this pathology were proposed [48]. High affinity anti-DNA Abs were shown to be the major components of the intrathecal IgG response. In addition, monoclonal anti-DNA Abs of multiple sclerosis (MS) patients and Abs specific to DNA derived from SLE patients interact efficiently with the surface of neuronal cells and oligodendrocytes [48]. Recognition of cell-surface by these Abs was DNA-dependent. The data indicate that Abs against DNA may be important for autoimmune and neuropathological mechanisms in chronic SLE and MS [48]. Interestingly, SLE and MS patients show some similarity in the same medical, biochemical, and immunological indexes including anti-DNA and other auto-Abs [13–22].

Anti-DNA and anti-RNA Abs with DNase and RNase activities were for the first time detected in sera of SLE patients [10, 11] and then with other ADs [13–22]. The origin of natural Abzs is very complex. First, similar to artificial abzymes, they may originate against analogues of transition states of chemical reactions or against enzyme substrates acting as haptens [8–22]. Many antigens can change their conformation after association with various proteins, and in such complexes, their structure could mimic that of a transition state of chemical reaction substrate. For example, DNA is a bad antigen and immunization of animals with pure DNA or RNA leads to the production of abzymes with very low DNase and RNase activities [49, 50].

Many anti-DNA auto-Abs in SLE are directed against DNA-histone nucleosomal complexes, resulting from internucleosomal cleavage during apoptosis [42]. Apoptotic cells and their different components are the primary antigens as well as immunogens in SLE and are important for the recognition, processing, perception, and/or apoptotic autoantigen presentation by antigen-presenting cells during development of autoimmune processes [42]. Therefore, immunization of mice with complex of DNA and histones or positively charged methylated bovine albumin, simulating positively charged histones, results in production of anti-DNA Abs and DNase abzymes with high activity [29–31, 49, 50]. It was shown that abzymes with different activities may be obtained with a significantly higher incidence in autoimmune mouse strains comparing to conventionally used control nonautoimmune mice [51, 52]. Immunization of autoimmune-prone MRL-lpr/lpr mice with DNA-protein complexes also results in significantly higher production of anti-DNA Abs and abzymes with DNase activity comparing with nonautoimmune CBA and BALB/c healthy mice [29–31]. At the same time, artificial antiidiotypic abzymes can be induced by immunization of animals with different enzymes [23–28]. It was first suggested that natural SLE DNase Abzs may be antiidiotypic abzymes to topoisomerase I [53]. Immunization of rabbits with DNase I led to the production of Abzs with DNase activity of antiidiotypic nature [54]. Idiotypic Abs first were obtained by immunization of animals with DNase I and then they were used to elicit a polyclonal antiidiotypic Abs hydrolyzing DNA; it indicates for the existence of internal Abs structure mimicking active centre of DNase I [54]. We have suggested that polyclonal DNase Abzs in autoimmune patients may be a cocktail of abzymes against complexes of proteins with DNA and RNA and antiidiotypic abzymes to different DNA-hydrolyzing enzymes. Therefore, we have immunized rabbits with DNase II, DNase I, pancreatic RNase A, DNA, and RNA [49, 50, 55–57]. In all cases, abzymes with intrinsic DNase and RNase activities were revealed. IgGs against DNase I with DNase activity also have an antiidiotypic nature [55]. Interestingly, 74–85% of the total polyclonal IgGs against RNase A possessing RNase and DNase activities belong to antiidiotypic Abs, while 15–26% of the Abzs cannot interact with affinity sorbent-bearing Abs against RNase A; they bind with DNA- and RNA-Sepharoses and may be antibodies to nucleic acids bound to RNase [56]. In addition, only ~10% of the polyclonal total IgGs demonstrating DNase and RNase activities from sera of rabbits immunized with DNase II have antiidiotypic nature, while the remaining 90% of Abzs did not interact with Sepharose-bearing Abs against DNase II, they may also be Abs to nucleic acids bound to DNase II [57]. The relatively low amount of antiidiotypic abzymes against DNase II hydrolyzing DNA and RNA may be a consequence of low immunogenicity of DNase II active site comparing with other antigenic determinants of this nuclease. Antibodies against DNA and RNA complexes with proteins and other antinuclear components were found in the blood sera of patients with several multisystem connective tissue diseases including SLE [58]. Interestingly, abzymes agains DNA and RNA bound with proteins are usually significantly more active in the hydrolysis of these substrates than antiidiotypic Abzs against enzyme active centres [17–22, 49, 50, 55–57]. Thus, RNase A, DNase I, DNase II, and other DNA- and RNA-dependent enzymes can themselves be antigens producing not only antiidiotypic abzymes with corresponding active sites, but these enzymes can interact with RNA and DNA and induce formation of anti-RNA and or anti-DNA abzymes possessing no affinity for these enzymes, but having higher catalytic activities than antiidiotypic Abzs. In addition, various proteins interacting with DNA and RNA can differ in their ability to produce antiidiotypic Abzs and the formation of abzymes against bound nucleic acids. Overall, it is clear that abzymes of patients with various autoimmune diseases can be very different cocktails of idiotypic antibodies directly against DNA, RNA, and against complexes of these antigens with different enzymes or proteins as well as antiidiotypic Abs against many DNA-dependent enzymes [17–22, 49, 50, 55–57].

3. Catalytic activities of SLE prone mice antibodies

It was shown that DNase Abzs of patients with SLE [59], MS [16], and DNA-hydrolyzing Bence-Jones proteins of patients with multiple myeloma [60] are cytotoxic, able to penetrate cell nucleus and cause fragmentation of nuclear DNA leading to cell apoptosis. A significant decrease in cell apoptosis in the case of ADs may be a very important factor providing the increase in the level of specific lymphocytes producing auto-Abs and abzymes, which are usually eliminated in different organs of healthy mammals [61, 62]. The cell apoptosis caused by Abzs with DNase activity leads to increase in the concentration of histones complexes with DNA fragments in the blood of mammals and, consequently, to production of antibodies against DNA and DNA-hydrolyzing abzymes. Thus, the appearance Abzs with DNase activity in the blood of mammals may be a very important factor in the strengthening of the autoimmune reactions [13–22]. The abzymes with DNase activity should be considered as very dangerous since they can stimulate development of autoimmune reactions. The overall level of autoimmune reactions may depend on the ratio of cytotoxic (harmful) and beneficial to organisms auto-Abs. Therefore, it was very interesting to elucidate what factors underlie in the AI processes development and how possible mechanisms of autoimmunity are associated with the production of abzymes. Some data suggest that various ADs can originate from defects in the hematopoietic stem cells (HSCs) [63]. Therefore, it was reasonable to analyze what defects or changes may be revealed in the HSCs during spontaneous and DNA-induced development of SLE in autoimmune prone MRL-lpr/lpr mice.

It is known that after spontaneous development of SLE, MRL-lpr/lpr mice are characterized by visual symptoms of autoimmune pathology (baldness of head and parts of the back, pink spots, general health deterioration, etc.). Appearance of pronounced visual symptoms usually well correlate with high proteinuria (≥3 mg/ml of protein concentration in urine) [64, 65]. It was shown previously that sera of spontaneously diseased MRL-lpr/lpr mice contain Abzs with high DNase activity correlating with high proteinuria and visual symptoms usually at age of 5–12 months [64, 65], which is a typical period of signs of deep SLE pathology of MRL-lpr/lpr mice [66]. Obviously, that the state of "health" in the case of autoimmune-prone mice should be considered quite conventional, the development autoimmune pathology nevertheless is spontaneous, and AI processes leading to deep pathology increase gradually. To distinguish different levels of SLE development, MRL-lpr/lpr mice without typical autoimmune symptoms and demonstrating no abzyme activities (similar to nonautoimmune healthy control mice) were independently of age tentatively designated as healthy mice, while the animals having no visual or biochemical SLE symptoms but demonstrating detectable activities of abzymes were provisionally named as prediseased MRL-lpr/lpr mice. Mice demonstrating all visual symptoms and biochemical indexes of SLE were designated as diseased animals. We have compared healthy (2–3 months of age) and spontaneously diseased MRL-lpr/lpr mice with all visible symptoms no older than 7 months [29–31]. For a more precise characterization of the various states of these mice, we have evaluated a variety of medical, biochemical, and immunological characteristics of their status including the relative levels of Abs to various autoantigens of abzymes demonstrating different catalytic activities.

The average anti-DNA Abs concentration in the case of (CBAxC57BL)F1 and BALB/c nonautoimmune control mice was estimated to be approximately 0.03–0.04 A_{450} units and was comparable with that for healthy autoimmune-prone MRL-lpr/lpr mice (0.032 A_{450} units) [29–31]. After spontaneous development of SLE in MRL-lpr/lpr mice (depending of individual mice during 4–7 months), it increases to 0.2 A_{450} units, but there were no remarkable change in the anti-DNA Abs titers in the case of control nonautoimmune mice during 7–8 months of the experiment [29–31]. After MRL-lpr/lpr mice immunization with complex of methylated-BSA with DNA (further marked as DNA), the average concentration of anti-DNA Abs increased to approximately 0.6 A_{450} units [29–31]. It should be mentioned that IgG antibodies from the sera of control 2–7 month-old nonautoimmune CBA and BALB mice and conditionally healthy 2–3 months old MRL-lpr/lpr mice were shown to be catalytically inactive [29–31]. At the same time, during spontaneous development of SLE and especially after MRL-lpr/lpr mice immunization with DNA the relative catalytic DNase activity was significantly increased. **Figure 1(A)** demonstrates hydrolysis of supercoiled (sc) plasmid DNA by IgGs from various mice after 2 h of incubation. To quantify the DNase activity, a concentration of each electrophoretically and immunologically homogeneous IgG preparation (containing no any canonical enzymes) converting scDNA to relaxed DNA during 0.2–4 h of incubation without formation of linear or fragmented DNA was used (for example, lanes 1–3, **Figure 1A**). The relative efficiency of DNA hydrolysis was estimated from the relative percentage of DNA in the band of sc and relaxed DNA; the relative amount of DNA in these two bands for DNA incubated without IgGs or with Abs from healthy mice was taken into account. The measured relative activities (RAs) were normalized to standard conditions (0.1 mg/ml Abs, 2 h) and a complete hydrolysis of scDNA giving hydrolyzed form was taken for 100% of DNase activity. The RAs of IgGs in the hydrolysis of ATP (**Figure 1B**) and maltoheptaose (MHO; **Figure 1C**) were also estimated using the same approach as in the case of DNase activity.

All data obtained are given in **Table 1**. One can see, that at 7 months of age before development of visible pathology markers (similar to mice of 1–3 months of age before deep MRL-lpr/lpr mice spontaneous pathology) MRL-lpr/lpr mice demonstrate no proteinuria (urine proteins <3.0 mg/ml). In addition, they are characterized by a relatively weak increase in the concentrations of Abs to native and denatured DNA. Moreover, the values of these parameters for some individual prediseased mice are comparable with the values observed for healthy mice. Interestingly, IgGs from sera of healthy MRL-lpr/lpr and control CBA, BALB mice possess well-determined amylase activity. This activity increased in the case of prediseased MRL-lpr/lpr mice, but the observed difference with healthy animals was not statistically significant. The changes in this parameter become statistically significant only for mice

http://dx.doi.org/10.5772/67790

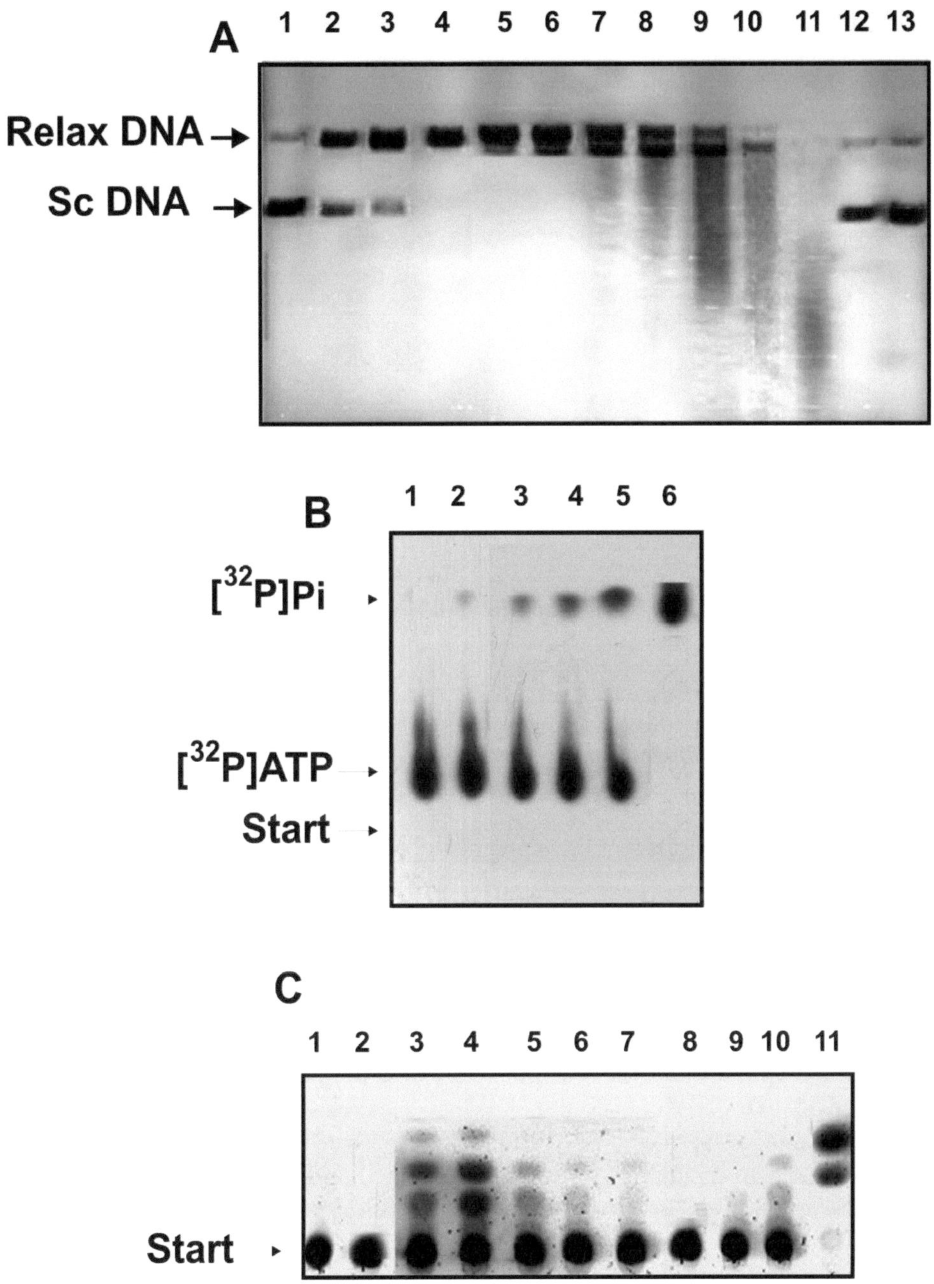

Figure 1. Determination of relative DNase (A), ATPase (B), and amylase (C) activities of catalytic IgGs (0.1 mg/ml) from different mice [29–31]. Analysis of DNA hydrolysis was performed using electrophoresis in 0.8% agarose gels. Before electrophoresis supercoiled pBluescript DNA (A) was incubated for 2 h at 30°C with IgGs from 11 different mice (lanes 1–11); lane 12, DNA incubated with Abs of healthy mouse; lane 13, DNA incubated alone. Hydrolysis of [γ-^{32}P]ATP (B) and maltoheptaose (C) was analyzed respectively by thin-layer chromatography on PEI cellulose and on Kieselgel plates. Reaction mixtures containing 0.2 mM ATP were incubated for 2 h at 30°C; lanes 2–6 correspond to IgGs from 5 different mice; lane 1 to ATP incubated alone. Standard reaction mixtures containing 0.15 mM maltoheptaose were incubated at 30°C for 12 h: lanes 2–11 correspond to IgGs from 10 different mice, lane 1, the substrate incubated alone.

Group description	Number of mice	Urine protein, mg/ml**	Abs to native DNA, A_{450}*	Abs to denatured DNA, A_{450}*	DNase activity, %*	ATPase activity, %*	Amylase activity, %*
	Control males and females						
(CBA × C57BL) F1 (3–7 mo.)	8 (4 f + 4 m)	0.12 ± 0.07	0.04 ± 0.01	0.02 ± 0.01	0***	0***	1.0 ± 0.5***
BALB/c (3–7 mo.)	8 (4 f + 4 m)	0.1 ± 0.08	0.03 ± 0.01	0.017 ± 0.004	0	0	1.1 ± 0.5
	MRL-lpr/lpr males						
Healthy (2–3 mo.)	5	0.38 ± 0.02	0.032 ± 0.01	0.09 ± 0.07	0	0	1.9 ± 1.2
Healthy, pre-diseased (7 mo.)	5	0.8 ± 0.3	0.11 ± 0.02	0.16 ± 0.05	**3.0 ± 1.0**[ξ]	**0.4 ± 0.25**	3.1 ± 1.4
Diseased (7 mo)	8	8.0 ± 3.1	0.18 ± 0 .08	0.23 ± 0.11	**22.0 ± 24.0**	**68.3 ± 9.8**	**3.7 ± 1.0**
Immunized	6	9.5 ± 1.7	0.6 ± 0.17	1.1 ± 0.16	**360.0 ± 230.0**	**1333 ± 530**	**17.6 ± 7.5**
	MRL-lpr/lpr females						
Healthy (2–3 mo)	5	0.31 ± 0.03	0.08 ± 0.03	0.12 ± 0.06	0	0	1.8 ± 1.1
Healthy, pre-diseased (7 mo)	5	0.9 ± 0.2	0.20 ± 0.06	0.08 ± 0.04	**6.1 ± 2.8**	**2.4 ± 1.7**	3.6 ± 1.4
Diseased (7 mo)	5	5.0 ± 3.8	0.16 ± 0.12	0.21 ± 0.12	**20.0 ± 21.0**	**65.0 ± 93.0**	**9.2 ± 5.4**

*For each mouse, the mean of three repeats is used.

**Proteinuria corresponds to ≥3 mg of total protein/ml of urine.

***100% relative activity corresponds to a complete transition of the substrate to its products after the hydrolysis in the presence of 0.1 mg/ml IgGs.

ξStatistically significant changes in parameters are given in bold.

Table 1. Autoimmune characteristics of AI-prone MRL-lpr/lpr and control non-autoimmune mice [31].

with deep pathology (**Table 1**). It is necessary to emphasize that IgGs of healthy MRL-lpr/lpr mice do not possess any DNase and ATPase activities and only the increase in these activities at a predisease stage should be considered as statistically significant indicator of the outset of spontaneous autoimmune disease of mice. After developing of deep SLE pathology, the RAs of DNase activity in the case of male and female mice increases 3.3- and 7.3-fold, respectively, comparing to prediseased mice, while increase in ATPase activity is significantly greater, 27- and 171-fold, respectively (**Table 1**). Thus, only these activities are the most important indicators of predisease state and deep pathology of MRL-lpr/lpr mice.

4. Possible role of brain stem cells and lymphocytes in development of SLE

4.1. Differentiation of bone marrow stem cells in SLE prone mice

The relationship between the relative activities of abzymes and the formation of following hematopoietic progenitors colonies has been analyzed: CFU-GM, granulocytic-macrophagic colony-forming unit; CFU-E, erythroid burst-forming unit (late erythroid colonies);

CFU-GEMM, granulocytic-erythroid-megacaryocytic-macrophagic colony-forming unit; and BFU-E, erythroid burst-forming unit (early erythroid colonies) [29–31]. In the bone marrow of healthy MRL-lpr/lpr males and females (3 months of age), normal distribution of committed progenitors was observed, and the blood serum IgGs in these mice as well as control CBA mice show no detectable DNase and ATPase activities (**Table 2**). In MRL-lpr/lpr males and females (7 months old) having no proteinuria and SLE clinical manifestations but demonstrating detectable activities of abzymes, the relative number of BFU-E and CFU-GEMM colonies increased ~2- and ~16.4–28.4-fold, respectively. For spontaneously deep diseased males and females showing high RAs of DNase and ATPase activities, the profile of HSC differentiation was changed significantly comparing with prediseased mice: BFU-E colonies number increased approximately two times, while the number of CFU-GEMM and CFU-GM colonies decreased by factors of 2.4–3.4 and ~2.6–4.0, respectively. After the development of SLE induced by the mice immunization with DNA, the highest rise in anti-DNA Abs, Abz activities, and proteinuria was observed [29–31]. In addition, a very specific differentiation profile of HSC was revealed (**Table 2**). The numbers of CFU-GEMM and BFU-E colonies were 4.3- and 3.6-fold lower than for spontaneously diseased mice, while the number of CFU-GM colonies was comparable. Interestingly, the profiles of bone marrow HSC differentiation for immunized mice and healthy mice were not much different (**Table 2**). The data of **Tables 1** and **2** are summarized in **Figure 2**.

One can see that in the condition of predisease a strong increase in the relative number of CFU-GM colonies is observed, and at this time, there is a reliable and statistically significant appearance of DNase and ATPase activities of IgG antibodies. At transition from predisease

Group description	Visual symptoms	Number of mice	Number of colonies*		
			BFU-E	CFU-GM	CFU-GEMM
CBA (3–7 mo)	No	8	3.0 ± 0.5**	7.3 ± 1.0**	0.25 ± 0.05**
	MRL-lpr/lpr males				
Healthy (2–3 mo.)	No	5	6.5 ± 1.5	7.0 ± 1.0	0.5 ± 0.1
Healthy, pre-diseased (7 mo)	No	5	12.7 ± 1.4	30.0 ± 1.3	9.2 ± 1.9
Diseased (7 mo)	Yes	5	25.3 ± 9.8	7.4 ± 0.4	3.9 ± 2.0
Immunized (3 mo)	yes, weak	5	7.0 ± 2.1	6.0 ± 2.6	0.9 ± 0.7
	MRL-lpr/lpr females				
Healthy (2–3 mo)	No	5	5.5 ± 0.5	11 ± 2.5	0.5 ± 0.2
Healthy, pre-diseased (7 mo)	No	5	11.5 ± 2.0	23.0 ± 3.0	8.2 ± 3.0
Diseased (7 mo)	Yes	5	22.1 ± 8.0	9.0 ± 3.9	2.4 ± 1.8

*For each mouse, the mean of four repeats is used.

**Mean ± confidence interval.

Table 2. Formation of bone marrow progenitor colonies in from control nonautoimmune and MRL-lpr/lpr mice [31].

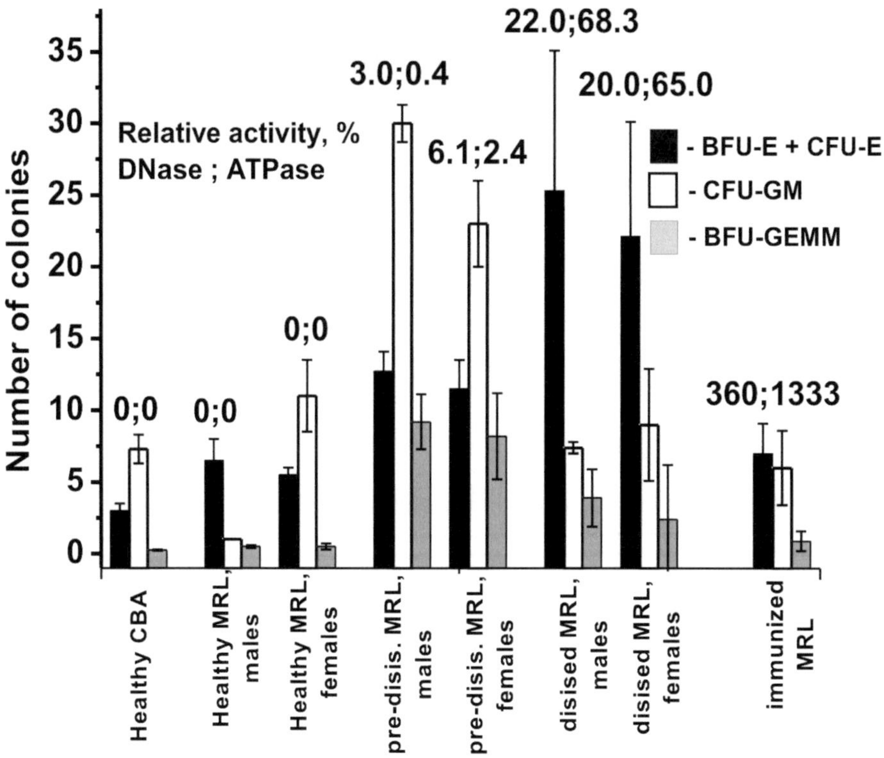

Figure 2. The relative profile of differentiation of bone marrow progenitors. Relative number of total erythroid cells (BFU-E+ CFU-E), CFU-GM, and CFU-GEMM colonies in the case of healthy CBA, conditionally healthy MRL-lpr/lpr mice at 3 months of age, after MRL-lpr/lpr mice development of pre-disease and deep SLE, as well as after mice immunization with DNA is shown [29–31]. The numbers above the bars show using a semicolon the relative average activity of mice serum IgGs in the hydrolysis of DNA and ATP, respectively.

condition to deep SLE pathology, there is additional change in profile differentiation of bone marrow HSC; the number of CFU-GM colonies is significantly decreased, but at the same time, a significant increase in BFU-E cells is observed. Such change in differentiation profile of bone marrow HSC is associated with significant increase in DNase and ATPase activities of IgGs. Healthy MRL-lpr/lpr mice 3 months of age treated with DNA show a very strong increase in DNase and ATPase activities, but differentiation profile of bone marrow HSC is almost same as for healthy male and female MRL-lpr/lpr mice. This could indicate that appearance of abzymes in healthy mice after their immunization with DNA is not associated with the change of differentiation profile of bone marrow HSC, and there may be some other ways of this phenomenon realization. Taking this into account, we analyzed lymphocyte proliferation in different organs of MRL-lpr/lpr mice [29–31].

4.2. Lymphocyte proliferation in SLE prone mice

Spontaneous development of SLE results in remarkable average increase in lymphocyte proliferation in all analyzed organs of males and females comparing with healthy control mice (**Figure 3**) [29–31].

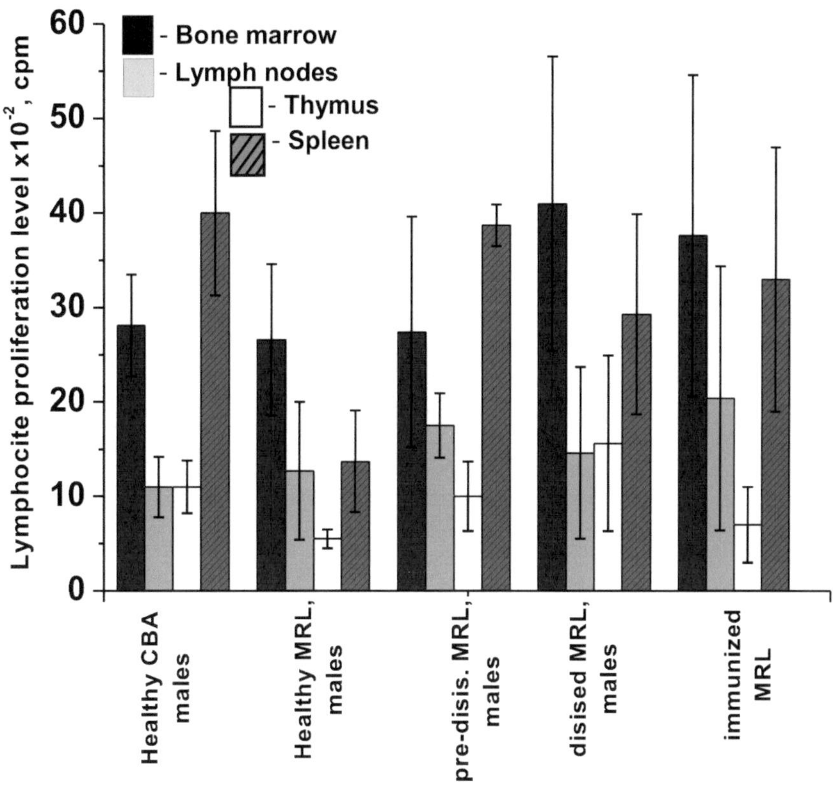

Figure 3. The relative level of lymphocyte proliferation in different organs of male healthy CBA, conditionally healthy MRL-lpr/lpr mice at 3 months of age, after development of pre-disease and deep SLE pathology MRL-lpr/lpr in mice, as well as after mice immunization with DNA is shown [29–31]. The designation of the various mouse organs is indicated in the figure.

Interestingly, the relative level of lymphocyte proliferation in the spleen of healthy control CBA mice is approximately threefold higher than that for healthy MRL-lpr/lpr mice (**Figure 3**). Transition from healthy to spontaneously prediseased mice leads to the increase in lymphocyte proliferation in spleen by ~2.8-fold in parallel with increase of average level of the proliferation 1.4- and 1.8-fold in lymph nodes and thymus, respectively [29–31]. While there is no remarkable difference in lymphocyte proliferation in bone marrow of healthy CBA, healthy and prediseased MRL-lpr/lpr mice, the diseased animals demonstrate increase in this parameter by a factor of ~1.5 (**Figure 3**). The spontaneous pathology of MRL-lpr/lpr mice develops slowly and most of the mice are showing signs of the deep disease only from 5 to 9 months of life. The average values of the lymphocyte proliferation of diseased MRL-lpr/lpr mice are significantly increased in all organs compared to healthy mice. Interestingly, immunization of healthy 3 months old MRL-lpr/lpr mice with DNA leads to the increase of lymphocyte proliferation in all organs except thymus at 20 days after their treatment (**Figure 3**). Thus, a significant increase in the relative level of lymphocyte proliferation in mice may be an important factor causing the development of abzymes with very high activity after their immunization with DNA. As mentioned above, mice immunized with DNA do not show significant changes in bone marrow HSC differentiation profile. However, DNA-treated mice demonstrate high level of bone marrow lymphocyte proliferation (**Figure 3**). This may be due to the fact that DNA has little effect on the profile of stem cells differentiation but effectively stimulates increase in the proliferation and changes the profile of mouse bone marrow lymphocyte differentiation.

In this regard, data comparing relative Abz activities from serum and cerebrospinal fluid (CSF) of the same MS patients with multiple sclerosis should be noted [67–69]. It was shown that IgGs from sera and cerebrospinal fluid of MS patients are active in the hydrolysis of DNA, MBP, and oligosaccharides. In addition, the specific RAs of these abzymes from the CSF of MS patients are dependently on their different activities were approximately 30- to 60-fold higher comparing to serum Abzs from the same patients [67–69]. It means that during spontaneous or induced development of ADs as a result of specific differentiation of lymphocytes in cerebrospinal fluid there may be formation of cells producing different catalytic antibodies directly in cerebrospinal fluid. Thus, one cannot exclude that the increased level of Abz activities in MRL-lpr/lpr mice immunized with DNA may be a consequence of specific additional differentiation of naive lymphocytes not only in different organs but also in the cerebrospinal fluid. Another important factor reducing the relative number of lymphocytes producing abzyme may be cell apoptosis.

4.3. Cell apoptosis in SLE prone mice

It is known that in norm (healthy mammals) harmful cells including lymphocytes are eliminated by apoptosis [61, 62]. The decrease in the lymphocyte apoptosis, producing Abzs harmful to mammals, can lead to increase in autoimmune reactions and acceleration of ADs development. The relative level of lymphocyte apoptosis in different organs and tissues of MRL-lpr/lpr mice was analyzed (**Figure 4**) [31].

In control CBA and healthy MRL-lpr/lpr mice, the cell apoptosis level in different organs on average was comparable (**Figure 4**). The prediseased mice demonstrated relatively low decrease in lymphocyte apoptosis in bone marrow, but its remarkable increase in spleen. Transition from predisease state to deep SLE led to a significant decrease in the cell apoptosis level in all organs comparing with healthy and prediseased mice and maximal decrease was observed for bone marrow lymphocytes (**Figure 4**). However, the statistically significant two- to threefold maximal decrease in the apoptosis level was observed for bone marrow, thymus lymph nodes, and spleen of the mice immunized with DNA, which correlates with a very strong increase in the specific Abz activities of treated mice comparing to the spontaneously diseased animals (**Figure 4**). Therefore, it should be assumed that in the case of mice predisposed to ADs, introduction of foreign antigen can inhibit the elimination of harmful lymphocytes including ones producing dangerous abzymes by apoptosis and stimulate the proliferation of such cells. Overall, immunization of healthy MRL-lpr/lpr mice with DNA leads to the production of abzymes with very high activities, but it is not associated with noticeable change in profile of HSC differentiation but mainly caused by increase in lymphocyte proliferation and specific suppression of lymphocyte apoptosis in different organs [35]. In this regard, it should be mentioned that these regularities may to some extent be common in

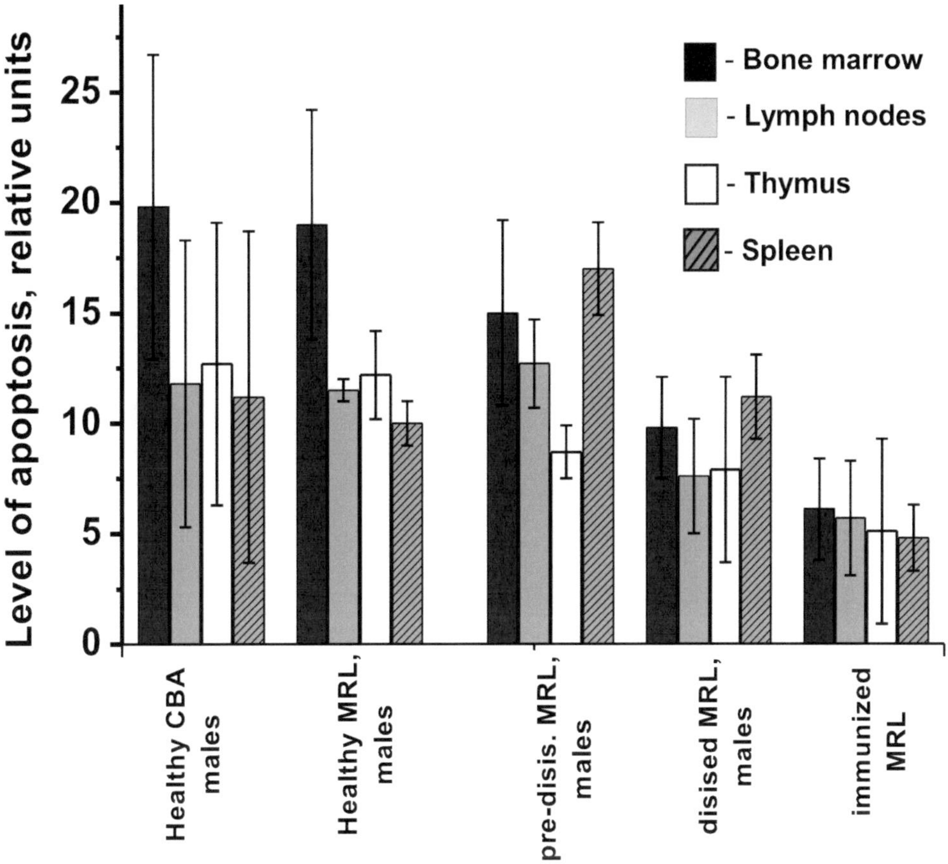

Figure 4. The relative level of lymphocyte apoptosis in different organs of male healthy CBA, conditionally healthy MRL-lpr/lpr mice at 3 months of age, after MRL-lpr/lpr mice development of pre-disease, and deep SLE pathology, as well as after mice immunization with DNA [29–31]. The designation of the various organs is indicated in the figure.

the development of various autoimmune diseases. For example, using experimental C57BL/6 autoimmune encephalomyelitis (EAE) mice (a model mimicking human MS), it was recently shown that spontaneous EAE development leads to the production of Abs to myelin basic protein (MBP) and DNA and to Abzs efficiently hydrolyzing these substrates, which associated with significant changes of the differentiation profile and level of lymphocytes proliferation of mice bone marrow HSC [32]. Immunization of these mice with MOG35 results in a very strong acceleration in the development of EAE and a very strong increase of the relative activities of abzymes hydrolyzing MOG, MBP, and DNA. The relative percent contents of total erythroid cells, CFU-GEMM and CFU-GM colonies at 3 months of age in healthy, nonautoimmune CBA, conditionally healthy, MRL-lpr/lpr and EAE C57BL/6 mice before and after development of these autoimmune pathologies were compared (**Figure 5**).

One can see that the relative content (percent of total number of different cells) of various bone marrow colonies after spontaneous achievement of deep pathologies by MRL-lpr/lpr and EAE mice is nearly the same. In addition, the level of lymphocyte proliferation as well

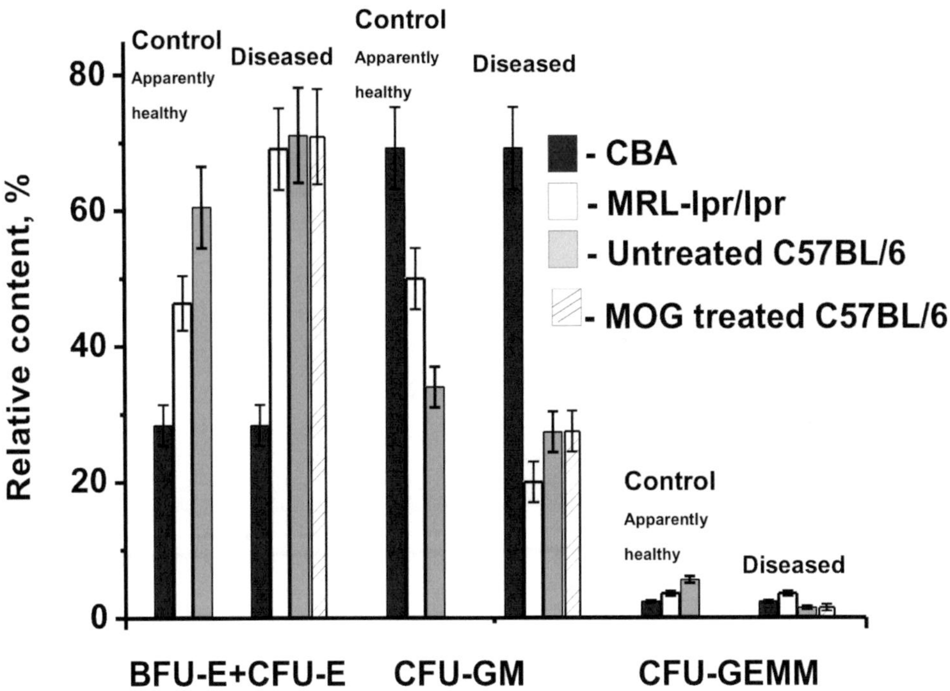

Figure 5. The relative content (%) of total erythroid cells (BFU-E+ CFU-E), CFU-GM, and CFU-GEMM colonies in the case of healthy CBA, conditionally healthy MRL-lpr/lpr and C57BL/6 mice at 3 months of age, and after development of, respectively, EAE and SLE is shown [32]. For C57BL/6 mice, the relative contents of progenitor colonies after spontaneous and MOG-stimulated development of EAE are given.

as cell apoptosis in different organs including bone marrow of healthy MRL-lpr/lpr and EAE mice, at stages of their prediseases and deep pathologies were also comparable [32]. In addition, it was shown that abzymes hydrolyzing MBP are formed in the early stages of human MS, unlike in later stages of SLE, while the reverse situation was observed for abzymes with DNase activity [70–87]. One gets the impression that SLE and MS differ greatly in their initial stages but become to some extent more similar at the later stages of these diseases. The blood of patients with SLE and MS after a long illness contains Abs to a variety of autoantigens and abzymes hydrolyzing nucleotides, oligosaccharides, lipids, DNA, RNA, MBP, and many other proteins [13–21, 70–93].

Clinically definite MS diagnosis is more often based on tomographic detection of brain-specific plaques appearing on late stages of this disease. But, similar brain plaques were also detected on the late stages of SLE [38, 41]. MS is a central nervous system disease resulting in the manifestation of different psychiatric and nervous disturbances. Neuropsychiatric disturbances occur also in about 50% of patients with SLE and carries a poor prognosis (reviewed in [41]). SLE affects mainly on the central nervous system and it supposedly more than any other inflammatory systemic disease causes various psychiatric disorders [41]. Peripheral nervous system involvement seems to be much less. Neural cell injury and rheological disturbances mediated by auto-Abs may be due to two of the main possible mechanism of tissue damage [41]. Interplay between these processes is determined by genetic factors, and may be modulated by hormones, complicated by a many of secondary factors, may explain the wide spectrum of features revealed in SLE [41]. Thus, not only specific changes in the profile of differentiation of bone marrow stem cells, increased levels of lymphocyte proliferation and suppression of apoptosis of harmful cells in different organs leading to the production of dangerous abzymes with various activities, but also some other indicators of different psychiatric and nervous disturbances in varying degrees, are common for some patients with SLE and MS.

5. Application of rigid criteria for analysis of antibodies catalytic activities

The sera of healthy humans and mammals contain usually autoantibodies to many different antigens, including RNA, DNA, proteins, and other antigens [13–22, 43, 44]. Natural abzymes from the sera of patients with different AI diseases are products of different immuno-competent cells and usually polyclonal in origin ([13–22] and refs cited here). Purification of natural abzymes containing no canonical enzymes is a very important task in their study; peculiarities of such antibodies isolation were discussed in detail in reviews [13, 19]. Electrophoretically and immunologically homogeneous IgG fractions with or without different catalytic activities from the sera of healthy donors and autoimmune patients described in this chapter were first purified using Protein G-Sepharose, while IgAs and IgMs by affinity chromatography on Protein A-Sepharose under conditions removing nonspecifically bound proteins. Then IgAs were separated from IgMs and IgGs from possible admixtures of canonical enzymes by FPLC gel filtration in acidic conditions (pH 2.6) destroying immuno-complexes [29–32, 49, 50, 55–57, 64–103]. Overall, ~900 kDa IgMs, 170 kDa IgAs, and 150 kDa IgGs did not contain possible contaminating proteins detected by acrylamide gel silver staining under reducing and nonreducing conditions.

The application of rigid criteria allowed the authors of the first article describing natural abzymes hydrolyzing vasoactive intestinal peptide to obtain irrefutable evidence that this activity is an intrinsic property of IgGs from sera of patients with asthma [9]. Later several additional rigid criteria were proposed (reviewed in Refs. [13, 19]). We applied a set of these strict criteria [9, 13–22] for the analysis of DNase and RNase [11, 31, 64, 65, 70–75], MBP-hydrolyzing [76–79], ATPase [30], and amylase [29, 88–91] activities as intrinsic properties of IgG and/or IgM and IgA antibodies from sera of SLE patients and mice. Several more important of them may be summarized as follows: (1) all Abs were electrophoretically homogeneous; (2) FPLC gel filtration of these Abs under conditions destroying strong noncovalent complexes (acidic buffer, pH 2.6) did not abolish these activities, and activities peaks exactly coincided with peaks of intact Abs; (3) immobilized mouse IgGs against the light chains of human Abs absorbed completely these activities; these activity's peaks coincided with the peaks of Abs eluted using acidic buffer; and (4) F(ab) and F(ab)2 fragments of Abs showed to some extent comparable levels of the activities comparing with intact Abzs. To exclude possible artifacts causing by hypothetical traces of canonical enzymes, Abs from sera of SLE patients were subjected to SDS-PAGE in a gel copolymerized with polymeric DNA or RNA and their nuclease activities were detected *in situ* by gel incubating in the standard reaction buffer. Staining of the gels after the electrophoresis with ethidium bromide (after refolding of Abs) showed sharp dark bands against a fluorescent background of nucleic acids. After incubation with DTT only light chains of SLE Abs demonstrated nuclease activities. After SDS-PAGE amylase, ATPase and MBP-hydrolyzing activities of SLE Abs were analyzed using extracts of

2- to 3-mm fragments of a longitudinal gel slice. Since SDS destroys all noncovalent protein complexes, the revealing of the analyzed activities in the gel zones of only intact IgGs and their separated light chains together with the absence of any other bands of the activities or proteins gave direct evidence that Abs from sera of SLE patients possess analyzed enzymatic activities. The fulfilment of these criteria was observed for SLE IgG, IgA, and IgM abzymes with all activities mentioned above. Some typical examples of rigid criteria application in the case of DNase, RNase, and MBP-hydrolyzing activities of SLE IgGs are given in **Figures 6** and **7**.

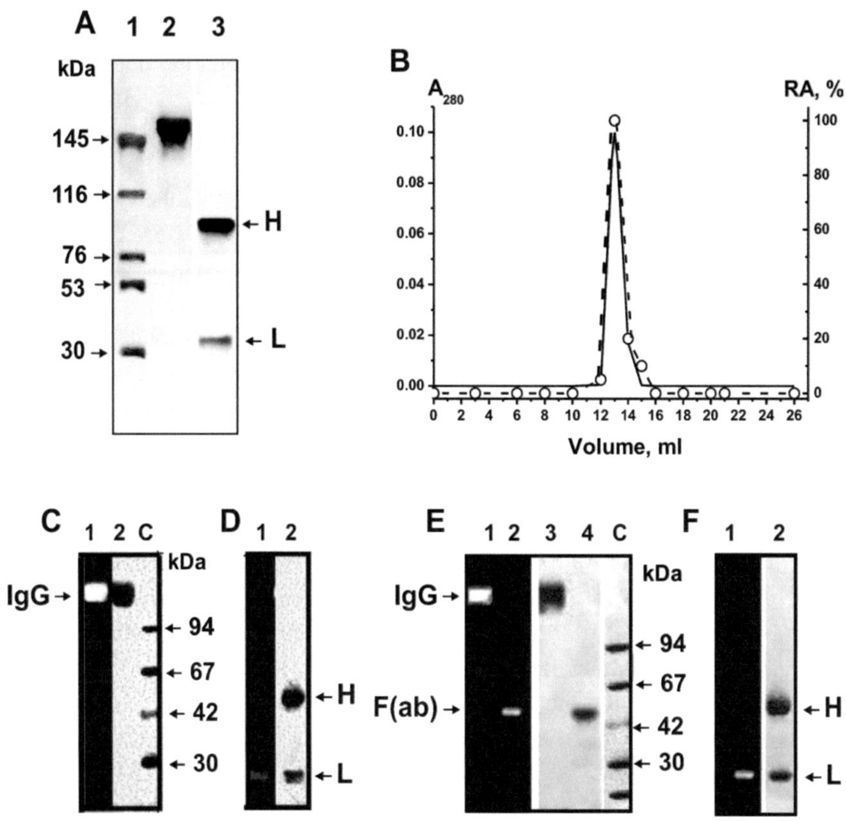

Figure 6. Analysis of the implementation of strict criteria of intrinsic enzymatic activities of IgGs from sera of SLE patients and mice. SDS-PAGE analysis of homogeneity of IgGmix (mixture of equal amounts of Abs from sera of 10 SLE patients) before (lane 2) and after (lane 3) Abs boiling with DTT; lane 1 shows positions of protein markers (A) [71]. FPLC gel filtration of IgGmix (mixture of 15 preparations) corresponding to diseased MRL-lpr/lpr mice on a Superdex 200 column in the acidic buffer (pH 2.6) destroying different immunocomplexes after IgGs incubation in the same buffer (B) [31]. *In situ* gel assay of DNase (C and D) and RNase (E and F) activities of IgGmix (10 preparations) corresponding to SLE patients using respectively gels containing polymeric DNA and RNA [71]. DNase and RNase activities were revealed by ethidium bromide staining as dark bands on the fluorescent background; lanes 1 (C and E) correspond to IgGs before, while lines 1 (D and F) after Abs mild treatment with DTT, lane 2 (E) to F(ab) fragments of IgG (negatives are given). Lanes 2 (C and D), 3 (E) and 2 (F) intact IgGs or their separated L and H chains, while lane 4 (E) corresponds to F(ab) fragments, positions of which were revealed by treatment of the gels with Coomassie R250. Lanes C (C and E) correspond to proteins with known molecular masses [71].

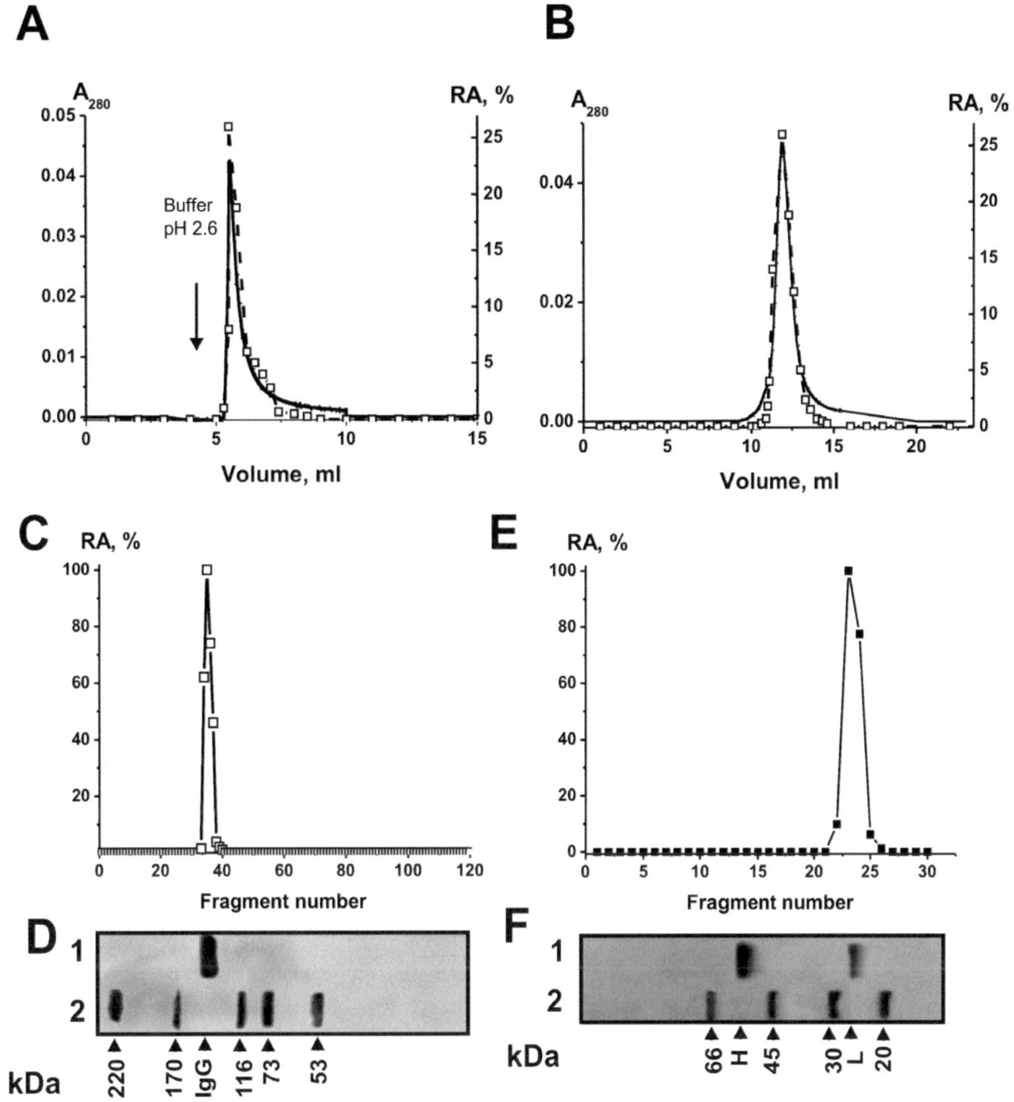

Figure 7. Application of the strict criteria to show that MBP-hydrolyzing activity is intrinsic property of IgGs from sera of SLE patients [76, 77]. Affinity chromatography of the IgGmix (Abs of 10 patients) using Sepharose bearing mouse Abs against human IgGs (A) and FPLC gel filtration IgGmix on column with Superdex 200 in acidic buffer (pH 2.6) after incubation of Abs in the same buffer (B): (—), absorbance at 280 nm (A280); (□), relative activity (RA) of IgGmix in the hydrolysis of human MBP (A and B). A complete hydrolysis of MBP (0.5 mg/ml) for 24 h at 37°C was taken for 100%. Analysis of MBP hydrolysis by IgGmix and its separated L and H chains after SDS-PAGE (C and E). After SDS-PAGE of IgGmix using nonreducing (C) and reducing (E) conditions, the gel was incubated under conditions for renaturation of Abs. The relative MBP-hydrolyzing activity (RA, %) was estimated using the extracts of 2- to 3-mm many gel fragments (C and E) of first longitudinal slices. The RA of IgGmix corresponding to a complete hydrolysis of MBP (0.5 mg/ml) after 24 h of standard mixture (30 μl) incubation with 20 μl of extracts was taken as 100%. The second control longitudinal slices corresponding to the same gels were treated with Coomassie R250 (lanes 1; D and F). Lane 2 (D and F) demonstrates position of protein molecular mass markers.

Similar rigid criteria were used by us for evidence of the catalytic activity belonging to the antibodies, hydrolyzing nucleotides, DNA, RNA, various peptides, proteins, oligosaccharides from blood with different autoimmune diseases, and animals immunized with different antigens [11, 13–22, 32, 49–57, 64–65, 67–103].

6. SLE patient's abzymes with DNase and RNase activities

6.1. Polyclonal DNase and RNase abzymes

Healthy humans do not demonstrate antibodies with detectable DNase and RNase activities, their levels are more often on the borderline of sensitivity of the detection methods [13–22]. The RAs of DNase and RNase abzymes from the sera of patients with SLE vary markedly from patient to patient [13–22].

We analyzed the possible heterogeneity of catalytic properties of polyclonal DNase and RNase IgGs from SLE patients and observed an extreme heterogeneity in kinetic and thermodynamic parameters, relative specific activities and substrate specificities, which are different very much from patient to patient. Chromatography on DNA-cellulose showed that only 10–30% of the total electrophoretically homogeneous IgGs and IgMs dependently on patient may be bound to the affinity sorbent. Interestingly, when Abs were eluted from DNA-cellulose by a NaCl gradient (0–3 M) and then acidic buffer (pH 2.6) the Abs and their DNase and RNase activities were distributed all over the chromatography profile (for example, **Figure 8A**) [70, 71]. The same situation was observed for Abs with nuclease activities from sera of MS patients [8, 80–82], and rabbits immunized with DNA, RNA, DNase I, DNase II, and pancreatic RNase [49, 50, 55–57]. The affinity of Abs fractions for these substrates was increased gradually with the increase in eluting salts concentrations. When IgGs eluted from DNA-cellulose were fractionated on Sepharose bearing immobilized monoclonal mouse Abs against anti-kappa or anti-lambda human IgGs, 60–70% of IgGs were adsorbed by Abs against lambda- and 30–40% by Abs against kappa-Abs (**Figure 8B**) [70, 71].

The fractions corresponding IgGs with kappa-light chain were about 30- to 50-fold more active in hydrolysis of both RNA and DNA than lambda-IgGs. SLE IgGs and IgAs with DNase activity [70, 71] similarly to Abs with nuclease activity from sera of patients (and mice) with other autoimmune diseases [80–82, 95, 99–103] efficiently hydrolyzed all single- and double-stranded DNA of different sequences and length. The substrate specificity of SLE IgGs with RNase activity, however, was unique within certain limits for Abs from every individual SLE patient [11]. In contrast to human RNases, SLE IgGs effectively hydrolyze the most resistant poly(A) substrate for all known human RNases [104–109]. SLE IgGs demonstrated a very slow hydrolysis of poly(C) [11], which is the best substrate for all mammalian RNases [104–106]. Therefore, for more detail analysis of IgGs of SLE patients ribo$(pA)_{13}$ was used. **Figure 8(C)** demonstrates pH dependence of $[5'-^{32}P](pA)_{13}$ hydrolysis by three of six SLE IgGs analyzed and by two human blood RNases. All six dependences showed individual features of pH dependencies. In contrast to all SLE abzymes, RNases

http://dx.doi.org/10.5772/67790

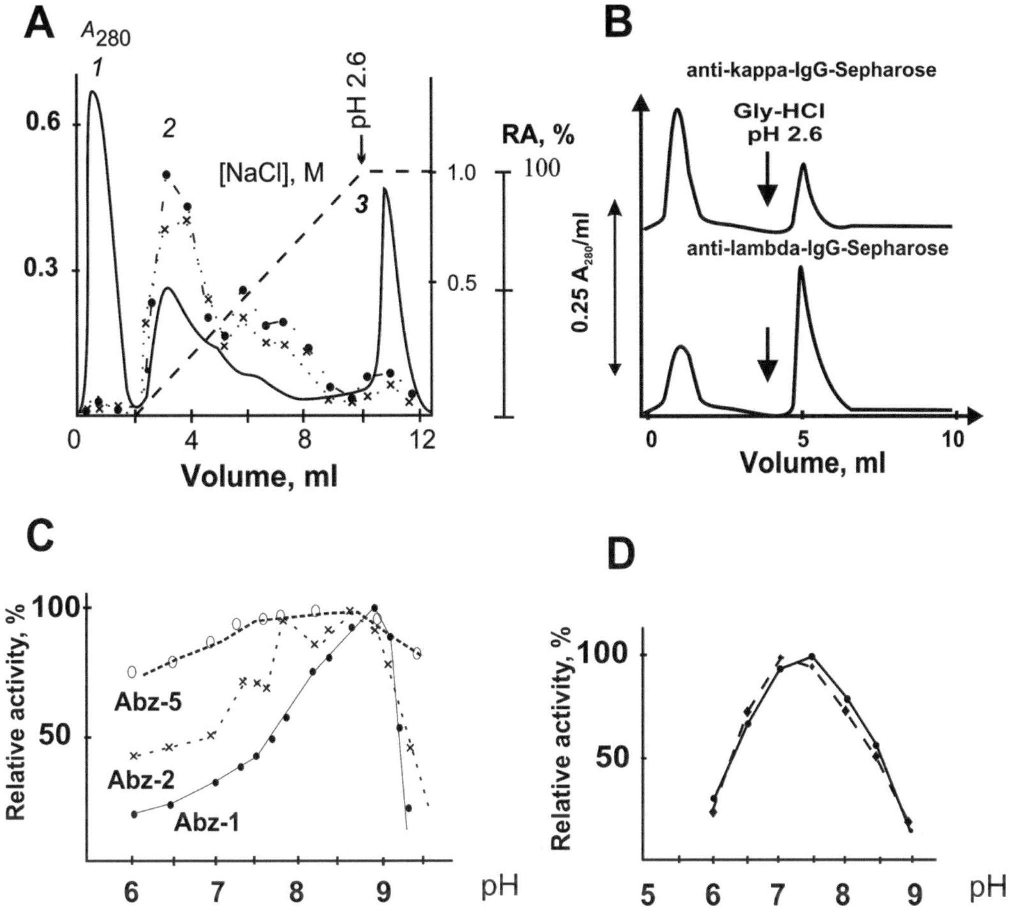

Figure 8. Separation of SLE IgMs having affinity to DNA by affinity chromatography on DNA-cellulose (A) [70]: (—) absorption at 280 nm, (•) and (x) RA of Abs in hydrolysis of respectively [5′-^{32}P](pA)$_{13}$ and [5′-^{32}P]d(pA)$_{13}$, 1–5 μl of each fraction was added to 100 μl of reaction mixture and maximal RNase and DNase activity was taken for 100%. Separation of anti-DNA IgGs containing light chains of kappa and lambda type by affinity chromatography on Sepharoses bearing immobilized Abs against human kappa- and lambda-IgGs [71]: (—) absorption at 280 nm (B). pH dependencies of the relative RNase activity of three SLE IgGs (C) and human serum RNases (RNase 3 (•) and RNase 4 (•)) (D) in the hydrolysis of [5′-^{32}P](pA)$_{13}$ [71].

have only one pH optimum (6.8–7.5) for hydrolysis of poly(A) [104–106] (**Figure 8D**). Polyclonal SLE abzymes more often shows high activity at pH from 6.0 to 9.5. For example, preparation Abz-1 demonstrates maximal activity at pH 8.8; Abz-2 shows three marked pH optima at pH 8.5, 7.7, and 7.2, while Abz-5 hydrolyzes RNA with comparable efficiency at pH values from 6.0 up to 9.5 (**Figure 8C**). Abz-3 and Abz-4 also demonstrated several pronounced optima at pH 6.0–9.5 similar with that for Abz-2, while Abz-6 showed no optimum, like Abz-5.

Interestingly, even at fixed pH 7.5 initial rates corresponding to increase in oligonucleotide concentrations were consistent with Michaelis-Menten kinetics only for all human RNases and Abz-1, for which was only one interception of curves in coordinates of Cornish-Bowden (**Figure 9A**) [71]. Three IgGs (Abz-2–Abz-4) demonstrated several apparent values of both K_m and V_{max} (for example, **Figure 9B**). The apparent K_m and k_{cat} values for Abz-5 and Abz-6 having comparable activity at pH from 6.0 to 9.0 demonstrated fan-like Cornish-Bowden dependencies showing smooth changes of the apparent K_m and V_{max} values with increase in substrate concentration, and there were no evident intersection points (**Figure 9C**). It means that Abz-5 contains a lot of monoclonal abzymes with comparable and different K_m and V_{max} values in their wide range. The data obtained are summarized in **Table 3** [71]. Similar pronounced heterogeneity was observed for SLE polyclonal DNase and RNase IgGs and IgAs [70, 71].

It should be mentioned that the same preparations of polyclonal Abzs hydrolyzed RNA approximately 10- to 300-fold faster than DNA [70, 71]. In addition, several monoclonal IgGs against B-DNA of different sequences (from SLE mice) efficiently hydrolyze single- and double-stranded RNA and DNA in a sequence-independent manner, the RNase activity was by a factor of 30–100 higher than of DNA [107]. Our findings indicate that a variety of anti-DNA and anti-RNA abzymes are able to hydrolyze both DNA and RNA [13–22]. In this respect, it should be mentioned that after immunization of rabbits with DNA, RNA, DNase I, DNase II, and pancreatic RNase I, antinuclease IgGs with different affinity to DNA were separated for several fractions by chromatography on DNA-cellulose [49, 50, 55–57]. IgGs of all fractions demonstrated DNase and RNase activity and RNase activity was 10- to 50-fold higher than DNase one. Only one small fraction in the case of abzymes obtained after immunization of rabbits with RNA demonstrated only DNase activity and was not able to hydrolyze RNA [50]. The data obtained testify in favor of the formation of abzymes with chimeric structure of the active centers, which are mostly able to hydrolyze both DNA and RNA.

Canonical RNases are usually specific for sequences (for example, RNase T1 is specific for guanosines, while RNase A for Py-A sequences) or for structural features (nuclease S1, for example, hydrolyzes only single-stranded domains of RNA). Abzymes of SLE and other autoimmune patients demonstrate novel RNase activities. Some of them may be stimulated by Mg^{2+}; they are not sequence-specific but sensitive to subtle and/or drastic folding changes of structurally well-characterized tRNA [72–75]. Two $tRNA^{Lys}$ [72, 74], one corresponding to human mitochondria, while the second $tRNA^{Lys}$ is a mutant revealed in patients with myoclonic epilepsy, in which A nucleotide at position 50 is changed for G nucleotide. Different canonical RNases including RNase A showed no difference in cleavage patterns of these $tRNA^{Lys}$ [72]. However, in the presence of Mg^{2+} RNase SLE abzymes produced new cleavage sites; the mutant $tRNA^{Lys}$ showed a significantly different sensitivity for abzymes in the substrate mutated region, and the hydrolysis was detected at new positions, showing local structural or conformational changes of $tRNA^{Lys}$.

Most of Mg^{2+}-dependent abzymes display usually no sequence specificity; they are more sensitive to structural features of different tRNAs specific for Gln, Phe, Asp, and Lys [72–75]. Abzymes of some AI patients demonstrate RNase A-type as a major specificity showing minor differences (preference for CpA and UpA sequences). However, some abzymes

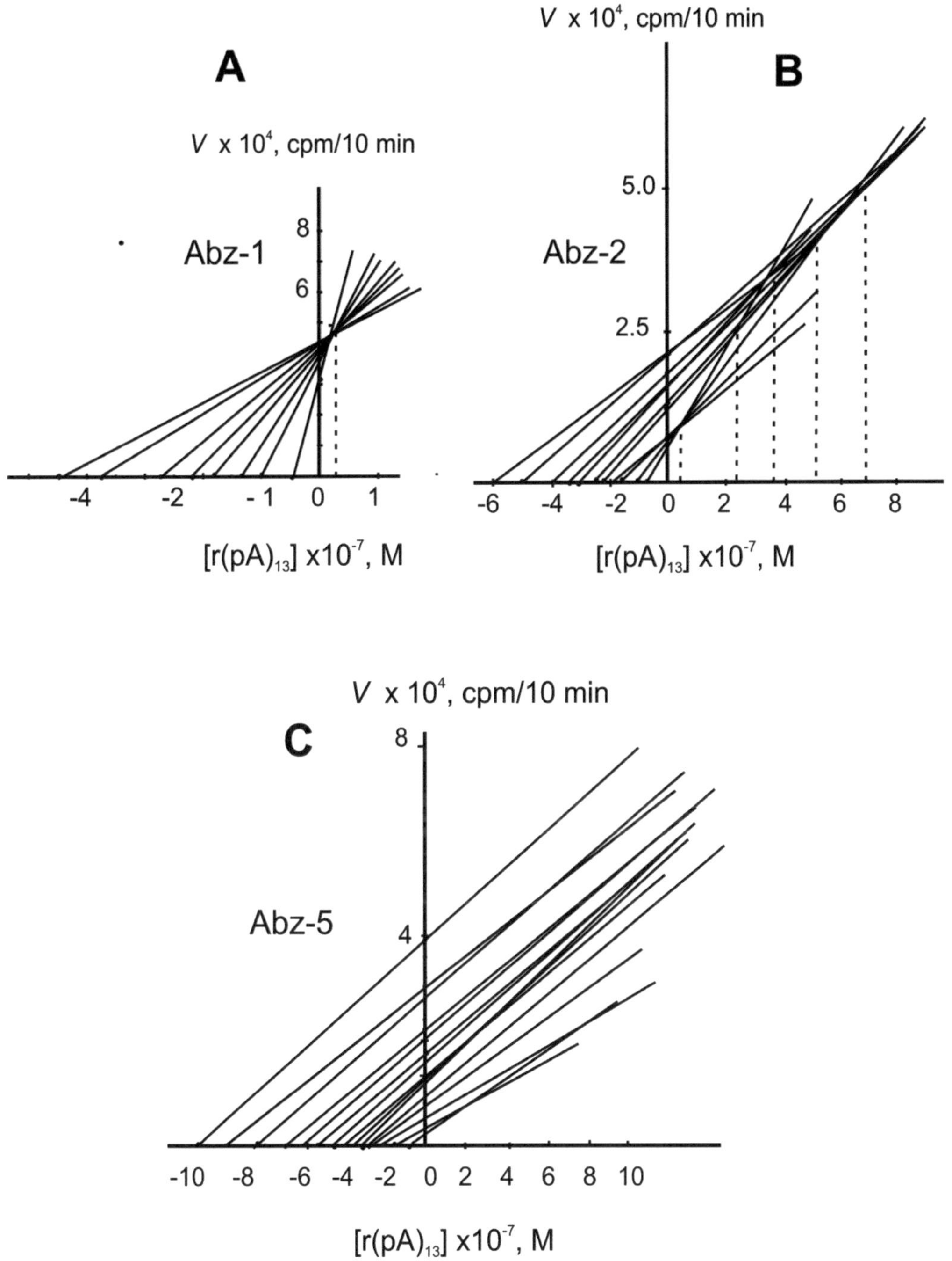

Figure 9. Initial rates of $[5'\text{-}^{32}P](pA)_{13}$ hydrolysis as a function of oligonucleotide concentration for three SLE IgGs [71]. The K_m and V_{max} values were determined using the Cornish-Bowden coordinates (A–C). The common intersection points give K_m and V_{max} values characterizing different abzymes; the absence of intersection points indicates that many different monoclonal abzymes with similar and different kinetic parameters catalyze the oligonucleotide hydrolysis.

Substrate	Preparation	$K_m{}^{\alpha}$ (M)	k_{cat} (min^{-1})
Antibodies			
$d(pA)_{13}$	Abz-1	7×10^{-8}	2.0×10^{-2}
$(pA)_{13}$		4×10^{-8}	1.4
$d(pA)_{13}$ $d(pA)_{13}$	Abz-2	4.7×10^{-8} to 3.0×10^{-7}	2.0×10^{-3} to 7.1×10^{-2}
$(pA)_{13}$		5.1×10^{-8} to 4.4×10^{-7}	0.12–0.84
$p(U)_{10}$		$9.0 \times 10^{-8} - 4.1 \times 10^{-7}$	$3.2 \times 10^{-3} - 1.3 \times 10^{-2}$
$(pA)_{13}$	Abz-3–Abz-4	1×10^{-8} to 2×10^{-6}	1.0×10^{-2} to 2.5
RNases			
$p(A)_{13}$	RNase A	3.4×10^{-6}	2.2×10^{-2}
$p(A)_{13}$	RNase 3	4.9×10^{-6}	1.7×10^{-2}
$p(U)_{10}$		2.1×10^{-6}	37
$p(A)_{13}$	RNase 4	7.2×10^{-6}	5.2×10^{-2}
$p(U)_{10}$		5.6×10^{-6}	26

[α]The errors of the values determination were within ± 10–30%.

Table 3. Kinetic parameters for hydrolysis of different oligonucleotides by catalytic SLE-IgGs, human serum RNases and pancreatic ribonuclease A [71].

contain a major subfraction demonstrating T1-type of RNase specificity. The Mg^{2+}-stimulated RNase IgGs had more often a cobra venom RNase V1-like specificity in cleavage of $tRNA^{Phe}$ with a unique Mg^{2+}-dependent specificity toward double-stranded regions [72, 74]. In spite of some similarities, SLE abzymes show specificities quite different from that of RNase V1, but this specificity remarkably differs from patient to patient. Overall, monoclonal SLE abzymes entering to total pool of Abzs can discriminate between subtle or large structural changes and nucleotide sequences. Interesting that IgGs from patients with different AI and viral diseases can demonstrate different patterns of various tRNAs cleavage [72–75].

Abzs from the sera of patients with MS [80–82], viral hepatitis [100], HIV-infected patients [95], with tick-borne encephalitis [101], Hashimoto's thyroiditis [102], and schizophrenia [103] also demonstrated DNase activity. All these diseases are characterized by different levels of the relative activity of abzymes, and DNase activity increases approximately in the following order: diabetes ≤ viral hepatitis ≈ tick borne encephalitis < polyarthritis ≤ Hashimoto's thyroiditis ≤ schizophrenia < AIDS ≤ MS < SLE [13–22, 80–82, 95, 101–103]. Overall, DNase and RNase polyclonal Abzs from sera of patient with SLE, MS, and other AI and several viral diseases may be characterized by a relatively small or extremely large content of polyclonal nuclease abzymes containing different relative amounts of kappa- and lambda-Abzs, demonstrating from one to several pH optima, having a different net charge, may be dependent or not on different metal ions, and demonstrate different substrate specificities.

6.2. Monoclonal nuclease SLE abzymes

The active centres of DNase, RNase, protease, and oligosaccharide-hydrolyzing abzymes from SLE, MS, and patients with other diseases are usually located on the light chains of these Abs [13–22]. The heavy chain is mainly responsible for specific antigen recognition and significantly increased antigen affinity for antibodies. The isolated light chains of IgGs cleavage vasoactive intestinal peptide with the activity 32-fold higher than Fab fragments [9]. Isolated by SDS-PAGE light chains of different abzymes were more active than the intact ones [13–22]. But, only multiple myeloma Bence-Jones proteins should be considered as natural human monoclonal abzymes [60].

A phagemid library of immunoglobulin kappa light chains derived from lymphocytes of peripheral blood of three SLE patients (106 variants) was cloned in pCANTAB5His6 vector. For amplification of the phage library *Escherichia coli* TG1 presenting monoclonal light chains (MLChs) on the surface of phage particles was used [111, 112]. Phage particles containing a pool of various MLChs having different affinity for DNA were separated by chromatography on DNA-cellulose (**Figure 10A**).

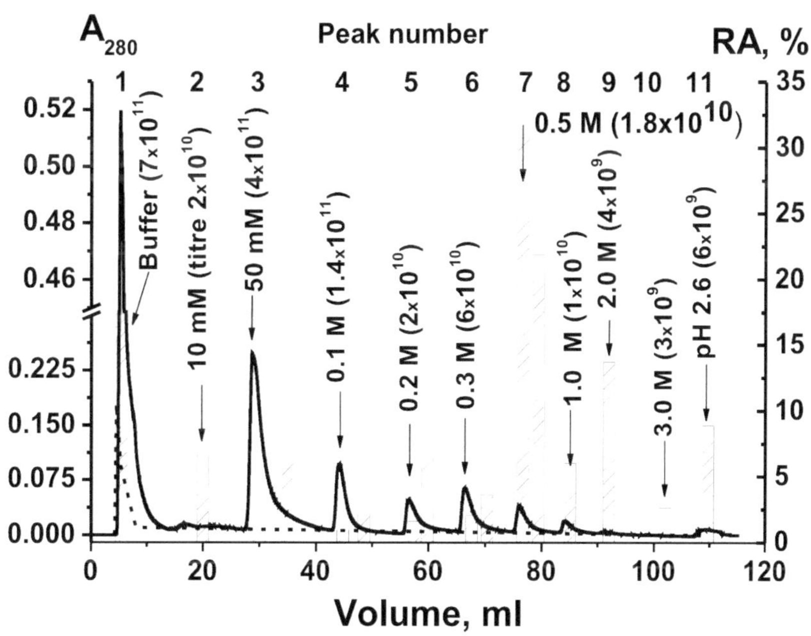

Figure 10. Affinity chromatography of phage particles on DNA-cellulose: (—) and (- - -), A280 values correspond respectively to the material of phage particles containing or not cDNA of kappa light chains [111]. The bars show the RAs of 16 fractions of 11 peaks eluted with various concentrations of NaCl and acidic buffer (pH 2.6). The titres of the particles of different peaks are given in the parenthesis.

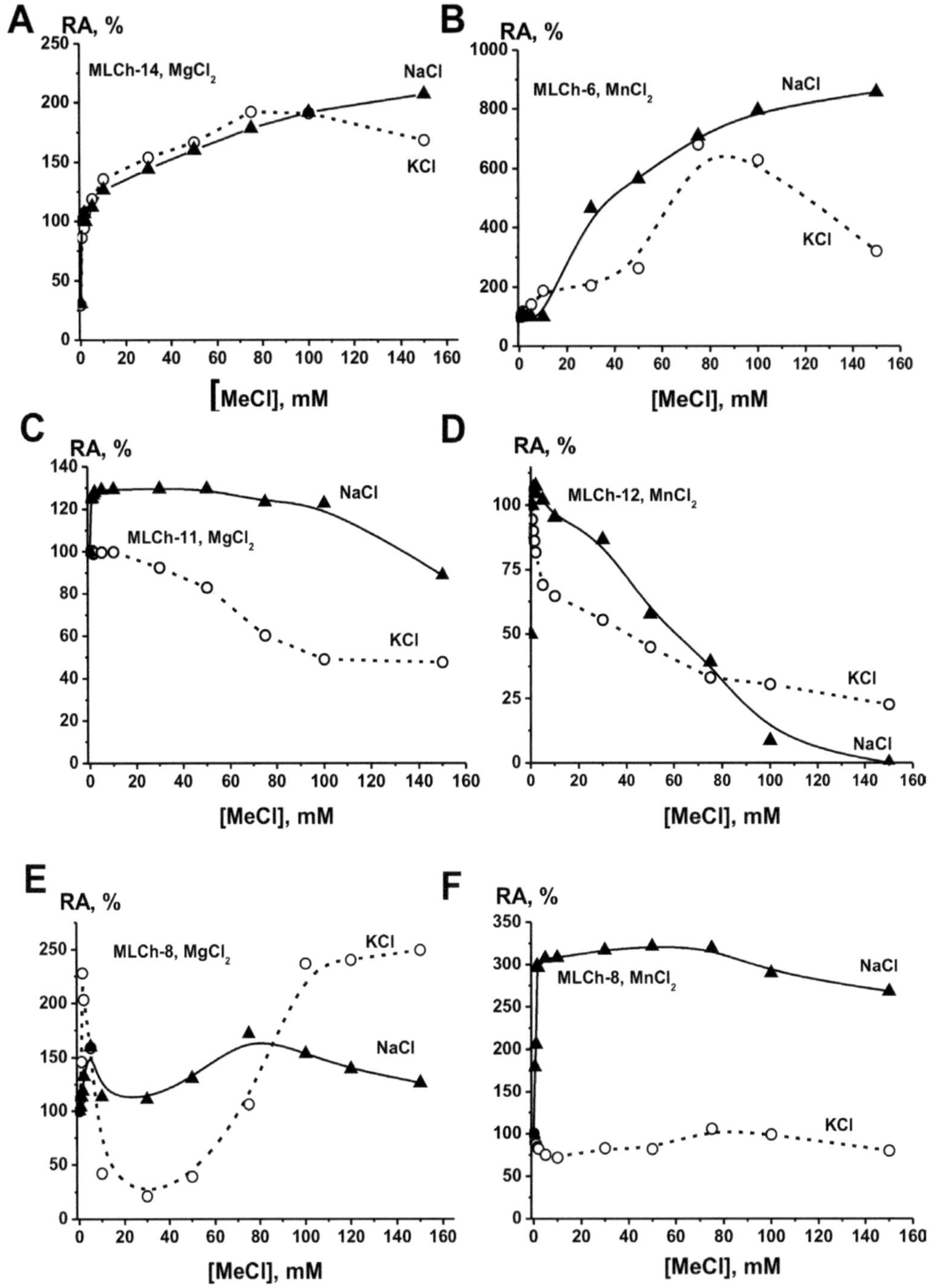

Figure 11. Dependences of the RAs of DNase activity for several MLChs upon the concentration of KCl and NaCl at 2 mM concentrations of $MgCl_2$ and $MnCl_2$ (A–F) [111]. The RAs in the absence of KCl and NaCl were taken for 100%. Numbers of MLChs (15 nM) and the used $MnCl_2$ or $MgCl_2$ are given on panels A–F.

The phage particles were distributed between 16 fractions of 11 peaks and all fractions corresponding to new small pools of anti-DNA MLChs demonstrated DNase activity (**Figure 10**). Thus, all small pools of MLChs of 16 fractions with different affinity of phage particles for DNA contained not only light chains without, but also with DNase activity. For preparation of individual colonies, *E. coli* HB2151 and phage particles eluted from DNA-cellulose with 0.5 M NaCl (peak 7) demonstrating high DNase activity were used. For study of DNase activity, 45 of 451 individual colonies from two Petri dishes were chosen in a random way; 15 of 45 single colonies (~33%) were capable to hydrolyze DNA.

MLChs of 15 single colonies were used for purification of individual MLChs using chromatography on Ni^{2+}-charged HiTrap chelating Sepharose and by following FPLC gel filtration [111]. The preparations of ~28-kDa MLChs were electrophoretically homogeneous, showed positive answer with mouse IgGs against human Abs light chains at Western blotting and positive ELISA answer using plates containing immobilized DNA; *in situ* analysis demonstrated DNase activity in the gel zone corresponding only to MLCh [111].

The dependences of DNase RAs for various MLCh preparations on the concentration of different metal ions were analyzed. It was shown that $MgCl_2$ and $MnCl_2$ are good activators of all 15 MLChs. Since K^+ and Na^+ ions can influence on the spatial structures of different enzymes, antibodies, and nucleic acids, we have analyzed dependencies of the RAs upon concentration of these ions at fixed concentrations of $MgCl_2$ and $MnCl_2$ (2 mM). All MLChs demonstrated very specific dependencies and optimal concentrations of NaCl and KCl (for example, **Figure 11**). Optimal concentrations of NaCl and KCl for 15 MLChs are given in **Table 4**. It was interesting to see whether optimal concentrations of $MgCl_2$ and $MnCl_2$ can depend on NaCl and KCl concentrations. **Figure 12** shows that for all MLChs in the presence of KCl and NaCl in different concentrations the dependencies reach plateau at 1.5–2.0 mM concentration of $MgCl_2$ and $MnCl_2$. Several MLChs demonstrated shape-bell dependencies; but the inhibition was usually observed at Mn^{2+} and Mg^{2+} concentrations higher than 2–4 mM (**Figure 12**) [111].

Various canonical DNases demonstrate usually different pH optima, but all of them have only one pH optimum [108, 109]. In contrast to known canonical DNases, polyclonal DNase Abzs from the sera of patients with SLE and other diseases can contain from one to many monoclonal abzymes demonstrating from 1 to 2–8 well pronounced pH optima in range from 5 to 10 [13–22, 72, 73, 82–84, 110]. pH optima of 15 MLChs in the presence of 2 mM $MgCl_2$ as well as for DNase II and DNase I were analyzed and several typical dependencies are given in **Figure 13**. DNase I has only one optimum at pH 7.0–7.2, while DNase II demonstrates one optimum at pH 4.9–5.0 (**Figure 13A**). Optimal pH for all 15 MLChs is given in **Table 5** [111].

Eight of 15 MLChs demonstrated only one pH optimum, while seven preparations shows two different pH optima (**Figure 13**). It was shown that Mn^{2+}, Co^{2+}, Ni^{2+}, and Ca^{2+} ions activate DNase I in significantly smaller degree than Mg^{2+} ions [108, 109]. The RAs of 15 MLChs in the presence of 6 various metal ions (2 mM) using optimal NaCl and KCl concentrations and optimal pH were estimated (**Table 6**). The maximal activity for various

Number of MLCh preparation	$MnCl_2$		$MgCl_2$	
	[KCl], mM	[NaCl], mM	[KCl], mM	[NaCl], mM
1	0–0.5; > 0.5 inhib.[a]	0–0.5; > 0.5 inhib.	30.0; > plateau[b]	100.0; >120.0 inhib.[a]
2	100; >120 inhib.	100; > 120 inhib.	75.0; >100 inhib.	15.0; >100.0 inhib.
3	5.0; > 10 inhib.	5.0; > 10.0 inhib.	0.0; > 0.0 inhib.	0.0; > 0.0 inhib.
4	2.5; > 4.0 inhib.	7.5; > 10.0 inhib.	5.0 > 10.0 inhib.	8.5; > 15.0 inhib.
5	5.0; > 10 inhib.	5.0; > 10.0 inhib.	0.0 > 0.0 inhib.	0.0; > 0.0 inhib.
6	1–2 and 75; >75 inhib.[c]	1–2 and 150	1.5–30 plateau; >40.0 inhib.	1–3 and 50.0; >100.0 inhib.
7	0.5; >1.0 inhib.	2.5; >3.0 inhib.	3.0; >4.0 inhib.	8.0; >10.0 inhib.
8	0–10 inhib.; 75; >80 inhib.	5–150 plateau	5.0 and 75.0; >80.0 inhib.	1.5; 2.0–75 inhib.; 100; >plateau[c]
9	20–25; >30 inhib.	2.0; >3.0 inhib.	10.0; >12.0 inhib.	5.0 and 75.0; >80.0 inhib.
10	2.5; plateau[b]	10.0; >15.0 inhib.	2.5; >5.0 inhib.	5.0; >7.0 inhib.
11	1–10 plateau; >10 inhib.	0.5–2.0 plateau; >2.0 inhib.	0–10.0 plateau; >10.0 inhib.	2–50 plateau; >60.0 inhib.
12	0.0; >0.0 inhib.	2.0 and 5–10; >10.0 inhib.	1–5; >10.0 inhib.	1–2 and 5–10; >10.0 inhib.
13	0.0; >0.0 inhib.	0.0 and 10.0; >10.0 inhib.	0.1–0.3; >0.7 inhib.	0–0.1; >0.1 inhib.
14	100–150 plateau	100–150 plateau	75.0; >100 inhib.	150.0
15	1.5; >2 inhib.	50.0; >50.0 inhib.	0.0 and 50.0; >50.0 inhib.	0–10 and 50.0; >50.0 inhib.

[a]For each value, a mean of two measurements is reported, optimal concentrations are given in bold; the mark (>value inhib.) means that the dependence demonstrates bell-shaped character and that at higher concentrations of the salt the inhibition of the reaction is observed.

[b]The mark (30 (or any other value in bold); >plateau) means that optimal concentration corresponds to 30 mM and there is no remarkable inhibition up to maximal concentration (100–150 mM) of NaCl or KCl used.

[c]The mark (1.5; 2.0–75 inhib.; 100; >plateau (or other similar values)) means that there are two optimal concentrations at 1.5 and 100 mM salt and a significant decrease in the activity of analyzed MLCh at concentrations in the region 2.0–75 mM.

Table 4. The optimal concentrations of KCl and NaCl in the case of individual recombinant MLChs in the presence of 2 mM $MgCl_2$ or 2 mM $MnCl_2$ [111].

MLChs was observed in the presence of different $MeCl_2$ salts, but in average the activity decreased in the following order: $MnCl_2$ > $CoCl_2$ > $MgCl_2$ > $NiCl_2$ ≈ $CaCl_2$ (**Table 6**). For all 15 MLChs, apparent k_{cat} values were estimated (**Table 6**) [111]. Overall, all 15 MLChs showed enzymatic properties very different from canonical DNases and each MLCh preparation demonstrated a very specific ratio in the RAs in the presence of different metal ions used (**Table 6**).

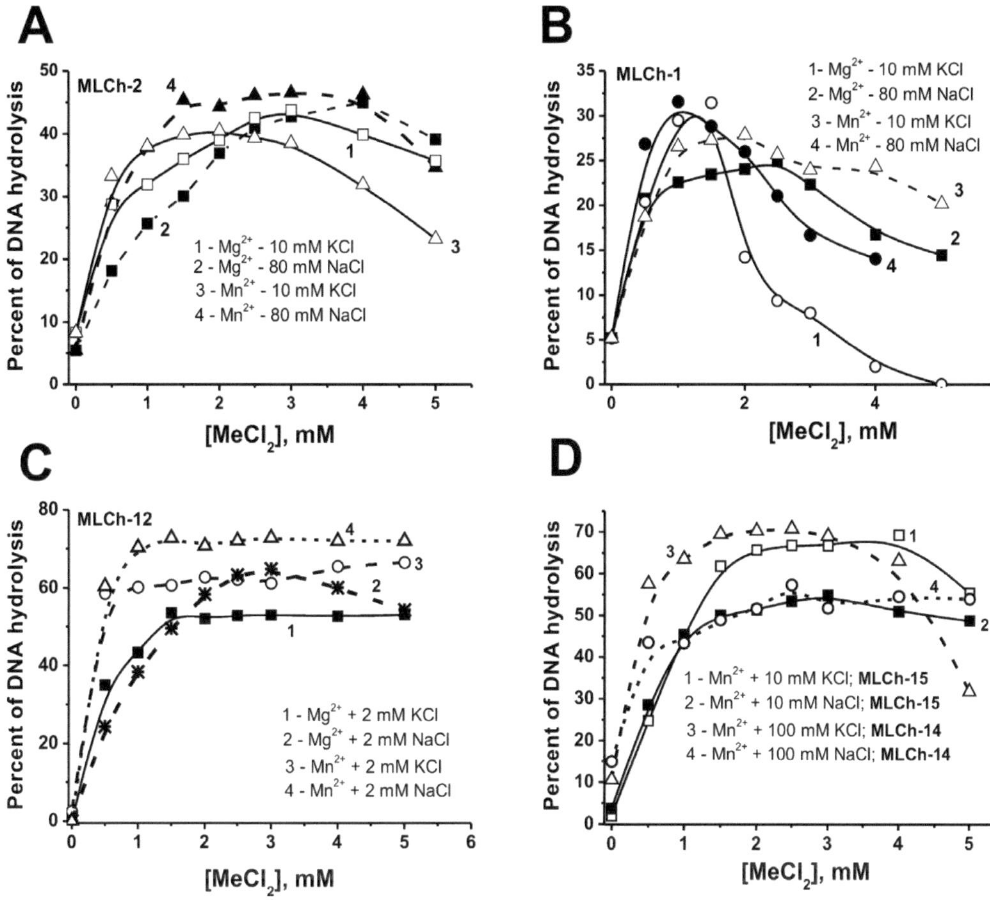

Figure 12. Dependences of the RAs of DNase activity for several MLChs (20 nM) on the concentrations of $MnCl_2$ and $MgCl_2$ at different fixed KCl and NaCl concentrations (A–D) [111]. Numbers of MLChs and concentrations of KCl and NaCl used are given on panels A–D. A complete hydrolysis of plasmid DNA was taken for 100%.

Our previous findings demonstrated that polyclonal abzymes from sera of patients with SLE, MS, and other autoimmune and/or viral diseases can contain many monoclonal DNase and RNase abzymes showing very different enzymatic properties [13–22]. At the same time, estimation of possible number of monoclonal abzymes in their total pools was very difficult, since they can have comparable or different affinity for DNA, significantly different optimal pHs, various k_{cat} values, and different dependencies on various Me^{2+} and Me^{+} ions.

In our study DNase activity only for 45 of 451 single colonies corresponding to only one (eluted with 0.5 M NaCl) of 16 fractions with different affinity for DNA-cellulose was analyzed, while MLChs of all these fractions effectively hydrolyze DNA [111]. Fifteen of 45 individual MLChs (~33%) were active in the hydrolysis of DNA. Taking into account the fact that only 45 of 451 colonies were analyzed, it should be assumed that even this fraction

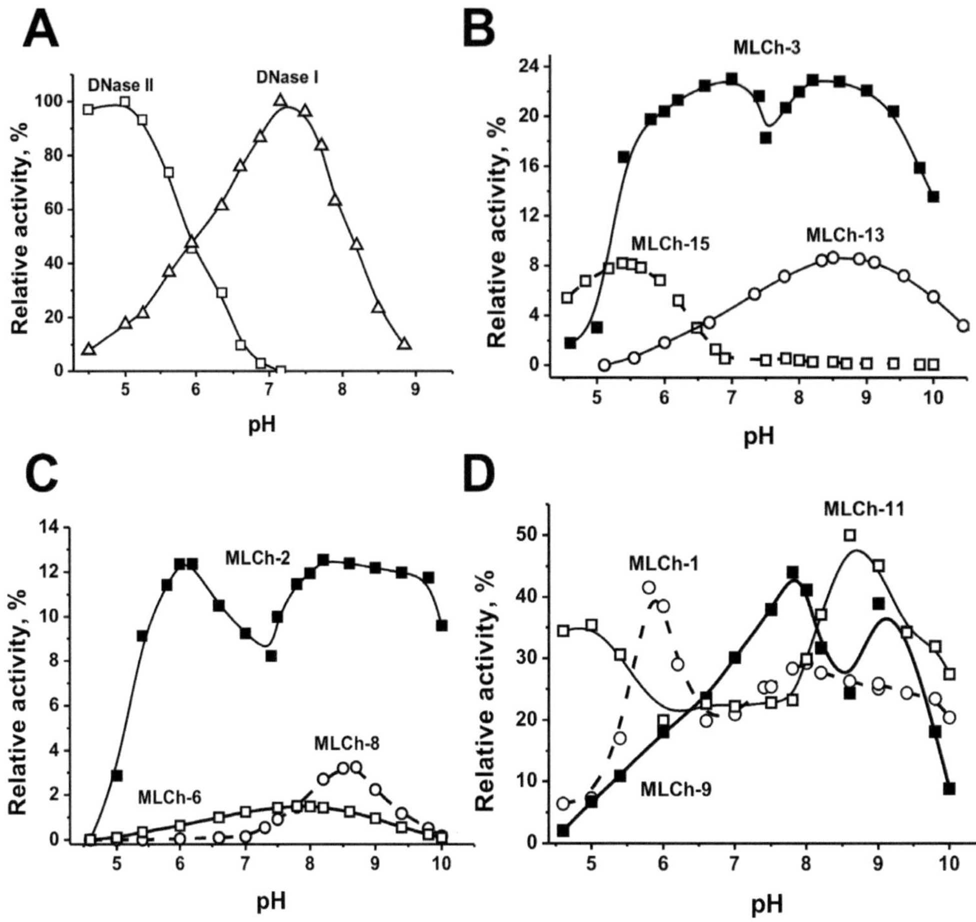

Figure 13. Dependences of the RAs of DNA-hydrolyzing activity of human DNase I and DNase II (A) and of nine MLChs (B–D) on pH of reaction mixtures [111]. The RAs for DNase II were estimated in the absence, while for DNase I, in the presence of $MgCl_2$ (10 mM). The RAs of nine MLChs were estimated using optimal $MeCl_2$ (2 mM), optimal concentration of KCl or NaCl (see **Table 6**). Reaction mixtures were incubated at 30°C for 0.4–5.0 h and then the data obtained were normalized to standard conditions; complete hydrolysis of scDNA for 30 min in the presence of various MLChs (10 nM) was taken as 100%.

contains much greater number of monoclonal abzymes with DNase activity. In this regard it should be mentioned the data of other article [112]. After separation of phage particles on DNA-cellulose, the fraction eluted by an acidic buffer (pH 2.6) was used for obtaining of MLChs (~28 kDa) with DNase activity. In this case, 33 of 687 individual colonies were chosen randomly for study of MLChs. Nineteen of 33 clones (58%) demonstrated DNase activity [112]. Detection of DNase activity *in situ* after SDS-PAGE of purified MLChs using gel containing DNA showed that they are not contaminated by canonical DNases. MLChs demonstrated from one to two pH optima. MLChs were inactive after the dialysis

http://dx.doi.org/10.5772/67790

DNase or number of MLCh preparation	Optimal pH	
	pH_1	pH_2
DNase I	7.0–7.2	No second optimum
DNAse II	4.9–5.0	No second optimum
1	5.7–5.9	7.9–8.1[b]
2	6.0–6.2	8.2–8.3
3	6.9–7.0	8.2–8.5
4	7.5–7.6	No second optimum
5	6.9–7.0	8.2–8.5
6	7.8–8.0	No second optimum
7	6.2–6.4	No second optimum
8	8.5–8.6	No second optimum
9	7.8–8.0	8.9–9.1
10	6.1–6.3	8.5–8.7
11	4.8–5.0	8.6–8.7
12	7.7–7.9	No second optimum
13	8.5–8.7	No second optimum
14	7.9–8.1	No second optimum
15	5.4–5.6	No second optimum

[a]For each value, a mean of two measurements is reported.
[b]For various MLChs one or two optimal pHs were revealed.

Table 5. The optimal pH values for DNase II, DNase I, and 15 different recombinant and individual MLChs[a] [111].

against EDTA but were activated by different metal ions; the ratio of RA in the presence of Mg^{2+}, Mn^{2+}, Ni^{2+}, Ca^{2+}, Zn^{2+}, and Co^{2+} was individual for each MLCh preparation. Na^+ and K^+ suppressed DNA-hydrolyzing activity of these MLChs at different concentrations [112]. Hydrolysis of DNA by all MLChs was consistent with Michaelis-Menten kinetics. These recombinant MLChs demonstrated high affinity for DNA (K_m = 3–9 nM) and high k_{cat} values (3.4–6.9 min^{-1}) [112]. Even if we assume that each of the above-mentioned 16 fractions can contain only about 20 MLChs with DNase activity, their total number may be close to 300, but it is obvious that this number is much larger and can be close from one to several thousands.

Number of MLChs	Mg^{2+}	Mn^{2+}	Zn^{2+}	Ni^{2+}	Co^{2+}	Cu^{2+}	Ca^{2+}	pH[c]	[NaCl] or [KCl], mM[d]	*App.* k_{cat}, min^{-1b}
1	92.7	100[a]	6.5	10.7	20.6	0.0	4.0	5.8[e]	100.0 Na^+	0.6 ± 0.04
	60.7	100.0	7.5	11.5	18.5	0.0	5.4	8.0[f]	100.0 Na^+	
2	69.6	100.0	55.4	83.8	73.0	0.0	10.1	6.1	80.0 Na^+	0.1 ± 0.01
	100.0	92.3	18.5	95.6	63.7	3.0	26.0	8.2	80.0 Na^+	
3	78.3	98.5	42.7	56.2	0.3	9.0	100.0	6.9	5.0 K^+	
	1.3	100.0	3.6	11.9	99.0	0.0	0.0	8.4	5.0 K^+	0.33 ± 0.03
4	51.0	100.0	80.0	56.0	24.0	5.0	26.0	7.5	7.5 Na^+	0.5 ± 0.04
5	78.3	98.5	42.7	56.2	0.0	9.0	100	6.9	5.0 K^+	0.3± 0.03
	1.3	100.0	3.6	11.9	99.0	0.0	0.0	8.4	5.0 K^+	0.34 ± 0.03
6	1.3	100.0	3.6	11.9	99.0	0.0	0.0	7.9	1.0 K^+	0.02 ± 0.003
7	75	70	80	85	100.0	5	21	6.3	2.5 Na^+	0.3 ± 0.04
8	58.5	100.0	18.3	19.7	0.0	0.0	16.2	8.5	5.0 Na^+	0.06 ± 0.07
9	100.0	85.2	15.9	0.0	85.4	0.0	75	7.8	1.5 Na^+	0.7 ± 0.08
10	25	20	15	100.0	17	2	39	8.6	10.0 Na^+	0.2 ± 0.02
11	80	85	43	24	100.0	0.0	8	8.6	5.0 K^+	0.7 ± 0.06
12	55.0	88.5	16.5	56.3	100.0	1.2	56.2	7.8	5.0 K^+	0.12 ± 0.01
13	34.5	25.0	16.9	83.3	100.0	4.8	41.9	8.6	0.1 K^+	0.13 ± 0.01
14	80.9	75.2	19.7	100.0	59.5	6.3	37.3	8.0	5.0 Na^+	0.11 ± 0.01
15	100.0	49.2	55.7	33.5	85.8	45.0	70.0	5.5	1.5 Na^+	0.12 ± 0.01

[a]The maximal RAs in the presence of one of seven metal ions used was taken as 100% and given in bold; the error of the values determination (two independent experiments) did not exceed 7–10%.

[b]The apparent k_{cat} values using optimal conditions were calculated as $k_{cat} = V_{max}$ (nM/min)/[MLCh] (nM).

[c]Optimal pHs were used for every of MLCh preparation.

[d]Optimal concentrations of KCl and NaCl in the case of different MLChs were used.

[e]The RAs for several MLChs were found in the case of two different pH optima.

Table 6. The RAs of different recombinant MLChs in the presence of various metal ions (2 mM) at optimal pHs and concentration of KCl and NaCl [111].

7. Abzymes with protease activity

7.1. Polyclonal abzymes hydrolyzing myelin basic protein

The increased level of antibodies to myelin basic protein and abzymes hydrolyzing MBP was revealed for the first time in the blood of patients with multiple sclerosis [83–87]. It was shown that Abs of healthy donors cannot hydrolyze MBP [13–22, 83–87]. The most widely accepted theory of multiple sclerosis pathogenesis assigns the major role in the destruction of myelin including MBP to the inflammation related to autoimmune reactions [43, 113–115]. Increased levels of Abs and oligoclonal IgGs in the cerebrospinal fluid together with clonal B cell accumulation in the CSF and lesions of MS patients are among the main evidences of MS [115].

ELISA was used for comparison of the relative levels of Abs against MBP in the sera of 12 healthy donors and 14 patients with SLE [77]. For healthy donors the concentrations of auto-Abs were not zero and varied from 0.02 to 0.16 A_{450} units; in average 0.09 ± 0.04 A_{450} units; similar value (0.09 ± 0.04 A_{450} units) was previously revealed for other 10 healthy volunteers [83]. Relative concentrations of anti-MBP Abs of SLE patients were changed from 0.27 to 0.54 A_{450} units, in average 0.38 ± 0.08 A_{450} units [77]. Using the same test system, it was previously revealed that the indexes of anti-MBP Abs for 25 MS patients are changed from 0.67 to 0.98 A_{450} units, in average 0.8 ± 0.1 A_{450} units [83, 84]. Thus, all SLE patients demonstrated in average ~4.2-fold higher level of anti-MBP Abs then healthy donors, but by a factor of ~2.1 lower level than MS patients.

Electrophoretically and immunologically homogeneous polyclonal IgGs were purified from the sera of SLE patients by sequential chromatography of serum proteins on Protein-G Sepharose using conditions removing nonspecifically bound proteins, followed by FPLC gel filtration in condition destroying immune complexes [77, 78] similarly to obtaining of MS IgGs [84–87]. It was shown that 150 kDa SLE IgGs are electrophoretically homogeneous and in contrast to Abs from healthy donors are active in the hydrolysis of MBP [55, 77]. To prove that MBP-hydrolyzing activity of SLE IgGs is their intrinsic property, we have checked the fulfilment of several known strict criteria described above including analysis of Ab protease activity after SDS-PAGE (**Figure 7**) [77]. In addition, it was shown that in contrast to canonical proteases, the SLE polyclonal IgGs separated using MBP-Sepharose specifically hydrolyzed only MBP (**Figure 14A**) but not many other tested control proteins (**Figure 14B**) [77].

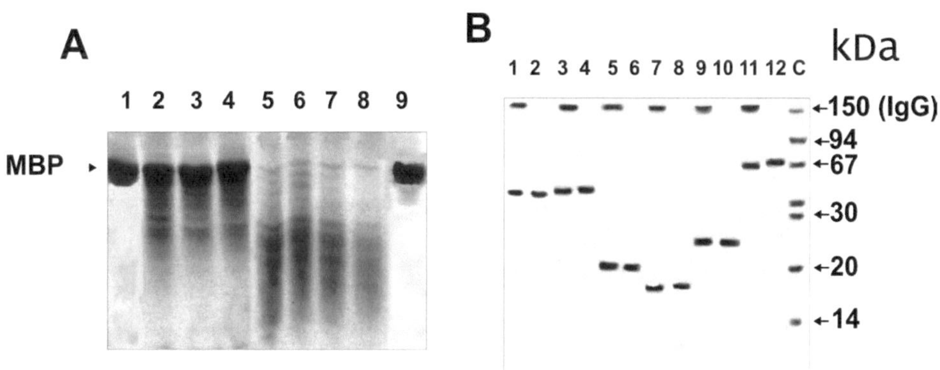

Figure 14. The hydrolysis of MBP (0.7 mg/ml) by 3 μg/ml IgGmix (mixture of IgGs of 12 SLE patients) separated by chromatography on MBP-Sepharose after incubation for 1 (lane 2), 2 (lane 3), 3 (lane 4), 14 (lane 5), 16 (lane 6), 18 (lane 7), and 24 h (lane 8) (A) [77]. Lanes 1 and 9 correspond respectively to MBP incubated during 24 h alone or in the presence of 0.2 mg/ml IgGmix from 12 healthy volunteers. SDS-PAGE analysis of the hydrolysis of different control proteins by the same IgGmix (B). Proteins were incubated for 24 h with 30 μg/ml IgGmix (odd numbers) or without antibodies (even numbers): BSA (lanes 1 and 2), human serum albumin (lanes 3 and 4), casein from human milk (lanes 5 and 6), lysozyme from hen eggs (lanes 7 and 8), bovine aldolase (lanes 9 and 10), and lactoferrin from human milk (lanes 11 and 12). Lane C corresponds to standard protein markers. SLE IgGs specifically hydrolyze only MBP (A), but not other proteins (B).

Protease IgGs from the sera of ~95–100% of patients with different autoimmune pathologies [9, 66, 116], human milk Abs hydrolyzing casein [96, 117], Abs from AIDS patients hydrolyzing HSA, casein, and HIV reverse transcriptase [95] are serine-like proteases, whose activity is strongly decreased after their preincubation with serine protease-specific inhibitors PMSF. In addition, a high metal-dependent MBP-hydrolyzing activity for MS IgGs [86] and casein-hydrolyzing of human milk sIgAs [96] were recently revealed. It was shown that antiintegrase IgGs and IgMs of HIV-infected patients can contain abzymes hydrolyzing viral integrase of four types, resembling serine, thiol, metal-dependent, and acidic proteases, the ratio of which may be individual for every AIDS patient [97, 98].

It was shown that preincubation of individual polyclonal SLE IgGs with specific inhibitor of thiol proteases iodoacetamide and of acidic proteases pepstatin A [77, 78] similarly to MS IgAs, IgGs, and IgMs [84–87] leads to a small effect (5–15%) on MBP hydrolysis by SLE IgGs. PMSF specifically inhibiting serine proteases and inhibitor of metalloproteases EDTA remarkably or significantly suppressed proteolytic activity of SLE IgGs (**Figure 15A**).

The inhibition of Abz activity by EDTA is significantly greater than by PMSF. Overall, all individual SLE abzymes possess specific ratio of RAs in the presence of PMSF and EDTA (**Figure 15A**). Interestingly, polyclonal SLE abzymes was more sensitive to EDTA than MS Abs [77]. Catalytic heterogeneity of polyclonal abzymes with several different activities from patients with various autoimmune diseases and animals was shown in many papers [65, 80–82, 92]. The above data also demonstrate extreme heterogeneity of SLE abzymes hydrolyzing MBP. In addition, polyclonal MBP-hydrolyzing abzymes of every patient are characterized with specific dependence of RAs upon pH; the pH profile of each IgG is unique (**Figure 15B** and **D**). The effect of several different metal ions on the MBP-hydrolyzing activities of dialyzed against EDTA individual 12 SLE polyclonal IgGs was analyzed (**Figure 16A** and **B**; B is a continuation of A).

All 12 IgGs demonstrated the individual ratios of RAs in the presence of eight various metal ions. To analyze the "average" effect of different metal ions on SLE and MS IgGs, we have used SLE IgGmix and MS IgGmix before (**Figure 16C**) and after (**Figure 16D**) their dialysis against EDTA. Ca^{2+} was shown to the best activator of SLE IgGmix the effect of different metals decrease in the following order: $Ca^{2+} > Co^{2+} \geq Ni^{2+} \geq Mg^{2+} \geq Mn^{2+} \geq Cu^{2+}$. Fe^{2+} did not activate SLE IgGmix, while Zn^{2+} inhibits its activity. MS IgGmix demonstrated a different order of the metal-dependent activity: $Mg^{2+} > Mn^{2+} \geq Cu^{2+} \geq Ni^{2+} \geq Co^{2+} \geq Ca^{2+}$, while Fe^{2+} and Zn^{2+} slightly inhibit MBP hydrolysis (**Figure 16C** and **D**).

In addition, the mixture of electrophoretically homogeneous IgGmix was separated to fractions of IgG1–IgG4 subclasses and to fractions of IgGs containing lambda- and kappa-type of light [76]. The immunological purity of IgGs of all types was revealed by ELISA; the preparations of IgG1, IgG2, IgG3, and IgG4 did not contain IgGs of other subclasses. The lambda - and kappa-IgGs and IgG1–IgG4 were active in the hydrolysis of MBP and their RAs and k_{cat} values are given in **Table 7**. Kappa-IgGs demonstrated 1.2-fold lower apparent k_{cat} (2.4×10^{-2} min^{-1}) than lambda-IgGs (2.8×10^{-2} min^{-1}). The apparent k_{cat} values of different subclasses IgG abzymes in the hydrolysis of MBP increased in the following order (min^{-1}): IgG4 (1.7) < IgG2 (2.7) < IgG3 (2.9) < IgG1 (3.0) (**Table 7**). The relative content of kappa-IgGs and lambda-IgGs

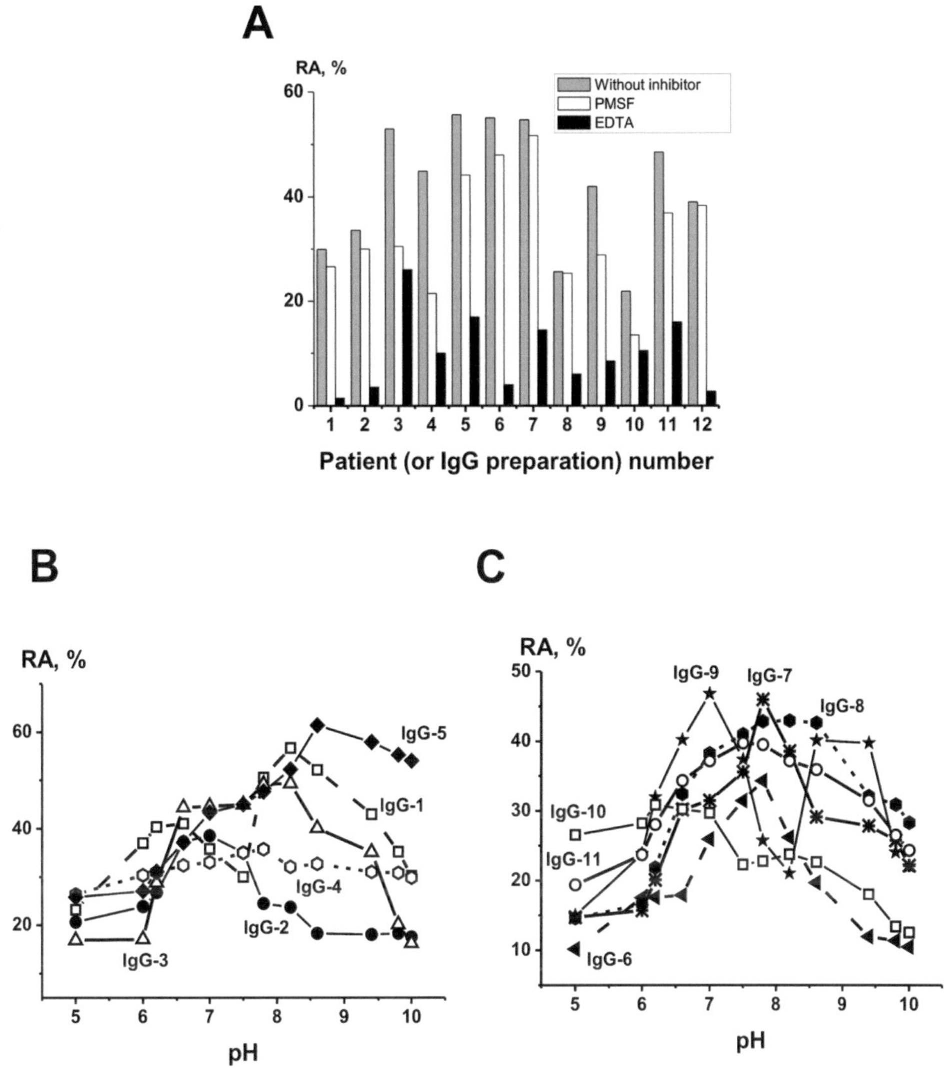

Figure 15. The relative proteolytic activities of 12 different individual SLE IgGs in the hydrolysis of MBP (0.5 mg/ml) before (gray columns), after their preincubation with PMSF (white columns) or 35 mM EDTA (black columns) (A) [77]. The pH dependences of the RAs of MBP-hydrolyzing activity of 11 individual SLE IgGs (B and C). The complete hydrolysis of MBP (0.5 mg/ml) was taken for 100%.

as well as IgG1–IgG4 in nonfractionated IgGmix was estimated (**Table 7**). Taking this content into account, the relative contribution of kappa-IgGs and lambda-IgGs into the total MBP-hydrolyzing activity of IgGmix was estimated as 48.4 ± 4.0% and 55.5 ± 4.3%, respectively (**Table 7**). The relative contribution of SLE IgGs of different subclasses to the total proteolytic activity of IgGmix was estimated in a similar way: IgG1 (73.0 ± 3.4%) > IgG2 (19.1 ± 1.8%) > IgG3 (6.7 ± 0.3%) > IgG4 (1.2 ± 0.2%). These data provided the first evidence that SLE IgGs of all types possess MBP-hydrolyzing activity, but they differ in the relative contribution into the total activity of proteolytic activity of polyclonal abzymes [76]. Kappa-IgGs and lambda-IgGs

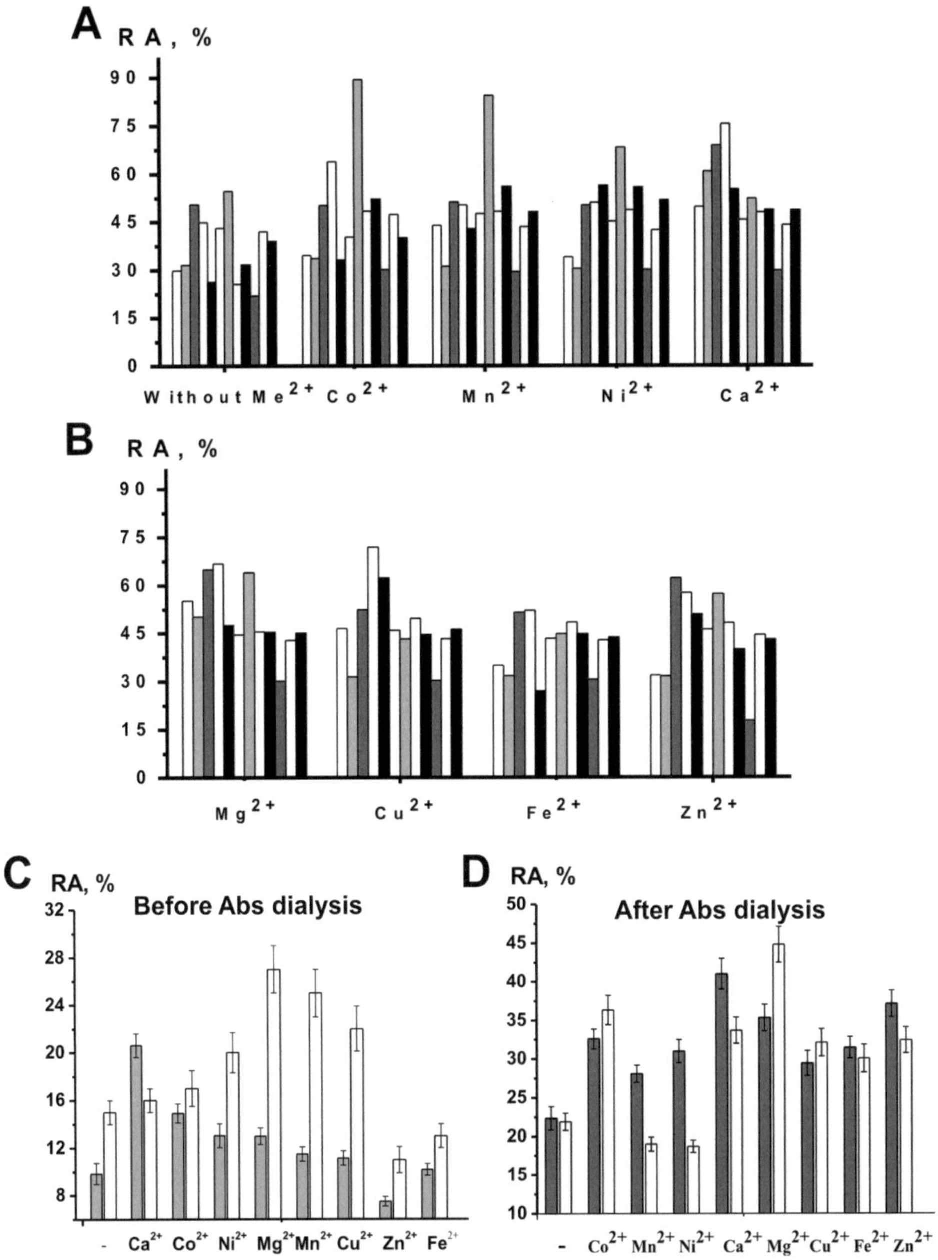

Figure 16. The RAs of 12 SLE IgGs dialyzed against EDTA in the hydrolysis of MBP [77]; 12 columns of different color of the first set (A) correspond to 12 individual Abs in the absence of external metal ions, while 8 other columns sets to the same 12 IgGs in the presence of 8 different metal ions marked on panels A and B. An average error did not exceed 10% (A and B). The RAs of SLE IgGmix (gray columns) and MS IgGmix (white columns) before (C) and after (D) these Abs dialysis against EDTA in the cleavage of MBP in the presence of different metal ions (2 mM). A complete hydrolysis of MBP (0.5 mg/ml) for 1 h in the presence of 0.01 mg/ml Abs was taken for 100%. Various metal ions are shown in panels A–D.

IgG	Content, %	RAs (mg MBP/1 h) / mg of IgGs**	Apparent k_{cat}, ×10² (min⁻¹)§	Contribution to the total activity, %#
IgG, nonfractionated	100	1.95 ± 0.05	2.6 ± 0.07	100
IgGs containing lambda- and kappa-types of light chains				
kappa-IgG	44.6 ± 4.0	2.1 ± 0.16*	2.8 ± 0.21	48.4 ± 4.0
lambda-IgG	55.4 ± 5.0	1.8 ± 0.15	2.4 ± 0.20	55.5 ± 4.3
IgGs of different subclasses				
IgG1	70.8 ± 2.0	2.3 ± 0.11	3.0 ± 0.14	73.0 ± 3.4
IgG2	20.6 ± 3.0	2.0 ± 0.2	2.7 ± 0.25	19.1 ± 1.8
IgG3	6.7 ± 1.5	2.2 ± 0.08	2.9 ± 0.10	6.7 ± 0.3
IgG4	1.9 ± 1.0	1.3 ± 0.07	1.7 ± 0.09	1.2 ± 0.2

*For each fraction, a mean of two repeats is used.

**Relative activities at fixed 0.75 mg/ml concentration of MBP were estimated.

§Apparent k_{cat} values were calculated as $k_{cat} = V$ (M/min)/[IgG] (M).

#Contribution of different IgGs to the total activity of nonfractionated Abs was calculated taking into account the relative content of these IgGs within polyclonal IgG_{mix} and their RAs in the hydrolysis of MBP.

Table 7. Relative specific MBP-hydrolyzing activities (RAs) of IgGs of different types and their relative contributions to the total activity of polyclonal IgG_{mix} [76].

hydrolyzed MBP within a wide range of pH values (5.3–9.5) and showed comparable pH dependencies, while the pH profiles for IgG1–IgG4 were unique (**Figure 17**).

These results clearly demonstrate that IgGs of all four subclasses are very heterogeneous and can consist of different sets of catalytic subfractions of polyclonal IgG having quite distinct pH dependencies. **Figure 17** shows the relative influence of PMSF and EDTA on the MBP-hydrolyzing activity of different IgGs. The nonfractionated IgGs and lambda-IgGs demonstrated lower inhibition by PMSF than that for EDTA (**Figure 17**). The inhibition of serine-like and metal-dependent activities of kappa-IgGs were comparable. PMSF suppressed MBP-hydrolyzing activity of IgG3, IgG2, and IgG1 by 13–17%, while the decrease of this activity by EDTA was significantly greater, 30–45%. There was no noticeable PMSF effect on the IgG4 activity, while EDTA decreased its activity by ~65% (**Figure 17**). Thus, IgG1–IgG4, kappa-IgGs, and lambda-IgGs are characterized by specific ratios of metal-dependent and serine-like proteolytic activities.

The cleavage site specificity of different IgG preparations in the case of four oligopeptides corresponding to four antigenic determinants of MBP was analyzed [76]. Overall, kappa-IgGs and lambda-IgGs, as well as IgG1–IgG4 demonstrated either different patterns of four oligopeptides cleavage, or at least stimulate the accumulation of the same products of the hydrolysis with different efficiency.

The dialysis of IgGs caused a more pronounced decrease in the activity of kappa-IgGs than of lambda-IgGs [76]. Addition to the reaction mixtures of Ca^{2+} + Mg^{2+} or Ca^{2+} + Co^{2+} led to

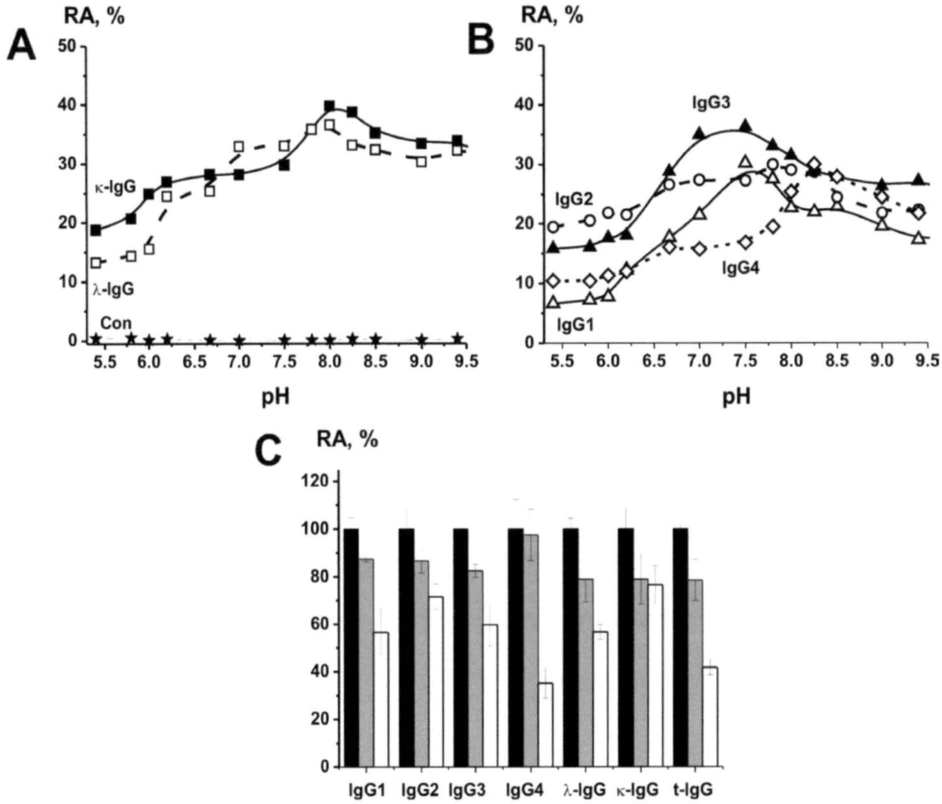

Figure 17. The pH dependence of RAs of MBP-hydrolyzing SLE kappa-and lambda-IgGs (A), as well IgG1, IgG2, IgG3, and IgG4 (B) [76]. Hydrolysis of MBP incubated without IgGs was used as control ("Con," A). The RAs of MBP-hydrolyzing activity of SLE IgG1, IgG2, IgG3, IgG4, and total IgGmix (t-IgG) (C). The RAs were determined before (black columns) and after IgGs preincubation with PMSF (gray columns) and EDTA (white columns). The RAs of all IgGs in the absence of the inhibitors were taken as 100%.

approximately comparable increase in the RAs of dialyzed lambda-IgG (1.6- to 1.7-fold), kappa-IgG (2.0- to 2.3-fold), and nonfractionated IgGs (1.7- to 1.8-fold). Ca^{2+}+Co^{2+} together cannot activate IgG1, while in the presence of Ca^{2+} + Mg^{2+} its activity increased by a factor of 1.6. Ca^{2+} + Co^{2+} increased the activity of IgG2 (~2.9-fold), IgG3 (~6.4-fold), and IgG4 (~6.0-fold). A significant increases in the RAs were revealed for Ca^{2+} + Mg^{2+} in the case of IgG3 (~3.5-fold), IgG4 (~4.4-fold), and IgG2 (~5.7-fold). While the Ca^{2+} + Mg^{2+} combination was the best for the activation of IgG2 and IgG1, IgG4, and IgG3 showed the highest activity in the presence of Ca^{2+} + Co^{2+}. The ratios of RAs of all IgG preparations before and after their dialysis against EDTA, as well as in the presence of different metal ions, were individual for every preparation analyzed. These data indicate for an extreme Me^{2+}-dependence diversity of different subclasses SLE IgGs hydrolyzing MBP.

The extraordinary diversity of polyclonal abzymes with DNase, RNase, and proteolytic activities was shown not only in the case of SLE, but also other diseases [13–22]. Very unexpected enzyme properties have been discovered in the case of monoclonal abzymes of patients with SLE.

7.2. Monoclonal SLE abzymes hydrolyzing myelin basic protein

For analysis of MBP-hydrolyzing activity of Abs, we have used the same phagemid library of kappa light chains [118–120] as for analysis of MLChs with DNase activity [111, 112]. The phage particles containing MLChs with different for MBP were separated by affinity chromatography on MBP-Sepharose (**Figure 18A**).

The pool of phage particles was distributed between 10 peaks eluted from the sorbent and all MLChs of fractions of 10 new small pools efficiently hydrolyzed MBP and four oligopeptides (OPs) corresponding to four immunodominant MBP sequences containing cleavage sites (**Figure 18B**). However, there were no any detectable particles peaks having considerable affinity for MBP after similar chromatography of phage particles with pCANTAB plasmid containing no cDNA of light chains (**Figure 18A**). Thus, the MLChs pools of all 10 phage particles fractions having different affinity to MBP contain both inactive and catalytically active light chains hydrolyzing MBP. Similar distribution all over the chromatography profiles was

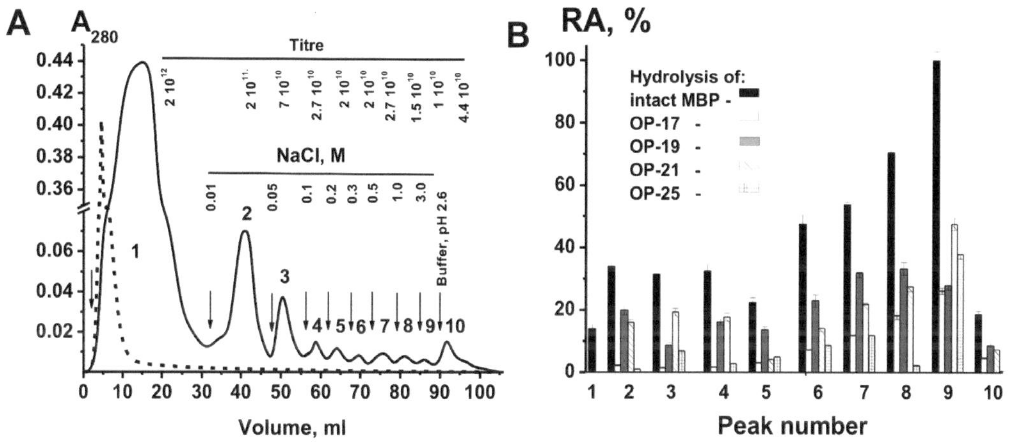

C

OP-21

AAQKRPSQRSK***YLASASTMDHARHGFLPR***RHRDTGILDSLGRFFGSDRGAPK

OP-17

RGSGKDGHHAARTTHYGSLPQKAQGHRPQD***ENPVVHFFKNIVTPRTP***PPSQG

OP-19

KGRGLS***LSRFSWGAEGQKPGFGYGG***RASDYKSAHKGLKGHD

OP-25

AOGTLSKIFKLGGRDSRSGSPMARR

Figure 18. Affinity chromatography on MBP-Sepharose of phage particles: (– –) and (—) absorbance at 280 nm of particles corresponding plasmid respectively without and with kappa light chains cDNA (A) [118]. Relative titres of phage particle and NaCl concentrations corresponding to various peaks are shown on panel A. The bars (B) indicate the RAs of 10 phage particles small pools of peaks 1–10 eluted from the MBP-Sepharose with different NaCl concentrations and acidic buffer (pH 2.6) (A); the reaction mixtures containing MBP (0.7 mg/ml) were incubated at 30°C for 12 h or different 1 mM OPs: OP17, OP19, OP21, and OP25 (see panel C) were incubated with 109 plaque-forming units/ml phage particles for 6 h and a complete hydrolysis of the substrates was taken as 100%. Complete MBP protein sequence and positions of four OPs sequences containing the protein cleavage sites (C).

observed for polyclonal IgGs from SLE and MS patients in the case of their chromatography on MBP-Sepharose [76, 77, 86, 87].

Phage particles eluted from MBP-Sepharose with 0.5 M NaCl (peak 7, **Figure 18A**) were used for preparation of individual colonies. Overall, 72 of 440 individual colonies choosing in a random way were used for study of MBP-hydrolyzing activity. MLChs of 22 of 72 single colonies (~30%) possess MBP-hydrolyzing activity. All 22 recombinant catalytically active MLChs containing a sequence of 6 histidine residues interacting with Ni^{2+} ions and 5 MLChs without activity were purified by chromatography on charged with Ni^{2+} ions HiTrap chelating Sepharose and by following FPLC gel filtration. Then a mixture of equal amounts of 22 catalytically active monoclonal MLChs (act-MLChmix) and second mixture of five preparations without activity (inact-MLChmix) were prepared. The electrophoretical homogeneity of ~26- to 27-kDa inact-MLChmix and act-MLChmix was shown by SDS-PAGE with silver staining (**Figure 19A**, lane 1).

MLChmix was subjected to SDS-PAGE; its proteolytic activity was revealed after extraction of proteins from the separated gel slices only in the band corresponding to the MLCh (**Figure 19A** and **B**). Act-MLChmix demonstrated activity in the hydrolysis of MBP (**Figure 19C**, lane 4), while inact-MLChmix had no activity (**Figure 19C**, lane 2). Moreover, in contrast to canonical proteases cleaving all proteins, act-MLChmix hydrolyzes only MBP (**Figure 19C**, lane 4) but no other control proteins (**Figure 19C**, lanes 5–8). All 22 act-MLChs and 5 inact-MLChs showed positive answer with mouse Abs (conjugated with horseradish peroxidase) against light chains of human Abs at Western blotting and positive ELISA response using plates with immobilized MBP.

The RAs in the hydrolysis of four different OPs were analyzed by TLC. **Figure 19(D)** and **(E)** demonstrates several typical examples of the OP19 and OP21 hydrolysis by different MLChs [118]. Initially, we have assumed that every of 22 MLChs corresponds to IgGs to one of four known specific MBP immunodominant sequences and that each MLCh can bind and hydrolyze only one of four OPs. At the same time, unexpected results were obtained. The RAs for 22 MLCh are summarized in **Figure 19(F)**. All 22 MLChs hydrolyzed only three or four OPs and with significantly different efficiency in the case of every OP. Hydrolysis of OP17 MBP was very weak (~1–1.5%) except seven MLChs: $15 \geq 10 \geq 12 \geq 1 \geq 16 \geq 20 \geq 8$ (1.6–7.1%) (**Figure 19F**). All MLChs except MLCh-22 hydrolyzed efficiently OP21 and several other OPs, while six other MLChs (8, 9, 10, 12, 13, and 14) demonstrated high activity only in the cleavage of OP21. Several MLChs (1–7, and 11) efficiently hydrolyzed OP19 and OP21, while MLCh-18 and 20 cleaved OP21 and OP25. Four recombinant MLChs (15, 17, 19, and 21) cleaved three OPs with relatively high efficiency, while MLCh-16 hydrolyzed all four OPs (**Figure 19E**). The ratios of the RAs in the hydrolysis of four OPs were specific for every MLCh (**Figure 19E**). OP21 and OP19 were shown to be the best substrates for most MLChs, while 15–22 MLChs better hydrolyzed OP25.

In contrast to MS IgGs [76, 77, 84–87], SLE polyclonal abzymes with MBP-hydrolyzing activity are less sensitive to PMSF than to EDTA. The effect of PMSF and EDTA on the RAs of 22 different MLChs was analyzed [118]. **Figure 20(A)** shows that the 12 MLChs (1, 2, 3, 5, 7, 8, 12, 13, 15, 16, 17, and 19) are metal-dependent proteases; they cannot not remarkably decrease

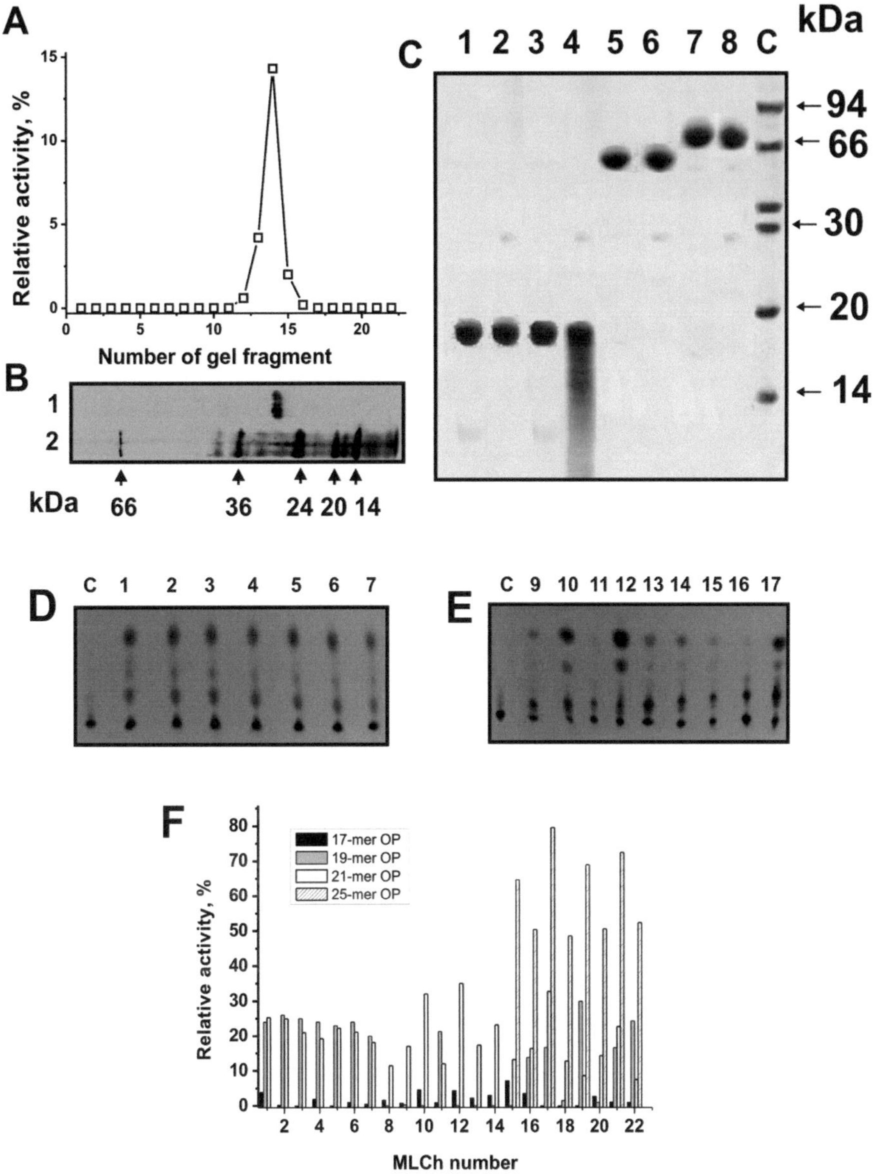

Figure 19. SDS-PAGE analysis of proteolytic activity (A) and homogeneity of act-MLChmix (7 μg) (B, lane 1) using a 5–16% gradient gel with following silver staining; the arrows indicate the positions of protein markers (B, lane 2) [118]. After electrophoresis the gel was incubated using special conditions for renaturation of act-MLChmix. The RAs in the hydrolysis of MBP (%) was determined using the extracts of 2- to 3-mm 22 gel fragments (A). The complete hydrolysis of MBP (0.7 mg/ml) after 24 h of mixture (20 μl) incubation with 15 μl of extracts was taken for 100%. SDS-PAGE analysis of MBP hydrolysis by 30 μg/ml inact-MLChmix (lane 2) and by act-MLChmix (lane 4) for 4 h; MBP incubated alone (lanes 1 and 3). The absence of detectable hydrolysis of control 0.7 mg/ml proteins by act-MLChmix is shown: human serum albumin (lane 6), human milk lactoferrin (lane 8); lanes 5 and 7 correspond to the proteins incubated alone. Lane C corresponds to standard protein markers. TLC analysis of OP19 (D) and OP21 (E) hydrolysis by different MLChs. The 1 mM OPs were incubated at 30°C for 24 h without MLChs (lanes C) or in the presence of 50 μg/ml of various MLChs (MLChs numbers are given on top of the panels) demonstrating relative activities in the hydrolysis of OP19 and OP21. Panel F shows the RAs of 22 various MLChs in the hydrolysis of OP25, OP21, OP19, and OP17.

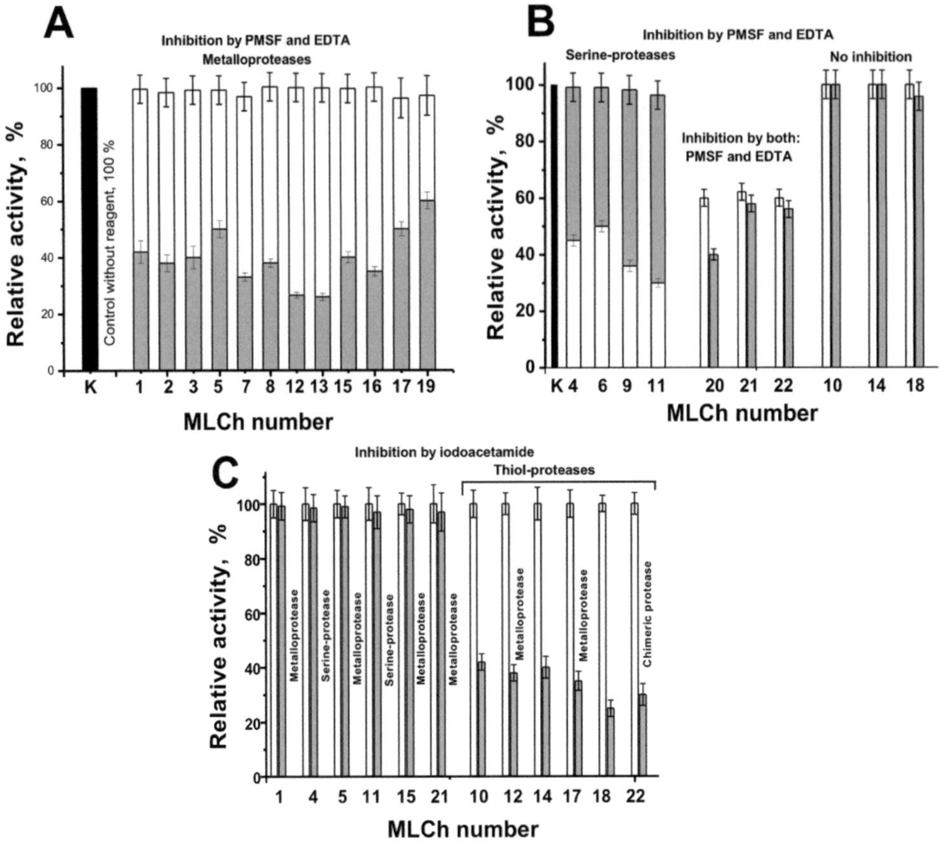

Figure 20. The RAs of 22 MLChs in hydrolysis of MBP after Abzs preincubation with specific inhibitors of proteases of different type. MLChs (0.1 mg/ml) were preincubated without of other components (black bars), with 50 mM EDTA (gray bars) or with 1 mM PMSF (white bars); then aliquots of these mixtures were added to standard reaction mixtures (A and B) [118]. Several examples (C) of the RAs of MLChs having metal-dependent activity (1, 5, 12, 15, and 21) and serine-protease-like activity (4 and 11), demonstrating no iodoacetamide-dependent activity; three MLChs (10, 14, and 18) showing negative response to EDTA and PMSF. MLCh-22 demonstrating positive effects of EDTA and PMSF, but significantly decreasing its activity after preincubation with iodoacetamide. White and gray bars show, respectively, the activity before (control) and after MLChs treatment with iodoacetamide (panel C). The RAs of all 22 MLChs before their treatment with different inhibitors were taken as 100%.

their proteolytic activity after incubation with PMSF, while EDTA significantly suppresses their MBP-hydrolyzing activity.

Four MLChs (4, 6, 9, and 11) demonstrate serine-like proteolytic activity; PMSF suppressed their activity, but there was no noticeable effect of EDTA (**Figure 20B**). PMSF suppressed protease activity of three MLChs (20, 21, and 22) by ~40%, and their inhibition by EDTA was to some extent comparable, 40–60% (**Figure 20B**). Thus, three MLChs (20–22) are characterized to some extent comparable ratios of metal-dependent and serine-like protease activities. A very intriguing situation was observed for three MLChs (18, 14, and 10); EDTA and PMSF do not remarkably decreased their proteolytic activity (**Figure 20B**). No significant suppression (5–15%) of MS and SLE polyclonal MBP-hydrolyzing abzymes by specific inhibitors of thiol proteases was revealed previously [76, 77, 84–87]. However, iodoacetamide inhibited integrase hydrolyzing activities of all polyclonal IgG and IgM preparations from HIV/AIDS patients by 12–99% [97, 98]. Proteolytic activities of three MLChs (18, 14, and 10) not inhibited by EDTA and PMSF were significantly suppressed by iodoacetamide, while there was no effect on the most of MLChs with metal-dependent and serine-like activities (for example, **Figure 20C**). Thus, these three MLChs (18, 14, and 10) are thiol proteases. Interestingly, but iodoacetamide significantly suppressed the activities of MLChs 17 and 12 (**Figure 20C**), which were also significantly inhibited by EDTA (**Figure 20A**). One can suppose that MLChs 17 and 12 may be MLChs, the active sites of which contain amino acid residues corresponding to metal-dependent and thiol proteases. A very surprising data were obtained for MLCh-22; its activity was significantly suppressed not only by EDTA and PMSF (**Figure 20B**), by also iodoacetamide (**Figure 20C**). The relative number of MLChs, which activity depend on iodoacetamide is only approximately 27% of all 22 MLChs, while at the same time, several of them possess metal-dependent and serine-like activities. Therefore, the relative contribution of thiol-like protease activity to a total MBP-hydrolyzing activity of polyclonal SLE and MS abzymes may be significantly lower than of Abzs with metal-dependent and serine-like proteolytic activities and, therefore, depending on the patient a relative contribution of thiol-like protease to the total activity may be about 5–15%, as found previously for polyclonal Abzs [76, 77, 84–87]. The effects of various metal ions on the protease activities of 22 MLChs were compared (**Figure 21A** and **B**; B is a continuation of A).

Seven different metal ions did not effect on the activity of MLChs with serine-like (9, 6, and 4) and thiol-dependent (18, 14, and 10) activities. Five MLChs (19, 17, 13, 8, and 2) were only slightly activated by several Me^{2+} ions, while Ca^{2+} was the best activator. Two MLCh preparations (5 and 3) were Co^{2+} dependent, but preparation 15 was better stimulated by Ni^{2+}, MLCh-16 and MLCh-20 were respectively Mn^{2+}- and Zn^{2+}-dependent (**Figure 21**). MLChs 22 and 12 were activated by two different metal ions, Zn^{2+} and Ca^{2+}. Two MLChs were activated by three different Me2 ions: MLCh-7 ($Ca^{2+} > Zn^{2+} > Co^{2+}$) and MLCh-1 ($Ca^{2+} > Ni^{2+} > Mg^{2+}$). In addition, MLCh-21 was activated by four ($Cu^{2+} > Ca^{2+} > Co^{2+} > Zn^{2+}$) metal ions. These data show the extreme Me^{2+}-dependence diversity of IgGs from SLE patients and their light chains in the hydrolysis of MBP [118].

All 22 MLCh preparations hydrolyzed efficiently MBP within a wide range of pHs (5.0–10), but in contrast to polyclonal SLE IgGs, they show mainly only one pH optimum [118]. Only the pH profile for preparation 4 demonstrates optimal pH at 5.7–5.9 and pronounced shoulder at pHs 6.5–7.5 (**Figure 21C**). The apparent k_{cat} values under optimal conditions for every MLCh were estimated. The data on several characteristics of 22 various MLCh preparations are summarized in **Table 8** [118]. One can see that all MLChs demonstrate very different physicochemical and enzymatic properties.

On the next step we analyzed in more detail three additional MLChs (numbers 23–25) corresponding to peak 7 eluted from MBP-Sepharose with 0.5 M NaCl (**Figure 18A**) [119, 120]. These three MLChs were purified and characterized in detail exactly similar to above described 22 preparations [118]. The DNA sequence of NGTA1-Me-pro demonstrated high

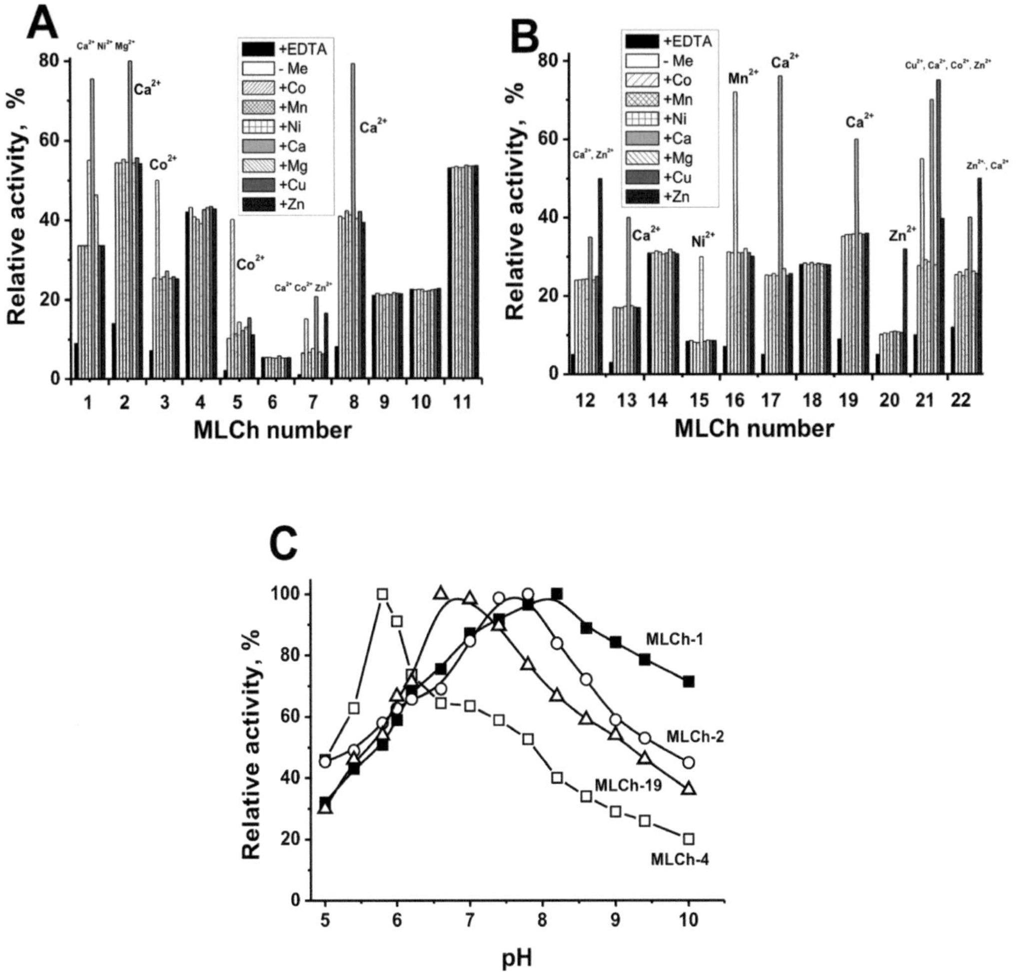

Figure 21. Effect of various metal ions on the RAs of 22 MLChs in the hydrolysis of MBP (A and B) [118]. Black first bars correspond to the RAs in the presence of EDTA, while white bars to MLChs without external metal ions. The MLChs numbers of and type of Me^{2+} ions, as well as best activators of various MLChs are shown on panels A and B. Typical examples of the dependences of four MLChs in MBP hydrolysis on pH of reaction mixtures are given (C).

identity to germline VL genes of IgLV8-61*02, IgLV8-61*01, and IgLV8-61*03IGKV1 (90% of identity) [120]. DNA sequence of NGTA2-Me-pro-Tr indicated high identity with germline VL gene IGKJ1*01 (100%), IGKJ4*01 (95.7%), IGKJ4*02 (91.2%), IGKV1-5*03 (87.9%), IGKV1-5*01 (86.2% of identity), and IGKV1-5*02 (85.6%) [119]. DNA sequence of NGTA3-pro-DNase has similarity with germline DNA sequence of light chains of several IgGs: IGKJ1*01 (100% of identity), IGKJ4*01 (95.7%), IGKJ4*02 (91.2%); IGKV1-5*03 (79.8% of identity), IGKV1-5*02 (78.4%), and IGKV1-5*01 (78.4%) [Timofeeva, Nevinsky, personal communication]. Thus, all three MLChs were shown to be typical light chain of Abs [119, 120, personal communication].

NGTA1-Me-pro was shown to be a specific metalloprotease; only EDTA efficiently inhibits its activity, while specific inhibitors of thiol-, serine-, and acidic-like proteases did not suppress its MBP-hydrolyzing activity (**Figure 22A**) [120].

MLCh number	Optimal pH[a]	Optimal Me^{2+} cofactor	Apparent k_{cat}, min^{-1a}
1	8.0–8.2	**Ca^{2+}**(Ni^{2+},Mg^{2+})[c]	0.14 ± 0.01[b]
2	7.6–7.8	**Ca^{2+}**	0.12 ± 0.01
3	7.6–7.8	**Co^{2+}**	0.09 ± 0.007
4	5.7–5.9	Me^{2+}-independent	0.12 ± 0.008
5	7.5–7.7	Co^{2+}	0.24 ± 0.02
6	7.0–7.2	Me^{2+}-independent	0.01 ± 0.001
7	7.2–7.4	**Ca^{2+}**(Zn^{2+},Co^{2+})	0.07 ± 0.004
8	7.4–7.6	**Ca^{2+}**	0.17 ± 0.003
9	7.2–7.4	Me^{2+}-independent	0.03 ± 0.001
10	8.1–8.3	Me^{2+}-independent	0.05 ± 0.002
11	7.7–7.8	Me^{2+}-independent	0.09 ± 0.006
12	7.8–8.0	**Zn^{2+}**(Ca^{2+})	0.19 ± 0.001
13	6.1–6.3	**Ca^{2+}**	0.16 ± 0.001
14	7.0–7.2	Me^{2+}-independent	0.06 ± 0.0003
15	7.0–7.2	**Ni^{2+}**	0.17 ± 0.007
16	6.9–7.1	**Mn^{2+}**	0.12 ± 0.001
17	8.2–8.4	**Ca^{2+}**	0.17 ± 0.001
18	6.2–6.4	Me^{2+}-independent	0.05 ± 0.0007
19	6.7–6.9	**Ca^{2+}**	0.1 ± 0.01
20	8.2–8.4	**Zn^{2+}**	0.09 ± 0.006
21	6.9–7.1	**Cu** (Ca^{2+}, Co^{2+}, Zn^{2+})	0.18 ± 0.007
22	7.8–8.0	**Zn^{2+}**(Ca^{2+})	0.11 ± 0.006

[a]For each value, a mean ± S.E. of two/three measurements is reported.

[b]Optimal pH of reaction mixtures and optimal metal cofactor (given in bold) were used for every of MLCh preparations; the apparent k_{cat} values under optimal conditions were calculated as $k_{cat} = V_{max}$ (M/min)/[MLCh] (M). MLChs were used in different concentrations (0.05–0.5 M) depending of their relative activity.

[c]The best metal activator is given in bold, while alternative cofactors demonstrating relatively high activation are given in parenthesis.

Table 8. The optimal pH values, optimal metal cofactors, and apparent k_{cat} values for 22 recombinant individual MLChs in the hydrolysis of MBP [118].

Seven various metal ions increase NGTA1-Me-pro activity in the following order: $Ca^{2+} > Mg^{2+} > Ni^{2+} \geq Zn^{2+} \geq Co^{2+} \geq Mn^{2+} > Cu^{2+}$ (**Figure 22B**). NGTA1-Me-pro demonstrated two different very well expressed pH optima at pH 6.0 and 8.5 (**Figure 22C**). **Figure 22(D)** indicates that at pH 6.0 MLCh has optimum at ~6 mM, when at pH 8.5 at 1 mM $CaCl_2$. The apparent values of K_m and k_{cat} for MBP in the presence of optimal $CaCl_2$ concentration at pH 6.0 (20 ± 2 μM;

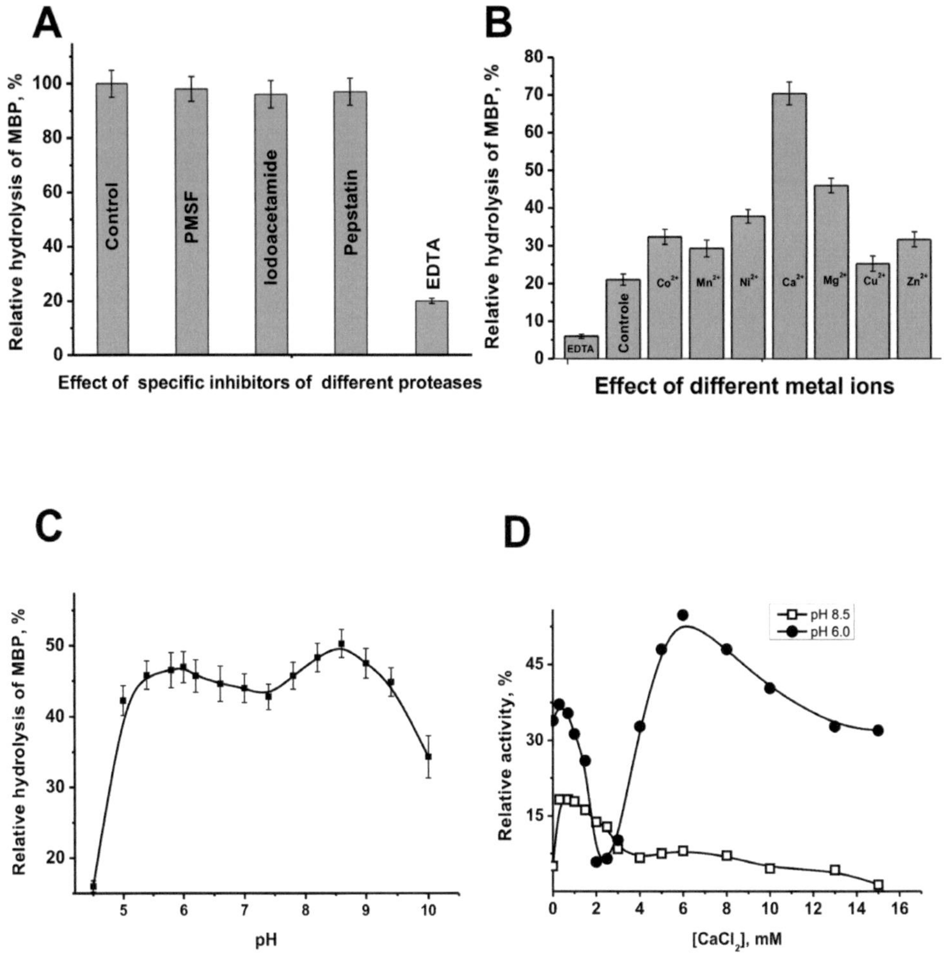

Figure 22. The RAs of NGTA1-Me-pro in the hydrolysis of MBP before and after its preincubation with specific inhibitors of various type proteases [120]. MLCh (0.1 mg/ml) was preincubated without other components (control), or the presence of EDTA, PMSF, pepstatin, and iodoacetamide; 1.0 μl of the mixtures were added to 29 μl of MBP-containing standard reaction mixtures (A). The RA before NGTA1-Me-pro preincubation with various inhibitors was taken as 100%. Effects of different Me^{2+} ions (2 mM) and EDTA on the RAs of MLCh are shown (B). Dependence of the RA upon pH of reaction mixture is shown (C). Dependence of NGTA1-Me-pro activity on CaCl2 concentration at pHs 6.0 and 8.5 (D).

0.22 ± 0.02 min^{-1}; 6.0 mM $CaCl_2$) and pH 8.5 (40 ± 3 μM; 0.07 ± 0.005 min^{-1}; 0.7 mM $CaCl_2$) were different. All data obtained unequivocally testified that NGTA1-Me-pro has two independent metal-dependent active centers [120].

MLCh NGTA2-Me-pro-Tr demonstrated two different activities: trypsin-like and metalloprotease. **Figure 23(A)** shows that NGTA2-Me-pro-Tr is not sensitive to pepstatin and iodoacetamide [119]. Preincubation of this MLCh with specific inhibitor of serine-like proteases results in a decrease of its activity for 42 ± 4%.

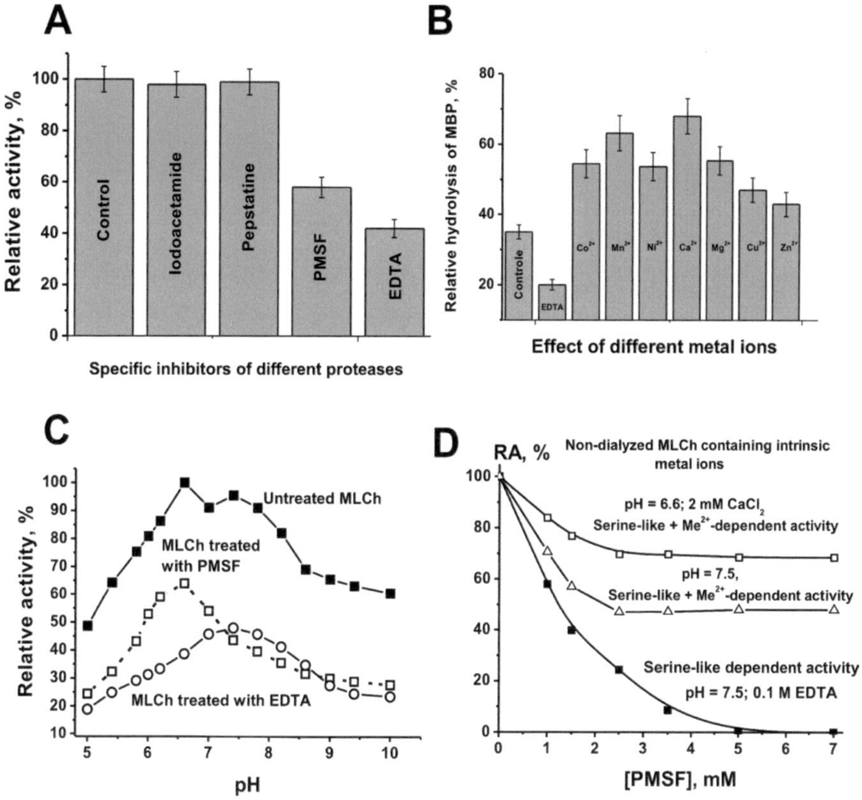

Figure 23. The RAs of the activity of NGTA2-Me-pro-Tr in the hydrolysis of MBP after its preincubation with specific inhibitors of different type proteases (A) [119]. MLCh (0.3 mg/ml) was preincubated alone (control), or the presence of iodoacetamide, PMSF, pepstatin, or EDTA; 1.0 μl of these mixture was added to 29 μl of MBP-containing standard reaction mixtures (A). The relative activity of NGTA2-Me-pro-Tr after preincubation with without different inhibitors (control) was taken for 100%. Effects of 10 mM EDTA and various Me^{2+} ions (2 mM) on the RAs of MLCh are shown (B). Dependences of the relative proteolytic activity of NGTA2-Me-pro-Tr before and after its treatment with PMSF and EDTA upon pH of reaction mixtures are shown (C). Dependence of the MBP-hydrolyzing activity on concentration of CaCl2 at pHs 6.0 and 8.5 (D).

Intact polyclonal Abs interact with various metal ions and they do not lose completely intrinsically bound ions during the standard purification procedures [121]. Addition of EDTA to NGTA2-Me-pro-Tr containing only intrinsically bound Me^{2+}-ions results in a decrease in its activity for 58 ± 5% (**Figure 23A**) [119]. Average serine-like activity of NGTA2-Me-pro-Tr containing only intrinsically bound Me^{2+} ions was ~1.4-fold lower than its Me^{2+}-dependent protease activity. Seven various external metal ions activate this MLCh in the following order: $Ca^{2+} \geq Mn^{2+} \geq Mg^{2+} > Co^{2+} > Ni^{2+} \geq Cu^{2+} \geq Zn^{2+}$ (**Figure 23B**). After NGTA2-Me-pro-Tr treatment with PMSF, its metalloprotease activity demonstrated pH optimum at 6.5–6.6 (**Figure 23C**). After dialysis of this MLCh against EDTA or in the presence of EDTA, serine-like protease activity showed pH optimum at 7.4–7.5. **Figure 23(D)** demonstrates that the increase in PMSF concentration results in a complete suppression of the activity at pH 7.5 in the presence of 50 mM EDTA, conditions corresponding to serine-like activity. NGTA2-Me-pro-Tr containing no intrinsic metal ions demonstrated in the absence of external metal ions at pH 7.5 K_m and k_{cat} (9.0 ± 1.0 μM, 8 ± 0.6 min^{-1}) different as in the presence of $CaCl_2$ at pH 6.5 (24.0 ± 2.0 μM, 15.2 ± 1.1 min^{-1}) [119]. Thus, NGTA2-Me-pro-Tr is the first example of recombinant MLCh having two combined serine-like and metalloprotease activities.

It should be emphasized that all recombinant MLChs were obtained using affinity chromatography of phage particles on MBP-Sepharose and all electrophoretically homogeneous preparations of MLChs have affinity for MBP-Sepharose; similar to phage particles homogeneous MLChs were eluded from the sorbet by 0.5 M NaCl. Taking this into account, a very unexpected result was obtained from the analysis of enzymatic activities of NGTA3-pro-DNase [Timofeeva and Nevinsky, personal communication].

The homogeneity of ~26–27-kDa NGTA3-pro-DNase was confirmed using SDS-PAGE with following silver staining (**Figure 24B**, lane 1). NGTA3-pro-DNase demonstrated positive answer with horseradish peroxidase conjugated with mouse IgGs against human Abs light chains at Western blotting and positive ELISA answer using plates with immobilized MBP and DNA.

After SDS-PAGE, MBP-hydrolyzing activity was revealed only in the band corresponding to the light chains in the presence of $CaCl_2$ (o) and in the absence of external metal ions (□); the positions of proteolytic (o, □) and DNase (x) activities of MLCh are coincided (**Figure 24A**). NGTA3-pro-DNase hydrolyzed specifically only MBP and not hydrolyzed foreign control proteins (**Figure 24C**).

Only one (NGTA3-pro-DNase) of 25 recombinant MLChs analyzed by us efficiently hydrolyzed not only MBP, but also DNA (for example, **Figure 24D**). DNase activity of NGTA3-pro-DNase was determined *in situ* after separation of proteins using SDS-PAGE gels copolymerized with calf thymus DNA (**Figure 24E**). Ethidium bromide staining of the gels after the electrophoresis of the NGTA3-pro-DNase revealed sharp dark bands against a fluorescent background of DNA in the gel zone corresponding only to the MLCh and there were no other peaks of proteins or DNase activity (**Figure 24E**).

NGTA3-pro-DNase containing intrinsic metal ions was not sensitive to treatment with iodoacetamide and pepstatin, while its preincubation with PMSF led to decrease in the activity for 67 ± 5% (**Figure 25A**).

The dialysis of NGTA3-pro-DNase containing only intrinsically bound Me^{2+} ions against EDTA or addition of EDTA to reaction mixture led to a decrease in its activity for 33 ± 3% (**Figure 25A**). And average Me^{2+}-dependent protease activity of MLCh containing only intrinsically bound Me^{2+} ions was approximately 2.0-fold lower (**Figure 25A**), but after addition of external Ca^{2+} ions became to be 2.2-fold higher than its serine-like activity (**Figure 25B**). Seven various external metal ions activate NGTA3-pro-DNase in the following order: $Ca^{2+} \geq Ni^{2+} > Co^{2+} \sim Mn^{2+} \geq Cu^{2+} \sim Zn^{2+} \geq Mg^{2+}$ (**Figure 25B**). An optimal concentration of $CaCl_2$, which is the best activator of this MLCh, was 3 mM. NGTA3-pro-DNase demonstrates two different optimal pHs (**Figure 25C**). After treatment of MLCh with PMSF, its metalloprotease activity was maximal at pH 8.6, while in the presence of EDTA, serine-like protease activity demonstrated pH optimum at 7.0 (**Figure 25B**). NGTA3-pro-DNase treated with PMSF in the presence of 3 mM $CaCl_2$ (pH 7.0) demonstrated K_m for intact MBP (15 ± 1.1 μM) and k_{cat} value 0.4 ± 0.03 min^{-1}, while in the presence of EDTA at pH 8.6, K_m and k_{cat} values were different (45 ± 1.1 μM and 0.2 ± 0.04 min^{-1}).

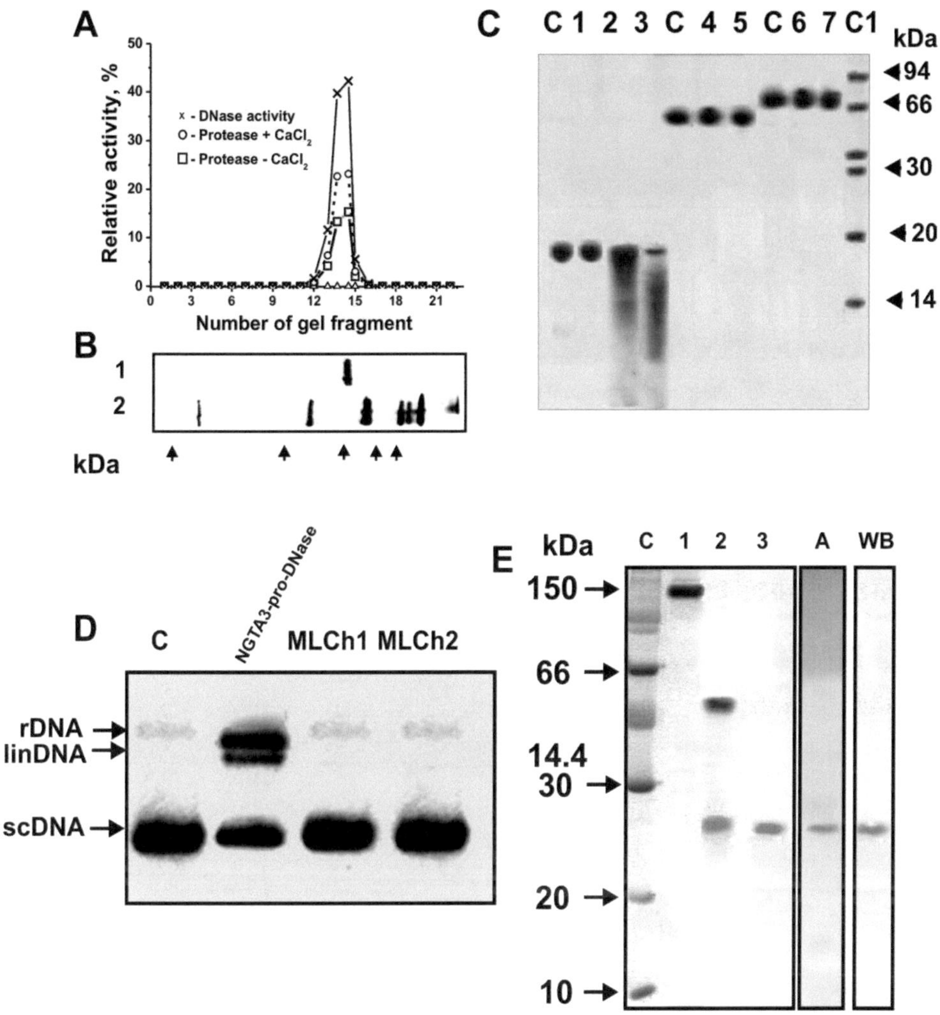

Figure 24. SDS-PAGE analysis of MBP- and DNA-hydrolyzing activities (A) and homogeneity of NGTA3-pro-DNase (7 μg) using a reducing 5–16% gradient gel followed by silver staining (B, lane 1); the arrows (B, lane 2) indicate the positions of protein markers. After SDS-PAGE the gel was incubated using conditions for renaturation of NGTA3-pro-DNase. The relative MBP- and DNA-hydrolyzing activity (%) was revealed using the extracts of 2- to 3-mm gel fragments (A). The activity of NGTA3-pro-DNase corresponding to a complete hydrolysis of 0.5 mg/ml MBP (or 18 nM scDNA) after 24 h of incubation of 25 μl reaction mixture containing 10 μl of the gel extracts was taken for 100%. SDS-PAGE analysis of hydrolysis of MBP by inact-MLChmix (lane 1) or NGTA3-pro-DNase (lanes 2 and 3, different time of incubation) (C). Hydrolysis of control proteins (0.5 mg/ml) by inact-MLChmix and NGTA3-pro-DNase was analyzed: human albumin (lanes 4 and 5) and lactoferrin from human milk (lanes 6 and 7) (C). The mixtures were incubated for 6 h with inact-MLChmix (lanes 4 and 6), or NGTA3-pro-DNase (lanes 5 and 7). All lanes C correspond to different proteins incubated alone without MLChs, while lane C1- to standard protein markers. DNase activity of NGTA3-pro-DNase and two control MLCh1 and MLCh2 (10 nM) was analyzed in the presence of 5 mM MgCl2 (D); lane C corresponds to scDNA incubated alone. *In situ* assay of DNase activity of the NGTA3-pro-DNase (8 μg) after treatment with DTT (lane A) (E). DNase activity was revealed by ethidium bromide staining as a dark band on the fluorescent background. A part of the gel was stained with Coomassie R250 to show the position of the SLE IgGs before (lane 1) and after incubation with DTT (lane 2), as well as NGTA3-pro-DNase (lane 3) (E). MLCh was analyzed by Western blotting to a nitrocellulose membrane using mouse IgGs against light chains of human Abs conjugated with horsedish peroxidase (lane WB) (E).

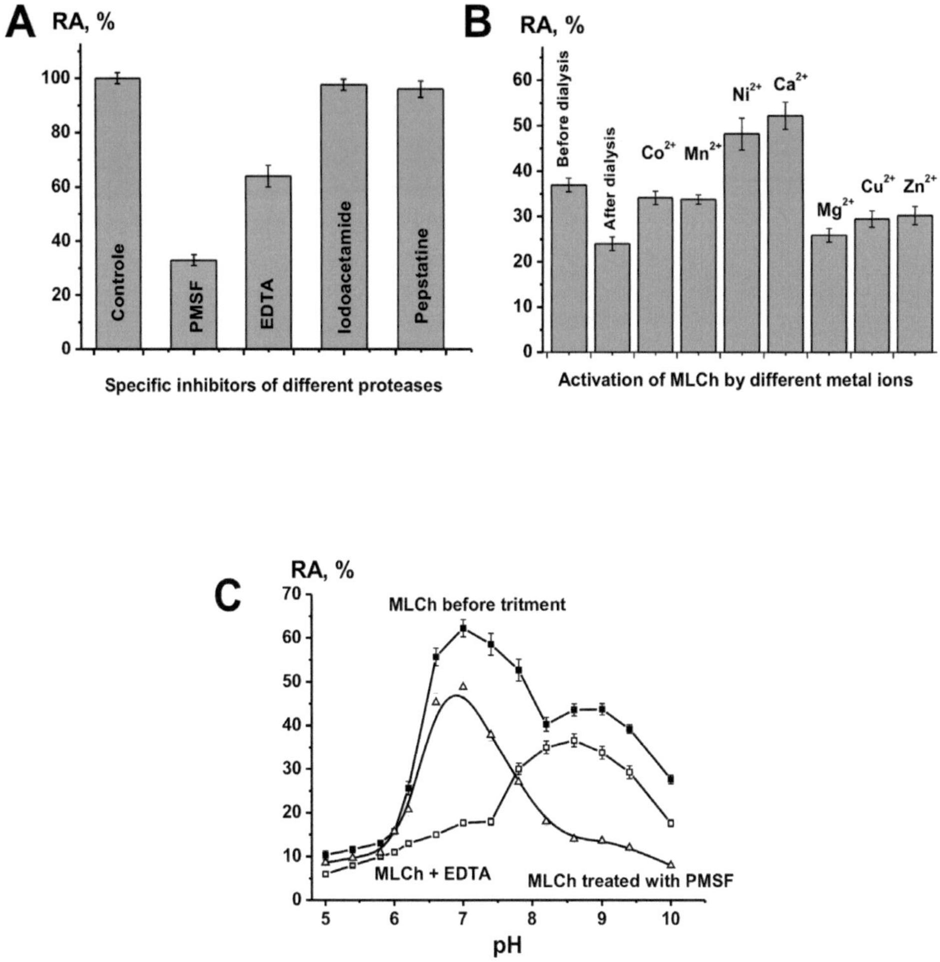

Figure 25. The RAs of MBP-hydrolyzing activity of NGTA3-pro-DNase after its preincubation with specific inhibitors of different types proteases (A). MLCh (0.1 mg/ml) was preincubated alone (control), in the presence of iodoacetamide, PMSF, pepstatin, or EDTA, and then 1.5 μl added to 29 μl of standard reaction mixture (A). The RA of NGTA1-Me-pro before its preincubation with various inhibitors was taken as 100%. Effect of EDTA and different metal ions (2 mM) on the RA of MLCh is shown (B). Dependence of RA of MBP-hydrolyzing activity of NGTA1-Me-pro on pH of reaction mixture before and after its treatment with EDTA and PMSF is given (C).

It is known that Mg^{2+} (10 mM) is optimal cofactor of DNase I, while other Me^{2+} ions very weakly activate DNase I [109, 110]. Optimal concentration for Mn^{2+}, Mg^{2+}, and Ni^{2+} in activation NGTA3-pro-DNase was ~4–5 mM, for Ca^{2+} and Zn^{2+} 2 mM, while Co^{2+} and Cu^{2+} activate MLCh up to 10 mM concentration. DNase activity increased in the presence of metal ions in the following order: $Mn^{2+} \approx Co^{2+} \geq Mg^{2+} > Cu^{2+} \approx Ni^{2+} \geq Ca^{2+} > Zn^{2+}$), which is completely different in comparing with that for DNases I and other recombinant MLChs analyzed.

DNase activity for NGTA3-pro-DNase in the presence of Mg^{2+} or Mn^{2+} at fixed concentration (5 mM) was increased at optimal concentrations of NaCl or KCl (30–40 mM) for only 27–28%.

In optimal conditions, NGTA3-pro-DNase demonstrated well expressed optima at pH 6.5–6.6. The K_m (2 ± 0.2 nM) and k_{cat} (1.1 ± 0.1) × 10^{-3} min^{-1} values for scDNA were estimated. The affinity of NGTA3-pro-DNase for supercoiled DNA is about 3.5 orders of magnitude higher than affinity of scDNA for DNase I (K_m = 46–58 μM [122].

8. Conclusion

In several articles, it was demonstrated that polyclonal RNA-, DNA-, MBP- integrase-, and oligosaccharide-hydrolyzing antibodies of different classes and subclasses from patients with SLE, MS, AIDS, and other diseases are very catalytically heterogeneous. These abzymes can contain lambda- and kappa- types of light chains, may be of different subclasses (IgG1–IgG4), can demonstrate different affinity for specific sorbents and free antigens-substrates, very different pH optima, and may be independent or dependent on metal ions. Different abzymes can catalyze the hydrolysis of MBP, HIV integrase, and other proteins as serine-, thiol-, and acidic-like or metalloproteases. Various IgGs of four subclasses (IgG1–IgG4) and/or IgAs and IgMs from the sera of patients with autoimmune and viral diseases are catalytically active in the hydrolysis of RNA, DNA, oligosaccharides, and various proteins with their different contribution to the total activity of the Abs in the hydrolysis of these substrates in the case of every individual patient.

At the same time, the analysis of polyclonal antibodies does not allow to obtain detail characteristics of monoclonal abzymes entering to small pools of polyclonal antibodies separated by affinity chromatography on sorbents with different immobilized antigens-substrates. As it was shown on the example of polyclonal IgGs with DNase and MBP-hydrolyzing activities from sera of SLE and MS patients, elution of Abs by a NaCl concentration gradient leads to their distribution all over the chromatography profiles. In this case, each eluted Ab fraction contains abzymes with comparable affinity for immobilized ligand, but demonstrating a significant diversity of various enzymatic properties described above. These data are strong evidence of exceptional diversity abzymes in the blood of some patients with SLE, MS, and other diseases. In this regard, it should be mentioned that theoretically immune system of human can produce up to 106 different Abs against one antigen. It is evident that all theoretically possible variants of antibodies are in reality not realized and much less than one million. However, in the case of some patients, a possible number of abzymes can be very large. In our studies, we used a cDNA library only kappa light chains of Abs from three patients with SLE [111, 112, 118–120]. We have analyzed only 45 of 451 single of colonies corresponding one peak eluted from DNA-cellulose with 0.5 M NaCl and 33 of 687 colonies of peak eluded with acidic buffer. In the first case 15 of 45 (~33%) [111] and in the second 19 of 33 MLChs (58%) demonstrated DNase activity [112]. For analysis of MBP-hydrolyzing activity, we have used 72 of 440 individual colonies corresponding to phage particles eluted from MBP-Sepharose with 0.5 M NaCl; 25 of 72 MLChs (~35%) effectively hydrolyzed MBP [118–120]. Since we analyzed abzymes corresponding only one or two of ≥10 phage particles, it is obvious that the number of MLChs with DNase and MBP-hydrolyzing activity with very different enzymatic properties may be at least ≥ 500–1000.

The question is why many abzyme with nuclease and protease activities exist in SLE and other AI patients. First, immunization of autoimmune mice leads to a dramatically higher incidence of Abzs with a higher activity comparing to conventionally used normal mouse strains [51, 52]. The immune response to RNA and DNA and their complexes with histones and other proteins only partially depends on the length and sequence of nucleic acid [123, 124]. In addition, antiidiotypic Abs against the active centres of different DNA- and RNA-dependent enzymes can also possess catalytic activity. We have shown that polyclonal nuclease abzymes of autoimmune patients are usually different cocktails of Abzs against DNA and RNA and their complexes with proteins as well as antiidiotypic Abzs to active centers of various DNA- and RNA-hydrolyzing enzymes [13–22].

It is possible to explain to some extent in a similar way the exceptional diversity of abzymes hydrolyzing MBP and other proteins. At the same time, possible ways of production of monoclonal abzymes having two or even three different catalytic centers have a special interest. It should be noted that the known antigenic determinants of different proteins are usually relatively long and the active centers of some abzymes with two activities can correspond at once to variable parts of the antibodies to different contiguous parts of these determinants. One cannot exclude that metal-dependent active centers may be against specific part of protein antigenic determinants bound with one or several metal ions.

The second question is why NGTA3-pro-DNase against MBP can hydrolyze DNA. It is believed that MBP and anti-MBP Abs cannot interact with DNA or RNA. However, it was recently shown that anti-MBP IgGs can efficiently interact with nucleic acids [125]. Using quenching of MBP tryptophan fluorescence emission, we have shown that MBP bind oligonucleotides showing two K_d values: 65 ± 5 and 250 ± 20 μM [Timofeeva and Nevinsky, personal communication]. Therefore, it is possible to suggest that 24 of 25 MLChs interacting only with MBP correspond to Abzs directly against this protein, while NGTA3-pro-DNase may be against the complex of MBP with DNA. In the latter case, it is impossible to exclude possibility of a formation of the chimeric MLChs possessing affinity for MBP and for DNA and also hydrolyzing these absolutely different substrates.

As mentioned above, DNA-hydrolyzing Bence-Jones proteins [60] and DNase abzymes of patients with SLE [59] and MS [16] are dangerous since they are cytotoxic, can penetrate to cell nuclear, and hydrolyze nuclear DNA resulting in cell apoptosis. Abzymes against vasoactive peptide are harmful since they decrease in the concentration of the peptide and have an important negative role in pathogenesis of patients with asthma [126]. RAs of DNase abzymes of patients with Hashimoto thyroiditis well correlate with different immunological and biochemical indices of this disease including a concentration of thyroid hormones, while decrease in their activity is related to decrease in thyroid gland damage and improvement of the clinical status [105]. Protease IgGs of patients with sepsis participate in the control of disseminated microvascular thrombosis and play important role in recovery from the disease [127]. Thus, various abzymes can play both a negative and positive role in the pathogenesis of SLE and other autoimmune or viral diseases. Meanwhile, it should be mentioned that in the later stages of SLE, MS, and other diseases, the blood of these patients contains abzymes not only with DNase and MBP-hydrolyzing activities, but also hydrolyzing other proteins, oligosaccharides, and lipids [13–22].

As it was shown in the example of Hashimoto thyroiditis production of harmful abzymes can be suppressed by using therapy with suppressing immune system drug plaquenil [102]. In MS and SLE, anti-MBP abzymes with proteolytic activity can attack MBP of the myelin-proteolipid sheath of axons. The established MS drug Copaxone was shown to be a specific inhibitor of abzymes with MBP-hydrolyzing activity [128]. One cannot exclude that the same drugs can be used for the treatment of SLE and other autoimmune diseases, which characterized by high level of abzymes with nuclease and MBP-hydrolyzing activities.

The presence of anti-DNA Abs is known as the main important diagnostic index for SLE. High-affinity anti-DNA Abs was recently shown to be major component of the intrathecal IgG in cerebrospinal fluid and brain of MS patients [48]. Moreover, DNase abzymes from SLE and MS patients are cytotoxic and induce cell death by apoptosis [16, 59]. The sera of patients with SLE and MS patients contain different free light chains [61, 62]. Therefore, we propose that exceptional diverse of intact antibodies and their free light chains hydrolyzing DNA, MBP, nucleotides, and polysaccharides may cooperatively all together promote important neuropathologic pathogenic mechanisms in SLE and MS.

Our data on the study of abzymes production in SLE patients associated with the change in profile differentiation of brain stem cells seem to be very important for understanding possible mechanisms of various autoimmune diseases development.

Acknowledgements

This research was made possible by grant from the Russian Science Foundation (no 16-15-10103 to G.A. Nevinsky).

Abbreviations

Abs	Antibodies
Abzs	Abzymes, or catalytically active antibodies
AI	Autoimmune
AD	Autoimmune disease
AIDS	Acquired immunodeficiency syndrome
a/u	Arbitrary units
BSA	Bovine serum albumin
HSCs	Hematopoietic stem cells
CBA	(CBAxC57BL)F1 mice
MBP	Human myelin basic protein

OP-17, OP-19, OP-21, and OP-25	17–25mer oligopeptides corresponding to four known MBP cleavage sites
MS	Multiple sclerosis
m-BSA	Methylated BSA
nat-DNA and den-DNA	Native and denatured DNA, respectively
OP	Oligopeptide
SLE	Systemic lupus erythematosus
SDS-PAGE	SDS-polyacrylamide gel electrophoresis
RA	Relative activity

Author details

Georgy A. Nevinsky

Address all correspondence to: nevinsky@niboch.nsc.ru

Institute of Chemical Biology and Fundamental Medicine, Siberian Division of Russian Academy of Sciences, Novosibirsk, Russia

References

[1] Pollack SJ, Jacobs JW, Schultz PG. Selective chemical catalysis by an antibody. Science. 1986;**234**:1570–1573.

[2] Tramontano A, Janda KD, Lerner RA. Catalytic antibodies. Science. 1986;**234**:1566–1570.

[3] Tramontano A, Janda KD, Lerner RA. Chemical reactivity at an antibody binding site elicited by mechanistic design of a synthetic antigen. Proc Natl Acad Sci USA. 1986;**83**:6736–6740.

[4] Lerner RA, Tramontano A. Antibodies as enzymes. Trends Biochem Sci. 1987;**12**:427–438.

[5] Stewart JD, Benkovic SJ. Recent developments in catalytic antibodies. Int Rev Immunol. 1993;**10**:229–240.

[6] Martin AB, Schultz PG. Opportunities at the interface of chemistry and biology. Trends Cell Biol. 1999;**9**:24–28.

[7] Nevinsky GA, Semenov DV, Buneva VN. Catalytic antibodies (abzymes) induced by stable transition-state analogs. Biochemistry (Moscow). 2000;**65**:1233–1244.

[8] Keinan EE, editor. Catalytic antibodies. Germany: Wiley-VCH Verlag GmbH and Co; 2005. 586 p.

[9] Paul S, Volle DJ, Beach CM, Johnson DR, Powell MJ, Massey RJ. Catalytic hydrolysis of vasoactive intestinal peptide by human autoantibody. Science. 1989;**244**:1158–1162.

[10] Shuster AM, Gololobov GV, Kvashuk OA, Bogomolova AE, Smirnov IV Gabibov AG. DNA hydrolyzing autoantibodies. Science. 1992;**256**:665–667.

[11] Buneva VN, Andrievskaia OA, Romannikova IV, Gololobov GV, Iadav RP, Iamkovoi VI, Nevinskii GA. Interaction of catalytically active antibodies with oligoribonucleotides. Mol Biol (Moscow). 1994;**28**:738–743.

[12] Suzuki H. Recent advances in abzyme studies. J Biochem. 1994;**115**:138–143.

[13] Nevinsky GA, Kanyshkova TG, Buneva VN. Natural catalytic antibodies (abzymes) in normalcy and pathology. Biochemistry (Moscow). 2000;**65**:1245–1255.

[14] Nevinsky GA, Buneva VN. Human catalytic RNA- and DNA-hydrolyzing antibodies. J Immunol Meth. 2002;**269**:235–249.

[15] Nevinsky GA, Favorova OO, Buneva VN. Natural catalytic antibodies—new characters in the protein repertoire. In: Golemis E, editor. Protein-Protein Interactions; A Molecular Cloning Manual. New York, Cold Spring Harbor: Cold Spring Harbor Lab Press; 2002. pp. 532–534.

[16] Nevinsky GA, Buneva VN. Catalytic antibodies in healthy humans and patients with autoimmune and viral pathologies. J Cell Mol Med. 2003;**7**:265–276.

[17] Nevinsky GA, Buneva VN. Natural catalytic antibodies-abzymes. In: Keinan E, editor. Catalytic Antibodies. Weinheim: Wiley-VCH Verlag GmbH and Co; 2005. pp. 503–567.

[18] Nevinsky GA, Buneva VN. Natural catalytic antibodies in norm, autoimmune, viral, and bacterial diseases. Sci World J. 2010;**10**:1203–1233.

[19] Nevinsky GA. Natural catalytic antibodies in norm and in autoimmune diseases. In: Brenner KJ, editor. Autoimmune Diseases: Symptoms, Diagnosis and Treatment. New York, USA: Nova Science Publishers; 2010. pp. 1–107.

[20] Nevinsky GA. Natural catalytic antibodies in norm and in HIV-infected patients. In: Fyson Hanania Kasenga, editor. Understanding HIV/AIDS Management and Care—Pandemic Approaches the 21st Century. Rijeka, Croatia: InTech; 2011. pp. 151–192.

[21] Nevinsky GA, Buneva VN. Autoantibodies and natural catalytic antibodies in health, multiple sclerosis, and some other diseases. Adv Neuroimmune Biol. 2012;**3**:157–182.

[22] Nevinsky GA. Autoimmune processes in multiple sclerosis: production of harmful catalytic antibodies associated with significant changes in the hematopoietic stem cell differentiation and proliferation. In: Conzalez-Quevedo A, editor. Multiple Sclerosis. Rijeka, Croatia: InTech; 2016. pp. 100–147.

[23] Izadyar L, Friboulet A, Remy MH, Roseto A, Thomas D. Monoclonal anti-idiotypic antibodies as functional internal images of enzyme active sites: production of a catalytic antibody with a cholinesterase activity. Proc Natl Acad Sci USA. 1993;**90**:8876–8880.

[24] Kolesnikov AV, KozyrAV, Alexandrova ES, Koralewski F, Demin AV, Titov MI, Avalle, B, Tramontano A, Paul S, Thomas D, Gabibov AG, Friboulet A. Enzyme mimicry by the antiidiotypic antibody approach. Proc Natl Acad Sci USA. 2000;**97**:13526–13531.

[25] Hu R, Xie GY, Zhang X, Guo ZQ, Jin S. roduction and characterization of monoclonal anti-idiotypic antibody exhibiting a catalytic activity similar to carboxypeptidase A. J Biotechnol. 1998;**61**:109–115.

[26] Friboulet A, Izadyar L, Avalle B, Roseto A, Thomas D. Abzyme generation using an anti-idiotypic antibody as the "internal image" of an enzyme active site. Appl Biochem Biotechnol. 1994;**47**:229–237.

[27] Debat H, Avalle B, Chose O, Sarde C-O, Friboulet A, Thomas D. Overpassing an aberrant V(kappa) gene to sequence an anti-idiotypic abzyme with (beta)-lactamase-like activity that could have a linkage with autoimmune diseases. FASEB J. 2001;**15**:815–822.

[28] Hifumi E, Morihara F, Hatiuchi K, Okuda T, Nishizono A, Uda T. Catalytic features and eradication ability of antibody light-chain UA15-L against Helicobacter pylori. J Biol Chem. 2008;**283**:899–907.

[29] Andryushkova AA, Kuznetsova IA, Orlovskaya IA, Buneva VN, Nevinsky GA. Antibodies with amylase activity from the sera of autoimmune-prone MRL/MpJ-lpr mice. FEBS Lett. 2006;**580**:5089–5095.

[30] Andryushkova AS, Kuznetsova IA, Orlovskaya IA, Buneva VN, Nevinsky GA. Nucleotide-hydrolyzing antibodies from the sera of autoimmune-prone MRL-lpr/lpr mice. Int Immunol. 2009;**21**:935–945.

[31] Andryushkova AS, Kuznetsova IA, Buneva VN, Toporkova LB, Sakhno LV, Tichonova MA, Chernykh ER, Orlovskaya IA, Nevinsky GA. Formation of different abzymes in autoimmune-prone MRL-lpr/lpr mice is associated with changes in colony formation of haematopoetic progenitors. J Cell Mol Med. 2007;**11**:531–551.

[32] Doronin VB, Parkhomenko TA, Korablev A, Toporkova LB, Lopatnikova JA, Alshevskaja AA, Sennikov SV, Buneva VN, Budde T, Meuth SG, Orlovskaya IA, Popova NA, Nevinsky GA. Changes in different parameters, lymphocyte proliferation, and hematopoietic progenitor colony formation in EAE mice treated with myelin oligodendrocyte glycoprotein. J Cell Mol Med. 2015;**20**:81–94.

[33] Wentworth P, Liu Y, Wentworth AD, Fan P, Foley MJ, Janda KD. A bait and switch hapten strategy generates catalytic antibodies for phosphodiester hydrolysis. Proc Natl Acad Sci USA. 1998;**95**:5971–5975.

[34] Tellier C. Exploiting antibodies as catalysts: potential therapeutic applications. Transfus Clin Biol. 2002;**9**:1–8.

[35] Zhou YX, Karle S, Taguchi P, Planque S, Nishiyama Y, Paul S. Prospects for immunotherapeutic proteolytic antibodies. J Immunol Meth. 2002;**269**:257–268.

[36] Zouali M. B cell tolerance to self in systemic autoimmunity. Arch Immunol Ther Exp (Warsz). 2001;**49**:361–365.

[37] Gabibov AG, Ponomarenko NA, Tretyak EB, Paltsev MA, Suchkov SV. Catalytic autoantibodies in clinical autoimmunity and modern medicine. Autoimmun Rev. 2006;**5**:324–330.

[38] Pisetsky D. Immune response to DNA in systemic lupus erythematosus. Isr Med Ass J. 2001;**3**:850–853.

[39] Earnshaw WC, Rothfield N. Identification of a family of human centromere proteins using autoimmune sera from patients with scleroderma. Chromosoma. 1985;**91**:313–321.

[40] Raptis L, Menard HA. Quantitation and characterization of plasma DNA in normals and patients with systemic lupus erythematosus. J Clin Invest. 1980;**66**:1391–1399.

[41] O'Connor KC, Bar-Or A, Hafler DA. Neuroimmunology of multiple sclerosis. J Clin Immunol. 2001;**21**:81–92.

[42] Founel S, Muller S. Antinucleosome antibodies and T-cell response in systemic lupus erythematosus. Ann Med Interne (Paris). 2002;**153**:513–519.

[43] Shoenfeld Y, Ben-Yehuda O, Messinger Y, Bentwitch Z, Rauch J, Isenberg DI, Gadoth N. Autoimmune diseases other than lupus share common anti-DNA idiotypes. Immunol Lett. 1988;**17**:285–291.

[44] Shoenfeld Y, Teplizki HA, Mendlovic S, Blank M, Mozes E, Isenberg DA. The role of the human anti-DNA idiotype 16/6 in autoimmunity. Clin Immunol Immunopathol. 1989;**51**:1989;51:313–325.

[45] Korovkina ES, Zonova EV, Buneva VN, Konenkova LP, Nevinsky GA. Interdependency analysis between antibody level to different antigenes and clinical data of systemic lupus erythematosus. Allergol Immunol (Russ.). 2006;**7**:498–507.

[46] Ershova NA, Garmashova NV, Buneva VN, Mogel'nitskii AS, Tyshkevich OB, Doronin B M, Konenkova LP, Boiko AN, Slanova AV, Nesterova VA, Gusev EI, Favorova OO, Nevinskii GA. Association between DNA antibodies levels in the blood of patients with multiple sclerosis and clinical presentation of the disease. Zh Nevrol Psikhiatr Im S. S. Korsakova (Russian). 2003;**2**:25–33.

[47] Ershova NA, Garmashova NV, Mogel'nitskii AS, Tyshkevich OB, Doronin BM, Konenkova LP, Buneva VN, Nevinskii GA. Antibodies to DNA in the blood of patients with multiple sclerosis. Russ J Immunol. 2007;**1**:229–245.

[48] Williamson RA, Burgoon MP, Owens GP, Ghausi O, Leclerc E, Firme L, Carlson S, Corboy J, Parren PW, Sanna PP, Gilden DH, Burton DR. Anti-DNA antibodies are a major component of the intrathecal B cell response in multiple sclerosis. Proc Natl Acad Sci USA. 2001;**98**:1793–1798.

[49] Krasnorutskii MA, Buneva VN, Nevinsky GA. Antibodies against DNA hydrolyze DNA and RNA. Biochem (Moscow). 2008;**73**:1547–1560.

[50] Krasnorutskii MA, Buneva VN, Nevinsky GA. Antibodies against RNA hydrolyze RNA and DNA. J Mol Recognit. 2008;**21**:337–346.

[51] Nishi Y. Evolution of catalytic antibody repertoire in autoimmune mice. J Immunol Methods. 2002;**269**:213–233.

[52] Tawfik DS, Chap R, Green BS, Sela M, Eshhar Z. Unexpectedly high occurrence of catalytic antibodies in MRL/lpr and SJL mice immunized with a transition-state analog: is there a linkage to autoimmunity?. Proc Natl Acad Sci USA. 2009;**92**:2145–2149.

[53] Bronshtein IB, Shuster AM, Gololobov GV, Gromova II, Kvashuk OA, Belostotskaya K M, Alekberova ZS, Prokaeva TB, Gabibov AG. DNA-specific antiidiotypic antibodies in the sera of patients with autoimmune diseases. FEBS Lett. 1992;**314**:259–263.

[54] Crespeau H, Laouar A, Rochu D. Polyclonal DNase abzyme produced by anti-idiotypic internal image method. CR Acad Sci III. 1994;**317**:819–823.

[55] Krasnorutskii MA, Buneva VN, Nevinsky GA. Immunization of rabbits with DNase I produces polyclonal antibodies with DNase and RNase activities. J Mol Recognit. 2008;**21**:233–242.

[56] Krasnorutskii MA, Buneva VN, Nevinsky GA. Anti-RNase antibodies against pancreatic ribonuclease A hydrolyze RNA and DNA. Int Immunol. 2008;**20**:1031–1040.

[57] Krasnorutskii MA, Buneva VN, Nevinsky GA. Immunization of rabbits with DNase II leads to formation of polyclonal antibodies with DNase and RNase activities. Int Immunol. 2009;**21**:349–360.

[58] Gottieb AA, Shwartz RH. Antigen-RNA interactions. Cell Immunol. 1972;**5**:341–362.

[59] Kozyr AV, Kolesnikov AV, Aleksandrova ES, Sashchenko LP, Gnuchev NV, Favorov PV, Kotelnikov MA, Iakhnina EI, Astsaturov IA, Prokaeva TB, Alekberova ZS, Suchkov SV, Gabibov AG. Novel functional activities of anti-DNA autoantibodies by proteases from sera of patients with lymphoproliferative and autoimmune diseases. Appl Biochem Biotechnol. 1998;**75**:45–61.

[60] Sinohara H, Matsuura K. Does catalytic activity of Bence-Jones proteins contribute to the pathogenesis of multiple myeloma?. Appl Biochem Biotechnol. 2000;**83**:85–94.

[61] Boiko AN, Favorova OO. Multiple sclerosis: molecular and cellular mechanisms. Mol Biol (Moscow). 1995;**29**:727–749.

[62] Gusev EI, Demina TL, Boiko AN. Multiple Sclerosis. Moscow: Oil and Gas; 1997.

[63] Ikehara S, Kawamura M, Takao F. Organ-specific and systemic autoimmune diseases originate from defects in hematopoietic stem cells. Proc Natl Acad Sci USA. 1990;**87**: 8341–8344.

[64] Dubrovskaya VV, Andryushkova AS, Kuznetsova IA, Toporkova LB, Buneva VN, Orlovskaya IA, Nevinsky GA. DNA-hydrolyzing antibodies from sera of autoimmune-prone MRL/MpJ-lpr mice. Biochem (Moscow). 2003;**68**:1081–1088.

[65] Kuznetsova IA, Orlovskaya IA, Buneva VN, Nevinsky GA. Activation of DNA-hydrolyzing antibodies from the sera of autoimmune-prone MRL-lpr/lpr mice by different metal ions. Biochim Biophys Acta. 2007;**1774**:884–896.

[66] Ponomarenko NA, Durova OM, Vorobiev II, Belogurov AA, Kurkova IN, Petrenko AG, Telegin GB, Suchkov SV, Kiselev SL, Lagarkova MA, Govorun VM, Serebryakova MV,

Avalle B, Tornatore P, Karavanov A, Morse HC 3rd, Thomas D, Friboulet A, Gabibov AG. Autoantibodies to myelin basic protein catalyze site-specific degradation of their antigen. Proc Natl Acad Sci USA. 2006;**103**:281–286.

[67] Parkhomenko TA, Doronin VB, Castellazzi M, Padroni M, Pastore M, Buneva VN, Granieri E, Nevinsky GA. Comparison of DNA-hydrolyzing antibodies from the cerebrospinal fluid and serum of patients with multiple sclerosis. PLoS One. 2014;**9**:e93001.

[68] Doronin VB, Parkhomenko TA, Castellazzi M, Padroni M, Pastore M, Buneva VN, Granieri E, Nevinsky GA. Comparison of antibodies hydrolyzing myelin basic protein from the cerebrospinal fluid and serum of patients with multiple sclerosis. PLoS One. 2014;**9**:e107807.

[69] Doronin VB, Parkhomenko TA, Castellazzi M, Cesnik E, Buneva VN, Granieri E, Nevinsky GA. Comparison of antibodies with amylase activity from cerebrospinal fluid and serum of patients with multiple sclerosis. PLoS One. 2016;**11**:e0154688.

[70] Andrievskaya OA, Buneva VN, Naumov VA, Nevinsky GA. Catalytic heterogeneity of polyclonal RNA-hydrolyzing IgM from sera of patients with lupus erythematosus. Med Sci Monit. 2000;**6**:460–470.

[71] Andrievskaya OA, Buneva VN, Baranovskii AG, Gal'vita AV, Benzo ES, Naumov VA, Nevinsky GA. Catalytic diversity of polyclonal RNA-hydrolyzing IgG antibodies from the sera of patients with systemic lupus erythematosus. Immunol Lett. 2002;**81**:191–198.

[72] Vlasov AV, Baranovskii AG, Kanyshkova TG, Prints AV, Zabara VG, Naumov VA, Breusov AA, Giege R, Buneva VN, Nevinskii GA. Substrate specificity of serum DNA- and RNA-hydrolyzing antibodies of patients with polyarthritis and autoimmune thyroiditis. Mol Biol (Moscow). 1998;**32**:559–569.

[73] Vlassov A, Florentz C, Helm M, Naumov V, Buneva V, Nevinsky G, Giege R. Characterization and selectivity of catalytic antibodies from human serum with RNAse activity. Nucl Acid Res. 1998;**26**:5243–5250.

[74] Vlassov AV, Helm M, Florentz C, Naumov V, Breusov AA, Buneva VN, Giege R, Nevinsky GA. Variability of substrate specificity of serum antibodies obtained from patients with different autoimmune and viral deseases in reaction of tRNA hydrolysis. Russ J Immunol. 1999;**4**:25–32.

[75] Vlasov AV, Helm M, Naumov VA, Breusov AA, Buneva VN, Florentz C, Giege R, Nevinskii GA. Features of tRNA hydrolysis by autoantibodies from blood serum of patients with certain autoimmune and virus diseases. Mol Biol (Moscow). 1999;**33**:866–872.

[76] Bezuglova AM, Konenkova LP, Buneva VN, Nevinsky GA. IgGs containing light chains of the k-and l-type and of all subclasses (IgG1-IgG4) from the sera of patients with systemic lupus erythematosus hydrolyze myelin basic protein. Int Immunol. 2012;**24**:759–770.

[77] Bezuglova AM, Konenkova LP, Doronin BM, Buneva VN, Nevinsky GA. Affinity and catalytic heterogeneity and metal-dependence of polyclonal myelin basic protein-hydrolyzing IgGs from sera of patients with systemic lupus erythematosus. J Mol Recognit. 2011;**24**:960–974.

[78] Bezuglova AM, Dmitrenok PS, Konenkova LP, Buneva VN, Nevinsky GA. Multiple sites of the cleavage of 17- and 19-mer encephalytogenic oligopeptides corresponding to human myelin basic protein (MBP) by specific anti-MBP antibodies from patients with systemic lupus erythematosus. Peptides. 2012;**37**:69–78.

[79] Timofeeva AM, Dmitrenok PS, Konenkova LP, Buneva VN, Nevinsky GA. Multiple sites of the cleavage of 21- and 25-mer encephalytogenic oligopeptides corresponding to human myelin basic protein (MBP) by specific anti-MBP antibodies from patients with systemic lupus erythematosus. PLoS One. 2013;**8**:e51600.

[80] Baranovskii AG, Kanyshkova TG, Mogelnitskii AS, Naumov VA, Buneva VN, Gusev EI, Boiko AN, Zargarova TA, Favorova OO, Nevinsky GA. Polyclonal antibodies from blood and cerebrospinal fluid of patients with multiple sclerosis effectively hydrolyze DNA and RNA. Biochemistry (Moscow). 1998;**63**:1239–1248.

[81] Baranovskii AG, Ershova NA, Buneva VN, Kanyshkova TG, Mogelnitskii AS, Doronin BM, Boiko AN, Gusev EI, Favorova OO, Nevinsky GA. Catalytic heterogeneity of polyclonal DNA- hydrolyzing antibodies from the sera of patients with multiple sclerosis. Immunol Lett. 2001;**76**:163–167 .

[82] Baranovskii AG, Buneva VN, Doronin BM, Nevinsky GA. Innunoglobulins from blood of patients with multiple sclerosis like catalytic heterogeneous nucleases. Russian J Immunol. 2008;**2**:405–419.

[83] Polosukhina DI, Garmashova NV, Tyshkevich OB, Doronin BM, Buneva VN, Nevinskii GA. Autoantibodies to myelin basic protein in patients with multiple sclerosis. Int J Immunorehabilatation. 2009;**11**:10–18.

[84] Polosukhina DI, Kanyshkova T, Doronin BM, Tyshkevich OB, Buneva VN, Boiko AN, Gusev EI, Favorova OO, Nevinsky GA. Hydrolysis of myelin basic protein by polyclonal catalytic IgGs from the sera of patients with multiple sclerosis. J Cell Mol Med. 2004;**8**:359–368.

[85] Polosukhina DI, Buneva VN, Doronin BM, Tyshkevich OB, Boiko AN, Gusev EI, Favorova OO, Nevinsky GA. Hydrolysis of myelin basic protein by IgM and IgA antibodies from the sera of patients with multiple sclerosis. Med Sci Monit. 2005;**11**:BR266–BR272.

[86] Polosukhina DI, Buneva VN, Doronin BM, Tyshkevich OB, Boiko AN, Gusev EI, Favorova OO, Nevinsky GA. Metal-dependent hydrolysis of myelin basic protein by IgGs from the sera of patients with multiple sclerosis. Immunol Lett. 2006;**103**:75–81.

[87] Legostaeva GA, Polosukhina DI, Bezuglova AM, Doronin BM, Buneva VN, Nevinsky GA. Affinity and catalytic heterogeneity of polyclonal myelin basic protein-hydrolyzing IgGs from sera of patients with multiple sclerosis. J Cell Mol Med. 2010;**14**:699–709.

[88] Savel'ev AN, Eneyskaya EV, Shabalin KA, Filatov MV, Neustroev KN. Antibodies with amylolytic activity. Prot Pept Lett. 1999;**6**:179–184.

[89] Ivanen DR, Kulminskaya AA, Ershova NA, Eneyskaya EV, Shabalin KA, Savel'ev AN, Kanyshkova TG, Buneva VN, Nevinsky GA, Neustroev KN. Human autoantibodies with amylolytic activity. Biologia. 2002;**11**:253–260.

[90] Savel'ev AN, Kulminskaya AA, Ivanen DR, Nevinsky GA, Neustroev KN. Human antibodies with amylolytic activity. Trends Glycosci Glycotechnol. 2004;**16**:17–31.

[91] Neustroev KN, Ivanen DR, Kulminskaya AA, Brumer IH, Saveliev AN, Saveliev AN, Nevinsky GA. Amylolytic activity and catalytic properties of IgM and IgG antibodies from patients with systemic lupus erythematosus. Hum Antibodies. 2003;**12**:31–34.

[92] Saveliev AN, Ivanen DR, Kulminskaya AA, Ershova NA, Kanyshkova TG, Buneva VN, Mogelnitskii AS, Doronin BM, Favorova OO, Nevinsky GA, Neustroev KN. Amylolytic activity of IgM and IgG antibodies from patients with multiple sclerosis. Immunol Lett. 2003;**86**:291–297.

[93] Ivanen DR, Kulminskaya AA, Shabalin KA, Isaeva-Ivanova LV, Saveliev AN, Nevinsky GA, Shabalin KA, Neustroev KN. Catalytic properties of IgMs with amylolytic activity isolated from patients with multiple sclerosis. Med Sci Monit. 2004;**10**:BR273–BR280.

[94] Odintsova ES, Kharitonova MA, Baranovskii AG, Siziakina LP, Buneva VN, Nevinsky GA. Proteolytic activity of IgG antibodies from blood of acquired immunodeficiency syndrome patients. Biochemistry (Moscow). 2006;**71**:251–261.

[95] Odintsova ES, Kharitonova MA, Baranovskii AG, Siziakina LP, Buneva VN, Nevinskii GA. DNA-hydrolyzing IgG antibodies from the blood of patients with acquired immune deficiency syndrome. Mol Biol (Moscow). 2006;**40**:857–864.

[96] Odintsova ES, Zaksas NP, Buneva VN, Nevinsky GA. Metal dependent hydrolysis of beta-casein by sIgA antibodies from human milk. J Mol Recognit. 2011;**24**:45–59.

[97] Baranova SV, Buneva VN, Kharitonova MA, Sizyakina LP, Calmels C, Andreola ML, Parissi V, Nevinsky GA. HIV-1 integrase-hydrolyzing antibodies from sera of HIV-infected patients. Biochimie. 2009;**91**:1081–1086.

[98] Baranova SV, Buneva VN, Kharitonova MA, Sizyakina LP, Calmels C, Andreola ML, Parissi V, Zakharova OD, Nevinsky GA. HIV-1 integrase-hydrolyzing IgM antibodies from sera of HIV-infected patients. Int Immunol. 2010;**22**:671–680.

[99] Galvita AV, Baranovskii AG, Kuznetsova IA, Vinshu NV, Galenok VA, Buneva VN, Nevinsky GA. A peculiarity of DNA hydrolysis by antibodies from patients with diabetes. Russ J Immunol. 2007;**1**:116–131.

[100] Baranovskii AG, Matushin VG, Vlassov AV, Zabara VG, Naumov VA, Buneva VN, Nevinskii GA. DNA- and RNA-hydrolyzing antibodies from the blood of patients with various forms of viral hepatitis. Biochemistry (Moscow). 1997;**62**:1358–1366.

[101] Parkhomenko TA, Buneva VN, Tyshkevich OB, Generalov II, Doronin BM, Nevinsky GA. DNA-hydrolyzing activity of IgG antibodies from the sera of patients with tick-borne encephalitis. Biochimie. 2010;**92**:545–554.

[102] Nevinsky GA, Breusov AA, Baranovskii AG, Prints AV, Kanyshkova TG, Galvita AV, Naumov VA, Buneva VN. Effect of different drugs on the level of DNA-hydrolyzing polyclonal IgG antibodies in sera of patients with Hashimoto's thyroiditis and nontoxic nodal goiter. Med Sci Monit. 2001;**7**:201–211.

[103] Ermakov EA, Smirnova LP, Parkhomenko TA, Dmitrenok PS, Krotenko NM, Fattakhov NS, Bokhan NA, Semke AV, Ivanova SA, Buneva VN, Nevinsky GA. DNA-hydrolysing activity of IgG antibodies from the sera of patients with schizophrenia. Open Biol. 2015;**5**:150064.

[104] Akagi K, Murai K, Hirao N, Yamanaka M. Purification and properties of alkaline ribonuclease from human serum. Biochim Biophys Acta. 1976;**442**:368–378.

[105] Blank A, Dekker CA. Ribonucleases of human serum, urine, cerebrospinal fluid, and leukocytes. Activity staining following electrophoresis in sodium dodecyl sulfate-polyacrylamide gels. Biochemistry. 1981;**20**:2261–2267.

[106] Sierakowska H, Shugar D. Mammalian nucleolytic enzymes. Prog Nucleic Acid Res Mol Biol. 1977;**20**:59–130.

[107] Andrievskaia OA, Kanyshkova TG, Iamkovoi VI, Buneva VN, Nevinskii GA. Monoclonal antibodies to DNA hydrolyze RNA better than DNA. Dokl Akad Nauk (Russian). 1997;**355**:401–403.

[108] Love JD, Hewitt RR. The relationship between human serum and human pancreatic DNase I. J Biol Chem. 1979;**254**:12588–12594.

[109] Suck D. DNA recognition by DNase I. J Mol Recognit. 1994;**7**:65–70.

[110] Parkhomenko TA, Legostaeva GA, Doronin BM, Buneva VN, Nevinsky GA. IgGs containing light chains of the kappa and lambda type and of all subclasses (IgG1-IgG4) from sera of patients with multiple sclerosis hydrolyze DNA. J Mol Recognit. 2010;**23**:486–494.

[111] Kostrikina IA, Buneva VN, Nevinsky GA. Systemic lupus erythematosus: molecular cloning of fourteen recombinant DNase monoclonal kappa light chains with different catalytic properties. Biochim Biophys Acta. 2014;**1840**:1725–1737.

[112] Botvinovskaya AV, Kostrikina IA, Buneva VN, Nevinsky GA. Systemic lupus erythematosus: molecular cloning of several recombinant DNase monoclonal kappa light chains with different catalytic properties. J Mol Recognit. 2013;**24**:450–460.

[113] Archelos JJ, Storch MK, Hartung HP. The role of B cells and autoantibodies in multiple sclerosis. Ann Neurol. 2000;**47**:694–706.

[114] Hemmer B, Archelos JJ, Hartung HP. New concepts in the immunopathogenesis of multiple sclerosis. Nat Rev Neurosci. 2002;**3**:291–301.

[115] Cross AH, Trotter JL, Lyons, J. B cells and antibodies in CNS demyelinating disease. J Neuroimmunol. 2001;**112**:1–14.

[116] Kalaga R, Li L, O'Dell JR, Paul S. Unexpected presence of polyreactive catalytic antibodies in IgG from unimmunized donors and decreased levels in rheumatoid arthritis. J Immunol. 1995;**155**:2695–2702.

[117] Odintsova ES, Buneva VN, Nevinsky GA. Casein-hydrolyzing activity of sIgA antibodies from human milk. J Mol Recognit. 2005;**18**:413–421.

[118] Timofeeva AM, Buneva VN, Nevinsky GA. Systemic lupus erythematosus: molecular cloning and analysis of 22 individual recombinant monoclonal kappa light chains specifically hydrolyzing human myelin basic protein. J Mol Recognit. 2015;**28**:614–627.

[119] Timofeeva AM, Ivanisenko NV, Buneva VN, Nevinsky GA. Systemic lupus erythematosus: molecular cloning and analysis of recombinant monoclonal kappa light chain NGTA2-Me-pro-ChTr possessing two different activities-trypsin-like and metalloprotease. Int Immunol. 2015;**27**:633–645.

[120] Timofeeva AM, Buneva VN, Nevinsky GA. Systemic lupus erythematosus: molecular cloning and analysis of recombinant monoclonal kappa light chain NGTA1-Me-pro with two metalloprotease active centers. Mol Biosyst. 2016;**12**:3556–3566.

[121] Tolmacheva AS, Zaksas NP, Buneva VN, Vasilenko NL, Nevinsky GA. Oxidoreductase activities of polyclonal IgGs from the sera of Wistar rats are better activated by combinations of different metal ions. J Mol Recognit. 2009;**22**:26–37.

[122] Gololobov GV, Chernova EA, Schourov DV, Smirnov IV, Kudelina IA, Gabibov AG. Cleavage of supercoiled plasmid DNA by autoantibody Fab fragment: application of the flow linear dichroism technique. Proc Natl Acad Sci USA. 1995;**92**:254–257.

[123] Kubota T. Lessons from a monoclonal antibody to double-stranded DNA. J Med Dent Sci. 1977;**44**:37–44.

[124] Mitsuhashi S, Saito R, Kurashige S, Yamashugi N. Ribonucleic acid in the immune response. Moll Cell Biochem. 1978;**20**:131–147.

[125] Vorobjeva MA, Krasitskaya VV, Fokina AA, Timoshenko VV, Nevinsky GA, Venyaminova AG, Frank LA. RNA aptamer against autoantibodies associated with multiple sclerosis and bioluminescent detection probe on its basis. Anal Chem. 2014;**86**:2590–2594.

[126] Paul S. Mechanism and functional role of antibody catalysis. Appl Biochem Biotechnol. 1998;**75**:13–23.

[127] Lacroix-Desmazes S, Bayry J, Kaveri S., Hayon-Sonsino D, Thorenoor N, Charpentier J, Luyt CE, Mira JP, Nagaraja V, Kazatchkine MD, Dhainaut JF, Mallet VO. High levels of catalytic antibodies correlate with favorable outcome in sepsis. Proc Natl Acad Sci USA. 2005;**102**:4109–4113.

[128] Belogurov AA, Kurkova IN, Friboulet A, Thomas D, Misikov VK, Zakharova M. Y, Suchkov SV, Kotov SV, Alehin AI, Avalle B, Suslova EA, Morse HC, Gabibov AG, Ponomarenko NA. Recognition and degradation of myelin basic protein peptides by serum autoantibodies: novel biomarker for multiple sclerosis. J Immunol. 2008;**180**:1258–1267.

Chapter 4

Elimination of Nucleoproteins in Systemic Lupus Erythematosus and Antinuclear Autoantibodies Production

Andrei S. Trofimenko

Additional information is available at the end of the chapter

http://dx.doi.org/10.5772/intechopen.68496

Abstract

The distinctive feature of systemic lupus erythematosus (SLE) is an immune reaction directed to diverse spectrum of autoantigens, which tends to change along with the disease spreading. The most common targets of the autoantibodies are protein and nucleoprotein components of cell nuclei: dsDNA, histones, nucleosomes, Sm antigen, and Ro and La antigens. Considering that the exact causes of this tolerance loss are unknown, a certain number of hypotheses are now discussed. One of the most promising is "waste disposal" concept, which makes a link between broken elimination of cellular debris, mononuclear phagocyte system dysfunction, and initiation of autoimmunity by the antigen presenting cells in SLE. This chapter concerns the ways nuclear antigens release from cells, necrosis, and apoptosis, as well as the key molecular mechanisms of transport and elimination of these antigens, its disturbances in SLE, and connection with innate immunity by mononuclear cells. Special attention is paid to nucleosomes and DNA degradation process, its principal factors (DNase I, C1q, SAP), blood DNA transportation by immune complexes, and immune stimulating action of DNA in SLE. Current pros and cons for the waste disposal concept and existing research trends in this field are discussed.

Keywords: systemic lupus erythematosus, autoantigens, DNA, nucleoproteins, DNase I, antigen cleavage

1. Introduction

Systemic lupus erythematosus (SLE) is a prototypic diffuse autoimmune disease of connective tissue with multiple organ involvement. The history of its exploration is not so long, compared with some other rheumatic diseases, such as osteoarthritis and gout. But, there is surprisingly few breakthrough advances in its basic conception since the 1950s, when this condition was established as a separate autoimmune disease and glucocorticoids became a groundwork in its treatment. The absence of integral and fully consistent theory of SLE etiopathogenesis appears to be the main problem for researchers, trying to improve the treatment mainly by empirical approach.

SLE etiology and pathogenesis are generally interpreted now as a multifactorially driven autoimmune process [1]. According to this conception, SLE is induced by multiple interactions of immunological, genetic, hormonal, microbial, and environmental factors. Meanwhile, first three ones apparently play the lead [2]. Genetic predisposition to SLE is suggested to be constituted mainly by definite HLA alleles, especially DR2 and DR3, by congenital deficiency of early complement components (C1, C2, C4) and by other genetic associations, including TNF, TCR, IL-6, and other genes [3]. There are genes of C-reactive protein (CRP), C1q, Fcγ-receptors, DNase I, serum amyloid P (SAP), and PDCD1 within seven loci, which are strongly linked with SLE [4]. Moreover, knocking out of these genes in mice induces autoimmune condition with glomerulonephritis [5, 6].

SLE occurs predominantly in women of childbearing age and, to a lesser extent, in prepuberta or menopause, whereupon a contribution of sex hormones could be assumed. Both men and women with SLE have high estrogen levels, the men also have low testosterone and high luteinizing hormone concentrations [7]. The connection between these deviations and SLE could be explained considering their influence on immune system cells, in particular, promotion of B cell proliferation and antibody synthesis under high estrogen levels [8].

Among all the events that can be proposed to initiate SLE onset, the leading one is suggested to be virus infection [9]. Although this "trigger agent" is not definitely identified, a wide spectrum of viruses, including Epstein-Barr virus, retroviruses, and herpesviruses, could make a substantial contribution [10]. Other influencing factors are insolation, drugs, and some pollutants.

The prominent immunological feature of SLE is the production of autoantibodies directed to a wide spectrum of self-antigens. According to Sherer et al. [11], more than 100 autoantigens, which could react with SLE-related antibodies, were mentioned in previously reported researches. However, antibodies to chromatin and its particular elements, nucleosomes, dsDNA, histones, components of DNA replication, and transcription apparatus are most representative for SLE. The second important cluster of antigens involves ribonucleoproteins and its constituents: RNA, small nuclear ribonucleoprotein (snRNP), Sm antigen, and Ro (SS-A) and La (SS-B) antigens. The third group, antiphospholipid antibodies, is common in SLE as well. Anti-DNA antibodies, and specifically anti-double-stranded DNA (dsDNA) antibodies, are thought to have most pathogenetic and diagnostic importance in SLE [12]. Their titers correlate with disease activity, and participation of anti-dsDNA antibodies in lupus nephritis is well established [13, 14].

The realization of anti-dsDNA pathogenic potential can occur by several ways. The most important contribution to systemic inflammation is generally attributed to the formation of immune complexes (IC), with both circulating and tissue-fixed antigens [15]. Nephritogenic action of ICs is mediated primarily by interaction with Fc receptors and Toll-like receptors, and, to a lesser extent, through classical pathway of complement activation [16]. In addition, autoantibodies could interfere in functioning of circulating, membrane, or even intracellular molecules [17].

However, pathogenic action is not an overall feature of anti-DNA antibodies. Both healthy individuals and SLE patients have at least two types of serum anti-DNA antibodies, unrelated directly with autoimmunity. First, there are low affinity antibodies, directed mainly against single-stranded DNA, which can be attributed to natural autoantibodies repertoire [18]. Another type consists of antibodies that are highly specific to microbial single-stranded DNA [19]. The essence of differences, influencing the pathogenic potential of these three types, is given in **Table 1**.

The way pathogenic anti-DNA antibodies appear in SLE is not well established until now. Several conjectures were made for explaining disturbed tolerance to autologous DNA. One of the hypotheses is implication of molecular mimicry, when immune response to autoantigens is induced by exogenous molecules with similar epitopes [24]. Epitope spreading mechanism may also participate in it, subsequently producing antibodies to hidden epitopes after initial reaction to major epitope [25]. Disturbance of T and/or B cellular function is third possible cause of it. Th2-polarization of $CD4^+$ T-cellular response and predominance of Th2-associated cytokines generally distinguish SLE [26]. In addition, there is low content of regulatory $CD4^+CD25^+$ T cells that restrict effector functions of $CD4^+$ and $CD8^+$ T cells and diminished suppressor activity of $CD8^+$T cells [27, 28]. Circulating B cells are usually low, mainly due to decrease of resting subpopulations, naïve and memory B cells, being in possible connection with high levels of mature plasmocytes in bone marrow [29]. Causes and mechanisms of the lymphocyte imbalance in SLE are incompletely disclosed now, as well as its pathogenetic relevance.

For the reviewing problem, information about structure of anti-dsDNA V genes, obtained from the mouse models and SLE patients, is of particular importance. Compared to their progenitors, mature genes were found to have multiple somatic hypermutations, which lead to very high avidity of these anti-dsDNA IgG [30]. Increase of arginine, asparagine, and lysine

Factor	Natural autoantibodies	SLE-associated autoantibodies	Antibodies, induced by immunization
Class	Mainly IgM	Mainly IgG	IgM or IgG
Avidity to DNA	Low	Moderate or high	High
Type of DNA to react	Preferentially with ssDNA	Usually both with ssDNA and dsDNA, more rarely—specific to dsDNA	Highly specific to ssDNA
Leading DNA epitope	No data	Deoxyribose-phosphate backbones	Immunogen-specific sequence of bases
Interaction with antigens, other than DNA	With wide spectrum of antigens	With restricted pattern of antigens	Extrinsic
Isotype switching and complement fixation	Extrinsic	Typical	Extrinsic
Somatic mutations of V gene	Few or absent	Typical	Typical
Ability to penetrate cells	In many idiotypes	In particular idiotypes	No data

Table 1. Tentative differences of pathogenic anti-DNA antibodies in SLE [20–23].

in the Complementarity-determining regions (CDR) due to hypermutations results in high isoelectric point of the antibodies, named cationic because of it [31]. Cationic anti-dsDNAs are more nephritogenic apparently through interaction with either negatively charged elements of glomerular basement membrane or DNA-containing antigens *in situ* [32].

Both somatic hypermutations and isotype switching are distinctive features of antigen-dependent B cell selection by T helper cells. High avidity of these autoantibodies points out the similarity of epitopes of the relevant autoantigen to dsDNA. Meanwhile, purified homologic DNA have been considered to be poorly immunogenic in health and in SLE models for a long time [33]. In view of this contradiction, there is emerging attention to different classes of endogenous nucleoproteins as anti-dsDNA inductors in SLE.

Besides anti-DNA antibodies, anti-nucleosome antibodies are also attributed to have a special pathogenetic significance in SLE [34]. Priority of anti-nucleosome immune response compared to anti-DNA and anti-histone ones is indirectly confirmed by revelation of earlier subtype of anti-nucleosome antibodies that do not interact with both DNA and histones [35]. There is close association of these antibodies with SLE activity and the kidney involvement [36]. But, unlike anti-dsDNA, anti-nucleosome antibodies do not develop glomerular deposits in the absence of nucleosomal antigens; further perfusion of nucleosome-containing ICs through the kidneys results in appearance of linear immunoglobulin deposits along glomerular basement membrane [37]. In addition, after interaction with antinuclear antibodies, nucleosome-containing apoptotic bodies, deposited on glomerular basement membrane or in mesangial space, turn into so-called electron-dense deposits, an attribute of IC-mediated nephritis. There is no immunoglobulin fixation in the kidneys outside these deposits [38].

In most SLE cases, serum anti-dsDNA and anti-nucleosome antibodies are presented at the same time [39]. Furthermore, chromatin immunization induces not only anti-nucleosome but also anti-dsDNA and anti-nucleosome antibodies, possibly through epitope spreading [40]. High avidity of anti-nucleosome antibodies is achieved by the same somatic hypermutations, as for anti-dsDNA production; reversion of these mutations to the initial sequence results in the loss of capability to interact with nucleoproteins and, interestingly, in obtaining antiphospholipid activity [41].

Altogether, increasing research data suggest that nucleosomes are just the best candidate antigen to induce and/or maintain production of anti-chromatin autoantibodies and to influence pathogenicity of preexisting immunoglobulins. In view of it, efficient elimination of endogenous nucleoproteins in SLE seems to be an important factor that counteracts the disease spreading.

2. Normal generation and clearance of extracellular DNA

Normal extracellular DNA concentrations are usually quite low, but the values may substantially differ depending on the detection approach and contamination of plasma with leukocytic DNA [42]. Circulating DNA is found to be not in free state but mainly as a part of mono- and oligonucleosomes; this conclusion is based upon its particular molecular weight and binding with histones [43]. Nucleosomes can release from cells during several physiological and pathological processes, namely apoptosis, necrosis, and formation of extracellular traps.

Apoptosis is considered to be predetermined death followed by the removal of damaged or unnecessary cells that is genetically, morphologically, and biochemically standalone of other kinds of cell destruction [44]. An essential condition for normal course of apoptosis is cleavage and utilization of chromosomal DNA. Internucleosomal fragmentation of chromatin is performed by specific apoptotic nucleases during early phase of the process [45]. Nuclear antigens, including nucleosomes, moved then to little bulbs of cell membrane, so-called apoptotic bodies [46]. Interestingly, in some virus infections, endogenous nucleoproteins are bundled together with virions and, thereby, can be jointly presented in apoptotic bodies [47].

The next phase includes transition of aminophospholipids, phosphatidylserine, and phosphatidylethanolamine to external side of cell membrane, and their opsonization by serum proteins, especially by C-reactive protein, C1q, and serum amyloid P (SAP) [48, 49]. This complex becomes a signal to mononuclear phagocytes for recognition and uptake. Interaction of phosphatidylserine and its circulating cofactors (C1q, β_2-glycoprotein I) with C1q receptor and Mer receptor of phosphatidylserine, expressed on macrophage surface, probably plays the lead in this complicated and insufficiently explored process [50, 51]. The ultimate destruction of engulfed nucleoproteins is provided by lysosomal enzymes, primarily by DNase II and cathepsins D, B, and L [52]. This way of clearance, which is supposed to be a major one, allows to keep the continuity of cell membrane as its distinctive feature and, thus, enables to prevent full-scale release of intracellular compounds to interstitial space [53]. Another peculiarity is the production of proinflammatory cytokines (TGF-β and IL-10), inhibiting antigen presentation by dendritic cells [54].

Appearance of circulating oligonucleosomes in apoptosis depends, to a large extent, on the activity of phagocytes [55]. Functional blocking of these cells in mice *in vivo* with clodronate is demonstrated to abolish plasma DNA spike after loading by apoptotic or necrotic cells [56]. Additional factor of substantial influence on DNA release is sex hormone balance, so far as above-mentioned DNA spike is much more higher in female mice compared to males and spays [57]. The causes of partial dissipation of DNA-containing substance during phagocytosis are now unsure. Tentative persistence of apoptotic cells, until their secondary necrosis and membrane disruption begin, is an alternative way of DNA release if elimination potential of mononuclear phagocytes is insufficient.

The second important source of extracellular DNA is cell necrosis. Unlike apoptosis, it is characterized by early cell membrane, proinflammatory effect as a result of different influences, and induction of dendritic cell maturation [58]. In necrosis, DNA is degraded at a later stage compared to apoptosis, with DNase I playing a considerable part in it [59].

The newly discovered and promising phenomenon, characterized by DNA release out of its natural compartment, is a formation of so-called extracellular traps. They were first found in neutrophils, thus being named neutrophil extracellular traps (NETs) [60]. NET are unusual extracellular structures, which are suggested to be a spare defense mechanism, activating when there are pathogens or particles, too big to be englobed by phagocytes [61]. In this case, large fibers, consisting of chromatin, serve as an external scaffold for immobilized enzymes, antimicrobial peptides, and ion chelators with locally high levels [62]. The components of NET, including dsDNA, histones, nucleosomes, and ribonucleoproteins, become bound to exogenous molecules when NET eliminates its target and thus may obtain new antigenic features.

In general, there is sustained release of nucleoproteins to extracellular space in health, and its rate can be considerably increased under certain conditions. Efficiency of its elimination strongly depends on circulating cofactor molecules, such as C1q, CRP, SAP, as well as DNase I and IgM [63]. They opsonize chromatin and keep it soluble, thus promoting digestion of long chromatin segments, transportation through circulation, and further recognition by macrophages [64]. The terminal points of this transfer are mononuclear phagocyte cells, primarily in the liver and spleen [65]. Overall efficiency of this elimination mechanism is quite high, since after injection of considerable amount of exogenous DNA, or after spontaneous release of endogenous nucleoproteins during hemodialysis, half-life of the DNA in circulation is within 4–15 min [66].

An alternative pathway of DNA elimination, that is just a subsidiary one in the absence of SLE, carries out by means of circulating immune complexes (CIC). Their clearance is determined principally by the activity of complement system. Binding of C1q with CIC results in the restriction of its further growth, prevention of precipitation, and induction of C3b and C4b occurrence [67]. Coupling of these molecules with CIC allows it to interact with CR1 complement receptor (CD35) of red blood cells [68]. Normal CIC transfer to macrophages of the spleen and liver presumably goes on in connection with erythrocytes, probably for prevention of CIC outflow from circulation, and the binding is more tight when CIC contains high molecular DNA (nearly 6000 kDa), then in case of shorter DNA segments (200–600 kDa) [69]. Both CIC and DNA, complexed with circulating opsonins, are captured by macrophages through Fcγ-receptors, the former alongside with CR1 cleavage [70]. However, elimination of DNA by means of CIC is much slower compared to CRP-SAP-linked DNA [71].

Apart from the elimination, binding of circulating ligands with DNA makes an obstacle for access of immune cells to nucleosome etitopes. This is especially important in view of chromatin immunology. It is generally considered that pure extracellular DNA have limited immunogenicity unless CpG motifs [72]. On the contrary, conjugation of protein with oligodeoxyribonucleotide can strongly promote interaction of the protein portion with antigen presenting cells, enhance antibody production, and presumably induce Th2-polarization [73]. From the other side, protein could serve as a carrier for oligonucleotide hapten. Circulating DNA ligands might also interfere in reaction of preexisting autoantibodies with apoptotic debris [74]. In light of all mentioned above, endogenous DNA elimination pathway, especially serum clearance mediators and mononuclear phagocytes, should be regarded in SLE.

3. DNA elimination pathway in SLE

Extracellular DNA levels in SLE patients tend to be appreciably elevated, their circulating DNA have predominantly low molecular weight and contain only human sequences [75]. It is also almost completely double-stranded and mainly included in oligonucleosomes, linked with serum proteins and immunoglobulins [76]. High plasma DNA concentration is usually associated with SLE flares and vascular involvement, being inversely correlated with anti-dsDNA titers, and decreases after efficient SLE treatment [77].

Functioning of the clearance mediators in SLE has some differences. Increase of disease activity does not generally combine with substantial elevation of plasma SAP and CRP levels; SAP molecular weight as well as its affinity to nucleosomes and heparin are also changeless [78]. Moreover, SAP-linked DNA levels are substantially decreased in SLE, despite elevation of total extracellular DNA; they reversely correlate with anti-dsDNA and disease activity [79]. On the contrary, plasma C1q concentrations tend to be lower in high SLE activity and in lupus nephritis, also directly correlating with CIC-linked DNA levels [80]. These changes taken one with another can be accounted for reallocation of plasma DNA pool to CIC in the presence of high-avidity anti-dsDNA. As C1q binds with both CIC and CRP-SAP-chromatin complex and participates in elimination of every type, simultaneous decrease of C1q and CIC-linked DNA is supposed to be a result of joint tissue deposition [81]. Some evidences were indeed revealed after analysis of DNA-containing CIC in SLE.

Compared to normal individuals, SLE patients commonly have elevated CIC-linked DNA concentration, which further increases along with disease activity, but its decrease is more inherent in extreme SLE flares and overt nephritis [82]. DNA from SLE CIC is double-stranded and mainly consists of fragments, which correspond to oligonucleosomes in their length, 150–250 and 370–460 bp, compared to 20 and 30–40 bp in normal controls [83]. It is revealed in SLE that in this DNA pool CpG motifs are 5–6 times more frequent than in human genome [84]. Apart from DNA and immunoglobulins, SLE CICs contain CRP, C1q, C3b, and C4b [85].

Clearance of CIC is reduced in SLE, and their half-life negatively correlates with SLE activity and extent of lupus nephritis manifestation [86]. This might be due to either impairment of CIC transportation or disturbance of phagocytosis. Furthermore, active SLE is known to have C3/C4 hypocomplementemia and low CR1 on red blood cells, probably because of its consumption [87]. It leads to persistence of CIC mostly out of erythrocytic pool, both free and connected with other blood cells [88]. This circumstance may be the cause of increased uptake of CIC by the liver macrophages and decreased one in the spleen, revealed by injection of labeled ICs to SLE patients [89]. Another unexpected finding from this experiment is substantial reversed release of partially digested ICs outside of phagocytes, which begins 40–60 min after the injection, coinciding with internalization period [90]. The causes and mechanisms of this phenomenon are now unknown. There is single publication about tentative disturbance of interaction between Fcγ receptors and intermediate filaments of mononuclear cells in SLE, what might affect internalization [91]. It is also known that knocking out of Axl/mer/tyro3 tyrosin kinase gene in Mer^{kd} mice is followed by disturbance of apoptotic debris internalization together with development of spontaneous autoimmunity. [92].

Delivery of endogenous nucleoproteins to the resident liver and spleen macrophages is thus realized in SLE presumably by way of CIC, while circulating protein mediators are responsible for this function in health. Pathogenetic importance of this shift is not restricted only to extravasation and tissue deposition of "free" DNA-containing CIC. Apart from phagocytosis, contact of CIC with macrophage Fcγ receptors initiates synthesis of proinflammatory signals, which can induce and maintain autoimmune responses [93]. Conversely, CRP-SAP-linked DNA promotes release of cytokines and chemokines, which suppress inflammation and autoimmunity as well as raise activation threshold of dendritic cells [94].

It is supposed that immune stimulating action of DNA-containing CIC in SLE is mediated by TLR9 Toll-like receptors, together with Fcγ receptors. After CIC internalization by phagocyte, TLR9 move from endoplasmic reticulum to phagosomes and then bind with CpG motifs of DNA-IgG-FcγRII complex [95]. According to the data reported by Lövgren et al. [96] and Means et al. [97], DNA-containing IC obtained from SLE patients promote macrophages and dendritic cells *in vitro* by means of TLR9 to produce α and γ interferons, IL-8, IL-1β, IL-6, IL-18, IL-12p40, TNF, and to generate chemokine signals to peripheral mononuclear cells, immature dendritic cells, T and NK cells. IC derived from patients with rheumatoid arthritis, Sjogren's disease, and DNA-lacking IC from SLE patients does not demonstrate these effects. Treatment of the IC from SLE patients with DNase I makes cytokine and chemokine induction down by 90–100% [98]. One may conclude that abundance of "free" DNA-containing CIC could amplify inflammation in SLE both directly and indirectly.

Using gene knockout approach, a possible relation between disturbance of cell debris removal and autoantibody synthesis is managed to establish. Mice with disabled SAP, C1q, Mer, secreted IgM genes develop spontaneous autoimmune disease with glomerular lesion and production of antinuclear antibodies [99]. This connection could also appear in human SLE.

As follows from the above, additional factors, that could digest extracellular DNA, mainly DNase I, become of special importance in SLE, when ordinary clearance pathway is disabled. Results of DNase I gene knockout had been published in 2000 [100], and since then the enzyme is considered to be a mediator of DNA clearance. Earlier data about low serum DNase I activity in SLE [101, 102] made this factor even more challenging for exploration of immunological tolerance to autologous DNA.

4. The DNase I riddle

DNase I is a DNA-specific endonuclease, which participates in DNA destruction in the presence of Mg^{2+} or Mn^{2+} cations. DNase I is able to destruct single-stranded, double-stranded, and protein-bound DNA; in the latter case, DNA breakdown is performed presumably in segments, free from protein, for example, in internucleosomal connectors of chromatin or in DNA segments where expression is going on [103]. Serum DNase I is usually supposed to be synthesized in gastrointestinal tract, and normal serum nuclease activity is provided almost completely by its function [104]. Proteases enhance DNase I effect on chromatin DNA, possibly due to removal of histones or liberation of basic amino acids, histidine, arginine, and lysine, which are known to be DNase I activators [105]. In general, little is known about physiological DNase I activators, including those, by which serum DNase I activity become significantly increased shortly after injection of purified DNA *in vivo* [106]. G-actin is widely considered to be a predominant physiological DNase I inhibitor [107].

Despite extensive examination, our knowledge about DNase I functions is quite superficial. Its digestive function as a participant of pancreatic secretion is the only universally recognized one. Other possible roles, including apoptotic chromatin degradation, cellular debris removal after necrosis, destruction of DNA genome viruses and some other, need to be fully established [108–110]. An important aspect of DNase I action is the loss of antigenic properties; it can be achieved for nucleoproteins and ICs, both circulating and *in situ* [111].

The rise of interest to DNase I in SLE became after the research performed by Napirei and colleagues had been published [100]. DNase I knockout in mice led to anti-dsDNA production, glomerular IC deposition, and lupus-like glomerulonephritis pathology. SLE patients and NZB/NZW F_1 lupus mice models were found to have low serum DNase I activity [112, 113]. Subsequently, it was shown with some preanalytic corrections that change of serum DNase I activity in SLE was bidirectional, with only about 30% of low enzyme activity, while other patients had moderately increased serum DNase I activity [114].

The origin of these changes is now unknown. The attempt to connect low DNase I activity with high serum actin concentrations was then rejected [114]. Numerous efforts to identify genetic changes, which can influence on the enzyme activity, resulted in very rare incidence of functionally significant gene alterations, about two per 1000 sequenced SLE patients [115–117]. Other important information, provided by geneticists, was markedly increased expression of DNase I gene in SLE [115]. One consistent explanation for it, enhanced DNase I inhibition in SLE, was challenged by Prince and colleagues [118]. Another hypothesis can be the inhibition of DNase I by specific autoantibodies, which were found by Yeh and colleagues [119]. Several factors are more likely to influence DNase I activity in SLE, as it was later shown, with about 50% cases of predominant inhibition by autoantibodies and/or actin, and the other half, impacted by unknown factor [114]. Without extensive research, this riddle is now difficult to solve.

5. Conclusion

If we could try to bring together all the facts, mentioned above, to puzzle them all into a single reasonable explanation, we will inevitably create so-called waste disposal hypothesis first published by Walport [120]. This concept defines that in SLE the most likely source of autoantigens and also leading autoimmunity inductor could be apoptotic bodies on the surface of apoptotic cells, containing almost all characteristic SLE antigens, or, as an alternative, necrotic cell debris. Another obligate condition for autoimmunity induction is postulated to be impaired clearance of the cellular "waste" and, as a consequence, antigen uptake by immature dendritic cells and their activation [121]. Several different impairments of the clearance pathway are proposed to induce SLE. Although this hypothesis seems to be consistent, and accounts for many clinical peculiarities and controversies of SLE, it has some weak points. There is no good inducible SLE model based on this concept. There is no explanation of late SLE onset, especially long after pregnancy, within this theory. The cases of spontaneous remission without glucocorticoid treatment are quite rare, despite obvious variability of "waste" generation rate.

Results of treatment with DNase I are generally discouraging. An enthusiast can, however, object to it that any correct theory usually has multiple discordances at the beginning of its life. So we shall wait a little and collect pros and contras for the final assessment of this hypothesis.

Author details

Andrei S. Trofimenko

Address all correspondence to: a.s.trofimenko@mail.ru

1 Research Institute for Clinical and Experimental Rheumatology, Volgograd, Russia

2 Volgograd State Medical University, Volgograd, Russia

References

[1] Crow MK. Etiology and pathogenesis of systemic lupus erythematosus. In: Firestein GS, Budd RC, Gabriel SE, McInnes IB, O'Dell JR, editors. Kelley and Firestein's Textbook of Rheumatology. 10th ed. Philadelphia: Elsevier; 2017. pp. 1329–1344

[2] Ferretti C, La Cava A. Overview of the pathogenesis of systemic lupus erythematosus. In: Tsokos GC, editor. Systemic Lupus Erythematosus: Basic, Applied and Clinical Aspects. Philadelphia: Elsevier; 2016. pp. 55–62. DOI: 10.1016/B978-0-12-801917-7.00008-5

[3] Deng Y, Tsao BP. Genes and genetics in human systemic lupus erythematosus. In: Tsokos GC, editor. Systemic Lupus Erythematosus: Basic, Applied and Clinical Aspects. Philadelphia: Elsevier; 2016. pp. 69–76. DOI: 10.1016/B978-0-12-801917-7.00010-3

[4] Ceccarelli F, Perricone C, Borgiani P, et al. Genetic factors in systemic lupus erythematosus: Contribution to disease phenotype. Journal of Immunology Research. 2015;**2015**:745647. DOI: 10.1155/2015/745647

[5] Botto M, Dell'Agnola C, Bygrave AE, et al. Homozygous C1q deficiency causes glomerulonephritis associated with multiple apoptotic bodies. Nature Genetics. 1998;**19**(1):56–59. DOI: 10.1038/ng0598-56

[6] Scott RS, McMahon EJ, Pop SM, et al. Phagocytosis and clearance of apoptotic cells is mediated by MER. Nature. 2001;**411**(6834):207–211. DOI: 10.1038/35075603

[7] Zen M, Ghirardello A, Iaccarino L, et al. Hormones, immune response, and pregnancy in healthy women and SLE patients. Swiss Medical Weekly. 2010;**140**(13–14):187–201

[8] Hughes GC, Choubey D. Modulation of autoimmune rheumatic diseases by oestrogen and progesterone. Nature Reviews Rheumatology. 2014;**10**(12):740–751. DOI: 10.1038/nrrheum.2014.144

[9] Nelson P, Rylance P, Roden D, Trela M, Tugnet N. Viruses as potential pathogenic agents in systemic lupus erythematosus. Lupus. 2014;**23**(6):596–605. DOI: 10.1177/0961203314531637

[10] Ascherio A, Munger KL. EBV and autoimmunity. Current Topics in Microbiology and Immunology. 2015;**390**(1):365–385. DOI: 10.1007/978-3-319-22822-8_15

[11] Sherer Y, Gorstein A, Fritzler MJ, Shoenfeld Y. Autoantibody explosion in systemic lupus erythematosus: More than 100 different antibodies found in SLE patients. Seminars in Arthritis and Rheumatism. 2004;**34**(2):501–537

[12] Ching KH, Burbelo PD, Tipton C, et al. Two major autoantibody clusters in systemic lupus erythematosus. PLoS One. 2012;**7**(2):e32001. DOI: 10.1371/journal.pone.0032001

[13] Gatto M, Iaccarino L, Ghirardello A, et al. Clinical and pathologic considerations of the qualitative and quantitative aspects of lupus nephritogenic autoantibodies: A comprehensive review. Journal of Autoimmunity. 2016;**69**:1–11. DOI: 10.1016/j.jaut.2016.02.003

[14] Floris A, Piga M, Cauli A, Mathieu A. Predictors of flares in systemic lupus erythematosus: Preventive therapeutic intervention based on serial anti-dsDNA antibodies assessment. Analysis of a monocentric cohort and literature review. Autoimmunity Reviews. 2016;**15**(7):656–663. DOI: 10.1016/j.autrev.2016.02.019

[15] Trofimenko AS, Gontar IP, Paramonova OV, Simakova ES, Zborovskaya IA. Experimental modeling of nucleoprotein disposal disorders in systemic lupus erythematosus. Biomeditsinskaya Khimiya. 2015;**61**(5):617–621. [in Russian] DOI: 10.18097/PBMC20156105617

[16] Sjöwall C, Olin AI, Skogh T, et al. C-reactive protein, immunoglobulin G and complement co-localize in renal immune deposits of proliferative lupus nephritis. Autoimmunity. 2013;**46**(3):205–214. DOI: 10.3109/08916934.2013.764992

[17] Song YC, Sun GH, Lee TP, et al. Arginines in the CDR of anti-dsDNA autoantibodies facilitate cell internalization via electrostatic interactions. European Journal of Immunology. 2008;**38**(11):3178–3190. DOI: 10.1002/eji.200838678

[18] Suurmond J, Calise J, Malkiel S, Diamond B. DNA-reactive B cells in lupus. Current Opinion in Immunology. 2016;**43**:1–7. DOI: 10.1016/j.coi.2016.07.002

[19] Haji-Ghassemi O, Müller-Loennies S, Rodriguez T, et al. Structural basis for antibody recognition of lipid A: Insights to polyspecificity toward single-stranded DNA. Journal of Biological Chemistry. 2015;**290**(32):19629–19640. DOI: 10.1074/jbc.M115.657874

[20] Seredkina N, Van Der Vlag J, Berden J, et al. Lupus nephritis: enigmas, conflicting models and an emerging concept. Molecular Medicine. 2013;**19**:161–169. DOI: 10.2119/molmed.2013.00010

[21] Yung S, Chan TM. Mechanisms of kidney injury in lupus nephritis: The role of anti-dsDNA antibodies. Frontiers in Immunology. 2015;**6**:475. DOI: 10.3389/fimmu.2015.00475

[22] Goilav B, Putterman C. The role of anti-DNA antibodies in the development of lupus nephritis: A complementary, or alternative, viewpoint? Seminars in Nephrology. 2015;**35** (5):439–443

[23] Witte T. IgM antibodies against dsDNA in SLE. Clinical Reviews in Allergy & Immunology. 2008;**34**(3):345–347. DOI: 10.1007/s12016-007-8046-x

[24] Aas-Hanssen K, Thompson KM, Bogen B, Munthe LA. Systemic lupus erythematosus: Molecular mimicry between anti-dsDNA CDR3 Idiotype, microbial and self-peptides as antigens for Th cells. Frontiers in Immunology. 2015;**6**:382. DOI: 10.3389/fimmu.2015.00382

[25] Rigante D, Esposito S. Infections and systemic lupus erythematosus: Binding or sparring partners?. International Journal of Molecular Sciences. 2015;**16**(8):17331–17343. DOI: 10.3390/ijms160817331

[26] Talaat RM, Mohamed SF, Bassyouni IH, Raouf AA. Th1/Th2/Th17/Treg cytokine imbalance in systemic lupus erythematosus (SLE) patients: Correlation with disease activity. Cytokine. 2015;**72**(2):146–153. DOI: 10.1016/j.cyto.2014.12.027

[27] Barreto M, Ferreira RC, Lourenço L, et al. Low frequency of CD4+CD25+ Treg in SLE patients: A heritable trait associated with CTLA4 and TGF-beta gene variants. BMC Immunology. 2009;**10**:5. DOI: 10.1186/1471-2172-10-5

[28] Mak A, Kow NY. The pathology of T cells in systemic lupus erythematosus. Journal of Immunology Research. 2014;**2014**:419029. DOI: 10.1155/2014/419029

[29] Zhao L, Ye Y, Zhang X. B cells biology in systemic lupus erythematosus-from bench to bedside. Science China Life Sciences. 2015;**58**(11):1111–1125. DOI: 10.1007/s11427-015-4953-x

[30] Bobeck MJ, Cleary J, Beckingham JA, et al. Effect of somatic mutation on DNA binding properties of anti-DNA autoantibodies. Biopolymers. 2007;**85**(5–6):471–480. DOI: 10.1002/bip.20691

[31] Guo W, Smith D, Aviszus K, et al. Somatic hypermutation as a generator of antinuclear antibodies in a murine model of systemic autoimmunity. Journal of Experimental Medicine. 2010;**207**(10):2225–2237. DOI: 10.1084/jem.20092712

[32] Kohro-Kawata J, Wang P, Kawata Y, et al. Highly cationic anti-DNA antibodies in patients with lupus nephritis analyzed by two-dimensional electrophoresis and immunoblotting. Electrophoresis. 1998;**19**(8–9):1511–1555. DOI: 10.1002/elps.1150190849

[33] Al Arfaj AS, Chowdhary AR, Khalil N, Ali R. Immunogenicity of singlet oxygen modified human DNA: Implications for anti-DNA antibodies in systemic lupus erythematosus. Clinical Immunology. 2007;**124**(1):83–89. DOI: 10.1016/j.clim.2007.03.548

[34] Yap DY, Lai KN. Pathogenesis of renal disease in systemic lupus erythematosus: The role of autoantibodies and lymphocytes subset abnormalities. International Journal of Molecular Sciences. 2015;**16**(4):7917–7931. DOI: 10.3390/ijms16047917

[35] Li T, Prokopec SD, Morrison S, et al. Anti-nucleosome antibodies outperform traditional biomarkers as longitudinal indicators of disease activity in systemic lupus erythematosus. Rheumatology (Oxford). 2015;**54**(3):449–457. DOI: 10.1093/rheumatology/keu326

[36] Bizzaro N, Villalta D, Giavarina D, Tozzoli R. Are anti-nucleosome antibodies a better diagnostic marker than anti-dsDNA antibodies for systemic lupus erythematosus? A systematic review and a study of meta analysis. Autoimmunity Reviews. 2012;**12**(2):97–106. DOI: 10.1016/j.autrev.2012.07.002

[37] Mjelle JE, Rekvig OP, Van Der Vlag J, Fenton KA. Nephritogenic antibodies bind in glomeruli through interaction with exposed chromatin fragments and not with renal cross-reactive antigens. Autoimmunity. 2011;**44**(5):373–383. DOI: 10.3109/08916934.2010.541170

[38] Olin AI, Mörgelin M, Truedsson L, et al. Pathogenic mechanisms in lupus nephritis: Nucleosomes bind aberrant laminin β1 with high affinity and colocalize in the electron-dense deposits. Arthritis & Rheumatology. 2014;**66**(2):397–406. DOI: 10.1002/art.38250

[39] Dieker J, Schlumberger W, McHugh N, et al. Reactivity in ELISA with DNA-loaded nucleosomes in patients with proliferative lupus nephritis. Molecular Immunology. 2015;**68**(1):20–24. DOI: 10.1016/j.molimm.2015.06.004

[40] Voynova EN, Tchorbanov AI, Todorov TA, Vassilev TL. Breaking of tolerance to native DNA in nonautoimmune mice by immunization with natural protein/DNA complexes. Lupus. 2005;**14**(7):543–550

[41] Wellmann U, Letz M, Herrmann M, et al. The evolution of human anti-double-stranded DNA autoantibodies. Proceedings of the National Academy of Sciences USA. 2005;**102**(26):9258–9263. DOI: 10.1073/pnas.0500132102

[42] Thierry AR, El Messaoudi S, Gahan PB, et al. Origins, structures, and functions of circulating DNA in oncology. Cancer and Metastasis Reviews. 2016;**35**(3):347–376

[43] Bryzgunova OE, Laktionov PP. Generation of blood circulating DNA: The sources, peculiarities of circulation and structure. Biomeditsinskaya Khimiya. 2015;**61**(4):409–426. [in Russian] DOI: 10.18097/PBMC20156104409

[44] Reed JC, Green DR, editors. Apoptosis: Physiology and Pathology. Cambridge: Cambridge University Press; 2011. p. 421

[45] Preedy VR, editor. Apoptosis. Enfield: Science Publishers; 2010. p. 654

[46] Yamamoto S, Azuma E, Muramatsu M, et al. Significance of extracellular vesicles: Pathobiological roles in disease. Cell Structure and Function. 2016;**41**(2):137–143

[47] Rosen A, Casciola-Rosen LA, Ahearn J. Novel packages of viral and self-antigens are generated during apoptosis. Journal of Experimental Medicine. 1995;**181**(4):1557–1561

[48] Paidassi H, Tacnet-Delorme P, Arlaud GJ, Frachet P. How phagocytes track down and respond to apoptotic cells. Critical Reviews in Immunology. 2009;**29**(2):111–130

[49] Kinchen JM. A model to die for: Signaling to apoptotic cell removal in worm, fly and mouse. Apoptosis. 2010;**15**(9):998–1006. DOI: 10.1007/s10495-010-0509-5

[50] Peter C, Wesselborg S, Herrmann M, Lauber K. Dangerous attraction: Phagocyte recruitment and danger signals of apoptotic and necrotic cells. Apoptosis. 2010;**15**(9):1007–1028. DOI: 10.1007/s10495-010-0472-1

[51] Biermann MH, Maueröder C, Brauner JM, et al. Surface code – biophysical signals for apoptotic cell clearance. Physical Biology. 2013;**10**(6):065007. DOI: 10.1088/1478-3975/10/6/065007

[52] Kawane K, Nagata S. Nucleases in programmed cell death. Methods in Enzymology. 2008;**442**:271–287. DOI: 10.1016/S0076-6879(08)01414-6

[53] Poon IK, Lucas CD, Rossi AG, Ravichandran KS. Apoptotic cell clearance: Basic biology and therapeutic potential. Nature Reviews Immunology. 2014;**14**(3):166–180. DOI: 10.1038/nri3607

[54] Biermann MH, Veissi S, Maueröder C. The role of dead cell clearance in the etiology and pathogenesis of systemic lupus erythematosus: Dendritic cells as potential targets. Expert Review of Clinical Immunology. 2014;**10**(9):1151–1164. DOI: 10.1586/1744666X.2014.944162

[55] Arandjelovic S, Ravichandran KS. Phagocytosis of apoptotic cells in homeostasis. Nature Immunology. 2015;**16**(9):907–917. DOI: 10.1038/ni.3253

[56] Jiang N, Reich CF 3rd, Pisetsky DS. Role of macrophages in the generation of circulating blood nucleosomes from dead and dying cells. Blood. 2003;**102**(6):2243–2250

[57] Pisetsky DS, Jiang N. The generation of extracellular DNA in SLE: The role of death and sex. Scandinavian Journal of Immunology. 2006;**64**(3):200–204. DOI: 10.1111/j.1365-3083.2006.01822.x

[58] Podolska MJ, Biermann MH, Maueröder C. Inflammatory etiopathogenesis of systemic lupus erythematosus: An update. Journal of Inflammation Research. 2015;**8**:161–171. DOI: 10.2147/JIR.S70325

[59] Krysko DV, D'Herde K, Vandenabeele P. Clearance of apoptotic and necrotic cells and its immunological consequences. Apoptosis. 2006;**11**(10):1709–1726

[60] Brinkmann V, Reichard U, Goosmann C, et al. Neutrophil extracellular traps kill bacteria. Science. 2004;**303**:1532–1535

[61] Zawrotniak M, Rapala-Kozik M. Neutrophil extracellular traps (NETs) - formation and implications. Acta Biochimica Polonica. 2013;**60**(3):277–284

[62] Gupta S, Kaplan MJ. The role of neutrophils and NETosis in autoimmune and renal diseases. Nature Reviews Nephrology. 2016;**12**(7):402–413. DOI: 10.1038/nrneph.2016.71

[63] Park B, Lee J, Moon H, et al. Co-receptors are dispensable for tethering receptor-mediated phagocytosis of apoptotic cells. Cell Death & Disease. 2015;**6**:e1772. DOI: 10.1038/cddis.2015.140

[64] Gregory CD, Pound JD. Microenvironmental influences of apoptosis *in vivo* and *in vitro*. Apoptosis. 2010;**15**(9):1029–1049. DOI: 10.1007/s10495-010-0485-9

[65] Prabagar MG, Do Y, Ryu S, et al. SIGN-R1, a C-type lectin, enhances apoptotic cell clearance through the complement deposition pathway by interacting with C1q in the spleen. Cell Death & Differentiation. 2013;**20**(4):535–545. DOI: 10.1038/cdd.2012.160

[66] Gauthier VJ, Tyler LN, Mannik M. Blood clearance kinetics and liver uptake of mononucleosomes in mice. Journal of Immunology. 1996;**156**(3):1151–1156

[67] Manderson AP, Botto M, Walport MJ. The role of complement in the development of systemic lupus erythematosus. Annual Review of Immunology. 2004;**22**:431–456

[68] Odera M, Otieno W, Adhiambo C, Stoute JA. Dual role of erythrocyte complement receptor type 1 in immune complex-mediated macrophage stimulation: Implications for the pathogenesis of *Plasmodium falciparum* malaria. Clinical & Experimental Immunology. 2011;**166**(2):201–207

[69] Horgan C, Burge J, Crawford L, Taylor RP. The kinetics of ^{3}H-dsDNA/anti-DNA immune complex formation, binding by red blood cells, and release into serum: Effect of DNA molecular weight and conditions of antibody excess. Journal of Immunology. 1984;**133**(4):2079–2084

[70] Karsten CM, Köhl J. The immunoglobulin, IgG Fc receptor and complement triangle in autoimmune diseases. Immunobiology. 2012;**217**(11):1067–1079. DOI: 10.1016/j.imbio.2012.07.015

[71] Rojko JL, Evans MG, Price SA, et al. Formation, clearance, deposition, pathogenicity, and identification of biopharmaceutical-related immune complexes: Review and case studies. Toxicologic Pathology. 2014;**42**(4):725–764. DOI: 10.1177/0192623314526475

[72] Hartmann G. Nucleic Acid Immunity. Advances in Immunology. 2017;**133**:121–169. DOI: 10.1016/bs.ai.2016.11.001

[73] Sano K, Shirota H, Terui T, et al. Oligodeoxynucleotides without CpG motifs work as adjuvant for the induction of Th2 differentiation in a sequence-independent manner. Journal of Immunology. 2003;**170**(5):2367–2373

[74] Squatrito D, Emmi G, Silvestri E, Prisco D, Emmi L. SLE Pathogenesis: From apoptosis to lymphocyte activation. In: Roccatello D, Emmi L, editors. Connective Tissue Disease: A Comprehensive Guide. Vol. 1. Heidelberg: Springer; 2016. pp. 23–34

[75] Chan RW, Jiang P, Peng X, et al. Plasma DNA aberrations in systemic lupus erythematosus revealed by genomic and methylomic sequencing. Proceedings of the National Academy of Sciences of the United States of America . 2014;**111**(49):E5302–E5311. DOI: 10.1073/pnas.1421126111

[76] Chen JA, Meister S, Urbonaviciute V, et al. Sensitive detection of plasma/serum DNA in patients with systemic lupus erythematosus. Autoimmunity. 2007;**40**(4):307–310

[77] Zborovskaya IA, Trofimenko AS, Gontar IP, et al. Prospects of extracorporeal biological therapy of systemic lupus erythematosus using the composite adsorbents. Kremlevskaya medicina. 2013;**3**:85–89 [in Russian]

[78] Firooz N, Albert DA, Wallace DJ, et al. High-sensitivity C-reactive protein and erythrocyte sedimentation rate in systemic lupus erythematosus. Lupus. 2011;**20**(6):588–597

[79] Voss A, Nielsen EH, Svehag SE, Junker P. Serum amyloid P component-DNA complexes are decreased in systemic lupus erythematosus: Inverse association with anti-dsDNA antibodies. Journal of Rheumatology. 2008;**35**(4):625–630

[80] Fenton K. The effect of cell death in the initiation of lupus nephritis. Clinical & Experimental Immunology. 2015;**179**(1):11–16. DOI: 10.1111/cei.12417

[81] Truedsson L, Bengtsson AA, Sturfelt G. Complement deficiencies and systemic lupus erythematosus. Autoimmunity. 2007;**40**(8):560–566. DOI: 10.1080/08916930701510673

[82] Nezlin R. A quantitative approach to the determination of antigen in immune complexes. Journal of Immunological Methods. 2000;**237**(1–2):1–17

[83] Nezlin R, Alarcón-Segovia D, Shoenfeld Y. Immunochemical determination of DNA in immune complexes present in the circulation of patients with systemic lupus erythematosus. Journal of Autoimmunity. 1998;**11**(5):489–493. DOI: 10.1006/jaut.1998.0231

[84] Sano H, Takai O, Harata N, et al. Binding properties of human anti-DNA antibodies to cloned human DNA fragments. Scandinavian Journal of Immunology. 1989;**30**(1):51–63

[85] Pradhan V, Rajadhyaksha A, Mahant G, et al. Anti-C1q antibodies and their association with complement components in Indian systemic lupus erythematosus patients. Indian Journal of Nephrology. 2012;**22**(5):353–357. DOI: 10.4103/0971-4065.103911

[86] Kavai M, Szegedi G. Immune complex clearance by monocytes and macrophages in systemic lupus erythematosus. Autoimmunity Reviews. 2007;**6**(7):497–502

[87] Julkunen H, Ekblom-Kullberg S, Miettinen A. Nonrenal and renal activity of systemic lupus erythematosus: A comparison of two anti-C1q and five anti-dsDNA assays and complement C3 and C4. Rheumatology International. 2012;**32**(8):2445–2451. DOI: 10.1007/s00296-011-1962-3

[88] Elkon KB, Santer DM. Complement, interferon and lupus. Current Opinion in Immunology. 2012;**24**(6):665–670. DOI: 10.1016/j.coi.2012.08.004

[89] Davies KA, Peters AM, Beynon HL, Walport MJ. Immune complex processing in patients with systemic lupus erythematosus. *In vivo* imaging and clearance studies. Journal of Clinical Investigation. 1992;**90**(5):2075–2083. DOI: 10.1172/JCI116090

[90] Davies KA, Robson MG, Peters AM, et al. Defective Fc-dependent processing of immune complexes in patients with systemic lupus erythematosus. Arthritis & Rheumatology. 2002;**46**(4):1028–1038

[91] Vázquez-Doval J, Sánchez-Ibarrola A. Defective mononuclear phagocyte function in systemic lupus erythematosus: Relationship of FcRII (CD32) with intermediate cytoskeletal filaments. Journal of Investigational Allergology and Clinical Immunology. 1993;**3**(2):86–91

[92] Jung JY, Suh CH. Incomplete clearance of apoptotic cells in systemic lupus erythematosus: Pathogenic role and potential biomarker. International Journal of Rheumatic Diseases. 2015;18(3):294–303. DOI: 10.1111/1756-185X.12568

[93] Toong C, Adelstein S, Phan TG. Clearing the complexity: Immune complexes and their treatment in lupus nephritis. International Journal of Nephrology and Renovascular Disease. 2011;4:17–28

[94] Rekvig OP, Van der Vlag J. The pathogenesis and diagnosis of systemic lupus erythematosus: Still not resolved. Seminars in Immunopathology. 2014;36(3):301–311. DOI: 10.1007/s00281-014-0428-6

[95] Tsokos GC, Lo MS, Reis PC, Sullivan KE. New insights into the immunopathogenesis of systemic lupus erythematosus. Nature Reviews Rheumatology. 2016;12(12):716–730. DOI: 10.1038/nrrheum.2016.186

[96] Lövgren T, Eloranta ML, Båve U, et al. Induction of interferon-alpha production in plasmacytoid dendritic cells by immune complexes containing nucleic acid released by necrotic or late apoptotic cells and lupus IgG. Arthritis & Rheumatology. 2004;50 (6):1861–1872

[97] Means TK, Latz E, Hayashi F, et al. Human lupus autoantibody-DNA complexes activate DCs through cooperation of CD32 and TLR9. Journal of Clinical Investigation. 2005;115(2):407–417

[98] Liao X, Reihl AM, Luo XM. Breakdown of immune tolerance in systemic lupus erythematosus by dendritic cells. Journal of Immunology Research. 2016;2016:6269157. DOI: 10.1155/2016/6269157

[99] Guo Y, Orme J, Mohan C. A genopedia of lupus genes - lessons from gene knockouts. Current Rheumatology Reviews. 2013;9(2):90–99

[100] Napirei M, Karsunky H, Zevnik B, et al. Features of systemic lupus erythematosus in Dnase1-deficient mice. Nature Genetics. 2000;25(2):177–181. DOI: 10.1038/76032

[101] Frost PG, Lachmann PJ. The relationship of desoxyribonuclease inhibitor levels in human sera to the occurrence of antinuclear antibodies. Clinical & Experimental Immunology. 1968;3(5):447–455

[102] Chitrabamrung S, Rubin RL, Tan EM. Serum deoxyribonuclease I and clinical activity in systemic lupus erythematosus. Rheumatology International. 1981;1(2):55–60

[103] Zborovskaya IA, Trofimenko AS, Gontar IP. Anti-DNase I antibody response in systemic lupus erythematosus: A possible way of the enzyme dysfunction. Nauchno Prakticheskaya Revmatologiya. 2007;**45**:64–68. [in Russian] DOI: 10.14412/1995-4484-2007-3

[104] Fujihara J, Yasuda T, Ueki M, et al. Comparative biochemical properties of vertebrate deoxyribonuclease I. Comparative Biochemistry and Physiology Part B: Biochemistry and Molecular Biology. 2012;163(3–4):263–273. DOI: 10.1016/j.cbpb.2012.07.002

[105] Shapot VS. Nucleases. Moscow: Meditsina Publishers; 1968. p. 212 [in Russian]

[106] Mazurik VK, Moskaliova EU. Aspartate carbamoyltransferase, DNA polymerase, and DNase activities in rat hemopoietic tissues after single DNA injection. Bulletin of Experimental Biology and Medicine. 1974;77(2):32–35 [in Russian]

[107] Yokota E. Isolation of actin and actin-binding proteins. Methods in Molecular Biology. 2017;1511:291–299. DOI: 10.1007/978-1-4939-6533-5_23

[108] Nikiforov ND, Mamontov SG, Ilnitsky Yu A, et al. Treatment of acute hepatitis B with deoxyribonuclease. Sovetskaia Meditsina. 1990;7:82–83 [in Russian]

[109] Peer V, Abu Hamad R, Berman S, Efrati S. Renoprotective effects of DNAse-I treatment in a rat model of ischemia/reperfusion-induced acute kidney injury. American Journal of Nephrology. 2016;43(3):195–205. DOI: 10.1159/000445546

[110] Koyama R, Arai T, Kijima M, et al. DNase γ, DNase I and caspase-activated DNase cooperate to degrade dead cells. Genes to Cells. 2016;21(11):1150–1163. DOI: 10.1111/gtc.12433

[111] Lefkowith JB, Kiehl M, Rubenstein J, et al. Heterogeneity and clinical significance of glomerular-binding antibodies in systemic lupus erythematosus. Journal of Clinical Investigation. 1996;98(6):1373–1380

[112] Macanovic M, Lachmann PJ. Measurement of deoxyribonuclease I (DNase) in the serum and urine of systemic lupus erythematosus (SLE)-prone NZB/NZW mice by a new radial enzyme diffusion assay. Clinical & Experimental Immunology. 1997;108(2):220–226

[113] Sallai K, Nagy E, Derfalvy B, et al. Antinucleosome antibodies and decreased deoxyribonuclease activity in sera of patients with systemic lupus erythematosus. Clinical and Diagnostic Laboratory Immunology. 2005;12(1):56–59. DOI: 10.1128/CDLI.12.1.56-59.2005

[114] Trofimenko AS, Gontar IP, Zborovsky AB, Paramonova OV. Anti-DNase I antibodies in systemic lupus erythematosus: Diagnostic value and share in the enzyme inhibition. Rheumatology International. 2016;36(4):521–529. DOI: 10.1007/s00296-016-3437-z

[115] Feng XB, Shen N, Qian J, et al. Single nucleotide polymorphisms of deoxyribonuclease I and their expression in Chinese systemic lupus erythematosus patients. Chinese Medical Journal (England). 2004;**117**(11):1670–1676

[116] Yasutomo K, Horiuchi T, Kagami S, et al. Mutation of DNASE1 in people with systemic lupus erythematosus. Nature Genetics. 2001;28(4):313–314. DOI: 10.1038/91070

[117] Bodaño A, González A, Ferreiros-Vidal I, et al. Association of a non-synonymous single-nucleotide polymorphism of DNASEI with SLE susceptibility. Rheumatology (Oxford). 2006;45(7):819–823. DOI: 10.1093/rheumatology/kel019

[118] Prince WS, Baker DL, Dodge AH, et al. Pharmacodynamics of recombinant human DNase I in serum. Clinical & Experimental Immunology. 1998;113(2):289–296

[119] Yeh TM, Chang HC, Liang CC, et al. Deoxyribonuclease-inhibitory antibodies in systemic lupus erythematosus. Journal of Biomedical Science. 2003;10(5):544–551

[120] Walport MJ. Complement and systemic lupus erythematosus. Arthritis Research. 2002;4(Suppl 3):S279–S293. DOI: 10.1186/ar586

[121] Mahajan A, Herrmann M, Muñoz LE. Clearance deficiency and cell death pathways: A model for the pathogenesis of SLE. Frontiers in Immunology. 2016;7:35. DOI: 10.3389/fimmu.2016.00035

Chapter 5

T Regulatory Cells in Systemic Lupus Erythematosus: Current Knowledge and Future Prospects

Konstantinos Tselios, Alexandros Sarantopoulos, Ioannis Gkougkourelas and Panagiota Boura

Additional information is available at the end of the chapter

http://dx.doi.org/10.5772/intechopen.68479

Abstract

Systemic lupus erythematosus (SLE) is one of the most diverse autoimmune diseases, regarding clinical manifestations and therapeutic management. Visceral involvement is often and is generally associated with increased mortality and/or permanent disability. Thus, a reliable assessment of disease activity is required in order to follow-up disease activity and apply appropriate therapy. Several serological indexes have been studied due to their competence in assessing disease activity in SLE. Apart from conventional and currently assessed serological indexes, regulatory T cells (Tregs), a CD4+ cellular population of the acquired immune compartment with homeostatic phenotype, are currently under intense investigation in SLE. In this chapter, Tregs ontogenesis and subpopulations are discussed focusing on their implications in immunopathophysiology of SLE. The authors present data indicating that this CD4+ population is highly associated with disease activity and response to treatment, concluding that Tregs are a promising biomarker in SLE. Future prospective includes Tregs implication in SLE therapeutic interventions.

Keywords: regulatory T cells, systemic lupus erythematosus, SLE immunopathphysiology, Treg therapy

1. Introduction

Systemic lupus erythematosus represents the prototype of autoimmune diseases and is characterized by an unparalleled variety of clinical and laboratory manifestations. From a pathogenetic perspective, a breakdown of immune tolerance will lead to the proliferation and functional differentiation of certain effector cells of the innate and adaptive immunity, such as neutrophils, dendritic cells (DCs), macrophages, and auto-reactive lymphocytes [1, 2]. The net result will be the production of pro-inflammatory cytokines and autoantibodies, formation of immune-complexes and, eventually, tissue damage driven by the deposition of these complexes onto certain tissues and the activation of the complement cascade; other mechanisms have also been described, such as autoantibody- and cell-mediated toxicity. Tissue damage will, in turn, provide the substrate for neo-epitope formation or the revealing of cryptic epitopes; this will further amplify the autoimmune response. Given the clinical diversity of SLE, several studies investigating the molecular mechanisms of the disease have yielded contradictory findings regarding multiple cellular subpopulations or soluble mediators. These findings seem to be influenced by disease duration, global disease activity, therapeutic variables, and other confounders [2]. Among them, an impairment of the mechanisms of the peripheral immune tolerance, mainly represented by the T regulatory cells (Tregs), has been universally documented in SLE and considered to be a crucial factor in disease pathogenesis.

1.1. T regulatory cells

Tregs represent a subpopulation of the CD4+ T lymphocytes which were first described in the 1970s [3] as suppressor cells since their primary function was the suppression of the immune response [4]. At that time, the term 'infectious tolerance' was introduced to describe the acquisition of suppressive capacity of non-suppressor cells from Tregs with an, as yet, unknown mechanism [5]. The study of this cellular subpopulation was initially abandoned due to technical difficulties with regard to the isolation and analysis of these cells because of the lack of specific surface markers [6, 7].

Research interest in suppressor T cells re-emerged in 1995, when Sakaguchi et al. described the intense expression of the α chain of the IL-2 receptor (IL-2Rα, CD25) on their surface [8]. These cells were then called regulatory T cells since their function was the multifaceted regulation of the immune response and the maintenance of immune homeostasis [9]. During the next few years, several investigators showed that these cells are characterized by a unique functional phenotype, which is marked, not only by the over-expression of the CD25, but also from decreased responsiveness after polyclonal stimulation of their T cell receptor (TCR) [10, 11]. These studies suggested that their regulatory/suppressive capacity against the effector T cells was irrespective of the antigen that generated the initial activation of the effector cells (non-antigen specific and, thus, non-MHC restricted).

The demonstration of the high surface expression of the CD25 molecule led to the characterization and distinction of Tregs from other subsets of T lymphocytes, as well as to the discovery of their thymic origin and initial functional differentiation [12]. However, it was later shown that CD25 is not exclusively expressed in Tregs. Other recently activated T lymphocytes and all T cells with regulatory function *in vitro* were also expressing this molecule [13]. As might be expected, Tregs do express the highest levels of CD25 ($CD25^{high}$) as compared to the conventional CD4+ T cells, in which its expression is transient and of low intensity. Based on flow cytometric analysis, it has been shown that, among CD4+CD25+ cells, only those at the upper 2% of CD25 expression possess suppressive capacity [14].

In 2001, the gene FOXP3 (Forkhead Box P3) was discovered in mice; its mutations were leading to the spontaneous development of autoimmune phenomena [15]. Mutations of the human

FOXP3 have been associated with two distinct systemic autoimmune syndromes, namely the IPEX (immune dysregulation, polyendocrinopathy, enteropathy, X-linked syndrome) and XLAAD (X-linked, autoimmunity, allergy, dysregulation) [16–18]. In 2003, it was proven that FOXP3 is the master regulator for the functional differentiation of Tregs and is required for their proliferation [19]. It is found in the X chromosome (Xq11.23-Xq13.3) and consists of 11 exons that code a 48-kDa protein with 431 amino acids [18]. FOXP3 is mainly expressed in the T lymphocytes (mainly those that bear the αβTCR), whereas it is hardly detectable in B cells, γδ T cells, NK, macrophages, and dendritic cells. It is considered the lineage-specification factor of the natural T regulatory cells (nTregs).

The respective transcription factor FOXP3 is highly expressed in the CD4+CD25^{high} T cells, while its early activation in the naive T cells drives their differentiation toward a regulatory phenotype. This is particularly detected under inflammatory conditions where CD4+CD25- T cells overexpress FOXP3, which in turn leads to the increased surface expression of other molecules, such as CTLA-4 (cytotoxic T lymphocyte-associated antigen 4, CD152) and GITR (glucocorticoid-induced TNF receptor-a family-related protein) [20, 21]. These cells now possess suppressive capacity; they secrete less IL-2 and proliferate slowly.

Further research revealed that, like CD25, the expression of FOXP3 is not confined to naturally occurring Tregs; actually, it could be induced in recently activated cells (in low intensity) and CD4+ T cells that acquire suppressive properties afterward [22]. However, based on its critical importance, all cells bearing the FOXP3 key regulator are considered to be regulatory in function. FOXP3+ Tregs are divided in natural and inducible cells, according to their origin (thymus and/or periphery, respectively). The most well-studied subgroups of the inducible Tregs (iTregs) are the Tr1, Th3, and CD8+ Tregs (**Figure 1**).

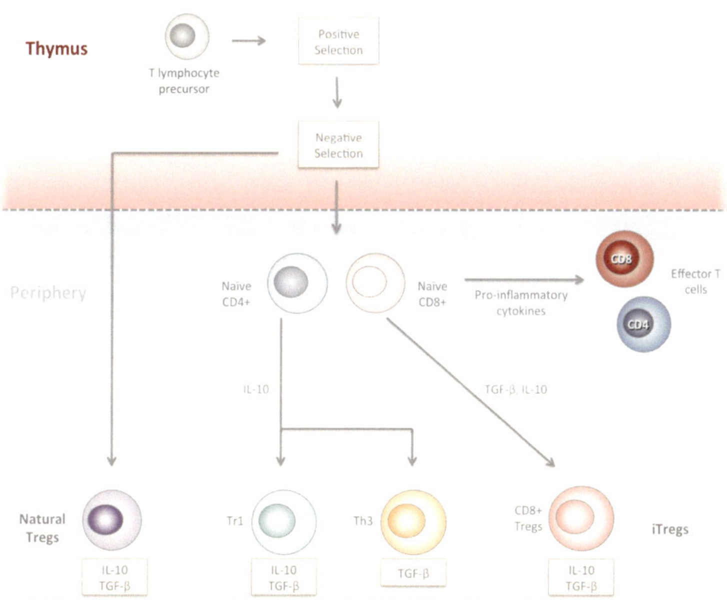

Figure 1. Natural (thymus derived) and inducible (peripheral) Tregs.

1.2. Natural Tregs (nTregs)

Thymic-derived Tregs or natural Tregs are characterized by the CD4+CD25^{high}FOXP3+ phenotype and range between 1 and 3% of the peripheral CD4+ T lymphocytes [13, 23]. They are considered to maintain an anergic state (based on the findings of decreased responsiveness to antigen stimulation and limited proliferation capacity), nTregs have remarkable proliferative potential, both *in vitro* and *in vivo*, upon antigen stimulation in the presence of dendritic cells [24]. Reciprocally, Tregs are able to induce tolerogenic DCs, further complicating their interactions with these cells [7, 12].

nTregs express the same αβTCR as the conventional T lymphocytes but they comprise a distinct clone [25]. They derive from pluripotent stem cells and differentiate in the thymic cortex through a positive selection process after the linkage of their TCR with self-antigens with intermediate affinity [26, 27]. These antigens are presented through MHC II molecules from the thymic cortical cells [28]. Co-stimulation via the CD28 molecule induces the FOXP3 promoter either directly or through other genes that increase its activation [29]. It seems that the selection of these CD25+ cells occurs according to a predefined ratio to the respective CD25− cells, which have been generated earlier. They are long-lived cells capable of producing anti-apoptotic molecules that protect them from the process of negative selection [26, 27].

Upon migration to the periphery, nTregs maintain their regulatory phenotype and suppressive capacity, which are mediated through cell-to-cell contact. This mechanism involves certain surface molecules, and it is independent of secreted cytokines [13, 26]. Survival in the periphery is facilitated by CD28 and its respective ligands (CD80, CD86), transforming growth factor β (TGF-β) and IL-2 [12].

Several surface molecules have been considered to allow the laboratory isolation from other cellular subpopulations and are crucial for their function. The most important such molecules are the CD4, CD25^{high}, CD127^{low}, CD45RO and CD45RB^{low}, providing a phenotype of activated memory cells [30].

Moreover, nTregs express other activation markers, such as CD28, CTLA-4, GITR and chemokine receptors, which are implicated in their migration and trafficking [30, 31]. They also express several Toll-like receptors (TLRs), TGF-β, neuropilin-1, perforin and granzymes, L-selectin (CD62L), LAG-3 (lymphocyte activation gene-3, CD223) and the folate receptor FR4 [32–35]. Multiple adhesion molecules are also abundantly expressed on their surface, such as CD11a, CD44, CD54, and CD103 [36]. All the aforementioned markers have been described in other cell types, which are not exclusively expressed in nTregs and cannot be used as differentiation markers.

Other markers that are thought to be highly specific for nTregs were discovered from the Ikaros gene family; the respective transcription factor is called Helios and is preferentially expressed in nTregs as compared to other CD4+ T cells [37].

Recently, it has been demonstrated that certain epigenetic mechanisms are implicated in the regulation and maintenance of FOXP3 expression [38]. In this regard, the methylation state of the Treg-specific demethylated region (TSDR, a conserved non-coding sequence in the

CNS2 region of the FOXP3 gene) plays a crucial role. Current isolation techniques require this method since only CD4+CD25+FOXP3+ T cells with demethylated TSDR were capable of strongly and permanently expressing FOXP3 and suppressing effector cells [39]. TSDR is incompletely hypomethylated in Tregs that are induced in the periphery and completely methylated in all other CD4+CD25+ T cells [38]. Helios+FOXP3+ Tregs have increased suppressive potential and are fully demethylated at the TSDR region [37].

1.3. Inducible or adaptive Tregs (iTregs)

These Tregs subgroups are not derived from the thymus but they are induced from naive CD4+ T cells in the periphery in response to the occasional micro-environmental conditions, **Figure 1** [40]. Inducible Tregs regulate the immune response against self and non-self antigens and are implicated in the pathophysiology of infections, neoplasias and organ transplantation. Their mechanism of action is usually dependent on the secreted cytokines and not on direct cellular contact. Their characterization is based on the aforementioned surface markers (CD25, CD127, CTLA-4, GITR, etc.), the intensity of intracellular FOXP3 expression as well as their suppressive capacity [13]. As mentioned above, their TSDR is incompletely hypomethylated; thus, FOXP3 expression is transient and unstable. The most important subgroups include the Tr1 and Th3 lymphocytes, the CD4+CD25+ Tregs that are induced from the CD4+CD25− activated T cells, CD103+ Tregs, CD8+ Tregs and the double negative Tregs (CD4−CD8−DN).

Tr1 cells are antigen-specific CD4+ T regulatory lymphocytes that are induced in the presence of IL-10 [41]. They derive from CD4+CD25− naive T lymphocytes after antigenic stimulation with certain costimulatory molecules, such as CD3 and CD46 [42, 43]. Apart from the epigenetic differences, they are phenotypically indistinguishable from natural Tregs, but they secrete large amounts of IL-10. The intensity of the surface expression of CD25 and intracellular FOXP3 is lower than that of nTregs; however, their suppressive capacity is as intense [44]. Their regulatory function is mediated mainly through IL-10 and, secondarily, through TGF-β. They play a major role in the pathophysiology of certain infections and the regulation of allergic reactions [45].

Th3 lymphocytes are CD4+ Tregs that were called helper T cells (T helper 3), although their function is primarily suppressive [46]. Their cardinal characteristic is the secretion of large amounts of TGF-β [47]. The *ex vivo* expansion of the Th3 cells was one of the first reports of clonal expansion of Tregs using an orally administered antigen in mice [48]. Th3 cells are generated and activated through an antigen-specific process but their suppressive function is not specific and mediated through TGF-β. Even in the absence of inflammation, TGF-β secretion induces the expression of FOXP3 in the activated T cells and maintains Tregs' survival in the periphery [49].

Other types of Tregs include the CD4+CD25+ Tregs deriving from CD4+CD25− T lymphocytes under specific conditions, the CD103+ Tregs (expressing integrin alpha-E beta-7), the CD8+CD28− Tregs and the CD4−CD8− double negative Tregs [13]. All these subpopulations express FOXP3 upon activation and are able to suppress immune responses in a non-antigen specific fashion.

Further research using certain surface markers revealed the existence of novel subpopulations of iTregs, including the CD4+CD25−FOXP3+ T cells, the CD4+CD45RA+FOXP3+ Tregs, the CD4+CD161+ Tregs, and the CD4+CXCR5+FOXP3+ Tregs [50–52]. Although the CD25–FOXP3+ T cells could suppress effector cells *in vitro,* it is still uncertain if they represent dysfunctional Tregs or, simply, activated T cells. The CD161+ Tregs represent an excellent paradigm of T cell plasticity, as they are capable of producing pro-inflammatory cytokines such as IL-2, IFN-γ, and IL-17, behaving like Th1 or Th17 cells under proper cytokine micro-environment [53]. In spite of their cytokine-producing properties, these cells also retain their regulatory functions and have the already mentioned demethylated TSDR in the FOXP3 locus, like the nTregs. Finally, the CXCR5+ Tregs are follicular T cells, which are able to gain access into the germinal centres (through the CXCR5) and directly suppress the B cells that undergo hypermutation and isotype switch at those sites. These cells are decreased in active and new onset SLE, seemingly allowing for the activation of B cells [54].

2. Mechanisms of action

The mechanisms of action of Tregs have been studied mostly in *in vitro* systems. Thus, it is not clear how accurately these studies may reproduce Treg activity *in vivo.* Tregs delete auto-reactive T cells and induce tolerance and dampen inflammation, while their cellular targets include CD4+CD25– T cells, CD8+ T cells, B cells, monocytes, DCs, and NK cells [55]. These cells appear to inhibit the target cells via IL-2 deprivation, cell-to-cell contact and cytolysis, secretion of inhibitory cytokines, metabolic disruption and modulation of DC maturation and function [56–60], **Figure 2**.

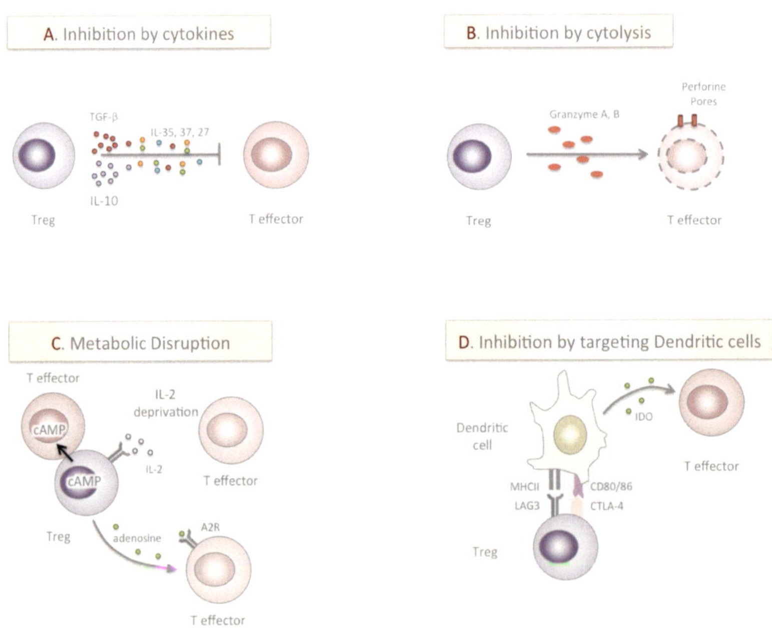

Figure 2. Treg mechanisms of action.

IL-2 is not required for the thymic development of nTregs; however, in the periphery, it acts as a growth factor, essential for their survival and functional integrity. Tregs have more requirements in IL-2 than conventional T cells. IL-2 drives the production of IL-10, CTLA-4, TGF-β, and the activation of FOXP3 [61]. Simultaneously, CD25 expression is induced, further amplifying the affinity of Tregs for IL-2. In co-cultures of Tregs and T effector cells, addition of exogenous IL-2 led to active proliferation and activation of Tregs [62]. In addition, Tregs inhibit the function of other T helper cells or cytotoxic cells by deprivation of other cytokines that share the common γ chain, such as IL-4 and IL-7; this leads to apoptosis of the effector cells [63]. Moreover, the prioritized usage of IL-2 may modify the function of Tregs by the increased IL-10 production [64].

The suppressive function of nTregs is mediated through direct cell-to-cell contact and is not dependent on the presence of inhibitory cytokines like IL-10 and TGF-β [13, 56, 57]. Surface molecules that are involved in this process include CTLA-4 [65, 66], membrane-bound TGF-β [67, 68], LAG-3 (lymphocyte activation gene-3, CD223) [69], GITR (glucocorticoid-induced TNFR-a family-related protein) [70, 71], PD-1 (programmed death-1, CD279) [72] and perforin and granzymes, which lead to cytolysis of the target cell [73].

Granzyme B, in particular, has been implicated as an effector mechanism in Treg-mediated suppression, since its up-regulation was associated with the killing of target cells in a granzyme B-dependent, perforin-independent manner [73]. Granzyme B-deficient Tregs display reduced suppressive activity [74]. Other studies proved that the activated Tregs could lyse CD4+, CD8+ T cells and B cells through granzyme A and perforin [56–58].

The intracellular signal transduction pathways have not been elucidated yet; however, it has been demonstrated that CTLA-4 induces the expression of ICER (inducible cAMP early repressor) and, subsequently, inhibition of IL-2 signals to target cells [75]. Membrane-bound TGF-β activates the Smad proteins and inhibits genes that are required for the functional differentiation of the effector cells [68].

Suppression by inhibitory cytokines is an important mode of action utilized by iTregs. The most important cytokines with regulatory/suppressive capacity are TGF-β [76, 77], primarily produced by the Th3 cells and IL-10 [78, 79] by the Tr1 cells. IL-10 activates the JAK/STAT intracellular pathway and the MAP kinases [78]. The net result is the inhibition of genes that control the synthesis and secretion of pro-inflammatory cytokines. Another regulatory cytokine that is produced from Tregs is the IL-35 [80]. This cytokine is assembled by two chains, IL-12α and EBI3, and is required for the suppressive capacity of Tregs *in vivo*, since inability to express these chains results in uncontrolled expansion of T effector cells in systemic autoimmune diseases [81]. Other anti-inflammatory cytokines that have been implicated in the mechanisms of action of Tregs include IL-27 and IL-37 [82]; more recently, it has been shown that fibrinogen-like protein 2 is also secreted by Tregs and mediates immune suppression [38].

Metabolic disruption of the target cells is another mechanism utilized by Tregs to regulate immune responses. nTregs possess large amounts of cAMP (cyclic adenosine monophosphate), which exerts potent inhibitory action against the proliferation and differentiation of the effector T cells and the expression of genes that control the synthesis of IL-2 and IFN-γ [83]. Gene expression is inhibited through the suppression of the protein kinase A of NF-κB or through activation of ICER. Tregs induce intracellular cAMP within the effector T cells with cell-to-cell cAMP transfer through the gap junctions. Neutralization of cAMP or blockage of the gap junctions led to significant weakening of Tregs' suppressive function [83]. In addition, co-expression of CD39 and CD73 on the surface of Tregs induces the secretion of large amounts of adenosine that suppresses T effectors [84]. The linkage of adenosine to its receptor A2A on Tregs induces TGF-β secretion and inhibits IL-6, generating appropriate circumstances for new Treg development [85, 86].

Tregs seem capable of limiting the capacity of DCs to stimulate effector cells. In this context, their interaction with the dendritic cells and the inhibition of their maturation is of particular importance [87, 88]. Tregs induce the production of regulatory molecules from DC, such as indoleamine-2,3-dioxygenase (IDO), IL-10 and TGF-β, through interactions between CTLA-4 and CD80/CD86 [89, 90]. The same investigators showed that Tregs reduce the expression of the costimulatory molecules CD80 and CD86 on DCs. Moreover, the catabolism of tryptophan and arginine through IDO leads to Tregs activation and induction of regulatory phenotype in naive T cells and T effector cell apoptosis [91].

3. Homeostasis of Tregs

3.1. Functional differentiation of Tregs in the periphery

Certain transcriptional factors are implicated in the process of maturation and functional specialization of the CD4+ T cells. The most important factors are T-bet for Th1 cells, GATA-3 for Th2 cells, RORγt for Th17 cells, Bcl6 for follicular T helper cells (Tfh), and FOXP3 for Tregs [92]. For Tregs, in particular, their functional integrity depends on the dynamic interaction of different transcriptional regulators, which is shaped by the occasional micro-environmental circumstances. These regulators include members of the nuclear factor of activated T (NFAT) cell family, the NF-κB, the activator protein-1 (AP-1) and STAT5 [93]. Furthermore, functional specialization of Tregs has been documented; for instance, these cells are using Th-related transcription factors during Th1, Th2 or Th17 immune responses. In this context, T-bet+ Tregs migrate into the inflamed tissue in cases of Th-1-mediated inflammation and suppress the Th1 effectors [94]. Accordingly, the expression of IRF4 in Tregs is required for the suppression of Th2 responses, while the deletion of STAT3 is linked to uncontrolled Th17 responses [95]. The precise mechanisms by which these transcription factors control Tregs differentiation are unknown. However, the experimental inhibition of these factors was associated with impaired expression of certain surface chemokine receptors, such as CXCR3 (for Th1), CCR8 (for Th2) and CCR6 (for Th17 immune response) [96]. Moreover, deletion of the respective genes of these chemokine receptors led to decreased Tregs activity and renders Tregs incapable of migrating into the site of Th-1-mediated inflammation [97]. Based on these data, it seems possible that phenotypically and functionally distinct Tregs may be active against different effector arms of the immune response.

3.2. Clonal expansion of Tregs

The question if nTregs numbers remain stable through life or if their pool is constantly enriched with new cells was based on the findings of stable numbers of CD4+CD25+ T cells in mice from the age of 2 weeks up to 1 year. In thymectomized mice with no T cells, adoptive transfer of Tregs was followed by an expansion of these cells to the extent of the nonthymectomized animals of similar age [98].

In humans, it has demonstrated that nTregs, after they leave thymus, are constantly proliferating after cytokine (TGF-β, IL-2, IL-10) stimulation and in the presence of tissue antigens. DCs can also induce Tregs in the presence of IL-2 [99].

3.3. Tregs recruitment at the site of inflammation

Natural Tregs are generated in the thymus and migrate into the periphery where their population will be enriched with inducible Tregs. The precise site of their clonal expansion (peripheral lymphoid organs or the site of inflammation) is not known. Apart from the thymus, Tregs have been found in the bone marrow, lymph nodes, intestine, liver, synovial fluid, skin, vessel wall, etc.

More than 25% of the total CD4+ T cells residing in the bone marrow have regulatory phenotype and properties [100]. In this regard, the bone marrow acts as a reservoir for Tregs that is able to release them upon inflammation. Bone marrow Tregs express CXCR4 (the CXCL12 receptor), which is crucial for their migration and their return to the bone marrow after suppression [100]. Integrins are also implicated in their migration; intense expression of CD62L and CCR7 along with poor expression of CD103 (integrin $\alpha E\beta 7$) allows for penetration into the lymph nodes. On the contrary, strong expression of CD103 is required for migrating into the inflamed tissues [94].

Integrins are crucial for the homeostasis of iTregs; integrin $\alpha 4\beta 7$ tissue expression (usually in the mucosal vessels) attracts Tr1 cells, whereas the $\alpha 4\beta 1$ (on the endothelium of inflamed tissues) engages the Th3 cells [101]. Furthermore, it has been showed that when Tregs migrate to the T-zone of lymph nodes, they utilize the CCL19/CCR7 ligation, while when they migrate to the B-zone, they utilize the CXCL13/CXCR9 interaction [102].

3.4. How effector cells escape Treg-mediated suppression

Tregs are also regulated by the immune system in a fashion that allows the control of their action either through negative feedback or through the development of escape mechanisms for the effector cells [103, 104]. The negative feedback is maintained through various mechanisms, such as TLR activation on DCs [104] and the direct regulation by cytokines like IL-21, IL-7, IL-15, TNF-α and IL-6. In particular, IL-21 increases the resistance of the effector T cells against Tregs in experimental diabetes [105]. DC-derived IL-6 renders CD4+ T cells resistant to Tregs suppression [106]. Additional mechanisms include the amplification of co-stimulatory molecule expression on the surface of T effectors and DCs, such as the CD80 and CD86 molecules, CD28, NFATc1, c2, c3 and TRAF6, which protect the integrity of intracellular signal transduction [10].

4. Tregs in systemic lupus erythematosus

4.1. A matter of numbers and function?

SLE is characterized by the breakdown of immune tolerance against self-antigens. The net result is the induction and proliferation of auto-reactive lymphocytes, the production pro-inflammatory soluble mediators, the formation of pathogenic autoantibodies and immuno-complexes that cause tissue damage [1]. Tregs are thought to play a critical role before and during this pathophysiological process. Most studies in lupus-prone mice and humans demonstrated quantitative and/or qualitative defects of these cells [14, 107–113]. Other reports present insignificant variations in Tregs numbers between lupus patients and healthy controls [50, 114, 115] or even higher numbers [116], probably as a result of significant differences in protocol designs. With regard to the functional capacity of these cells, studies are again controversial with reportedly defective [110, 111] or normal [14, 114, 115] function. In the latter case, T effectors showed decreased sensitivity to the suppressive function of Tregs [117].

In a seminal paper, Miyara et al. described the characteristics of Tregs kinetics and the strongly inverse the correlation with SLE disease activity [14]. They found that Tregs (CD4+CD25bright) were globally depleted from the periphery of active lupus patients. They provided evidence that these cells do not accumulate in involved organs (by kidney biopsies) or lymphoid tissue (by lymph node biopsies). In fact, Tregs were found to be more sensitive to Fas-mediated apoptosis although they were still functionally intact. Moreover, they were the first to show that Tregs are increased after the successful treatment of disease flare. FOXP3 expression was found in 85.6% of the CD4+CD25^{high} compartment.

The issue of functional integrity of Tregs within the lupus inflammatory microenvironment was questioned later by the findings of Valencia et al. [110] and Lyssouk et al. [111]. These groups reported that CD4+CD25^{high} Tregs were defective in terms of both proliferation and suppression against CD4+ and CD8+ T effector cells. They also showed that FOXP3 expression was decreased in Tregs from active lupus patients, generating doubt about the appropriate immunophenotype that should be used for cell isolation and study. These findings were confirmed later by using the mean fluorescence intensity (MFI) in newly diagnosed, untreated lupus patients [118].

At the same time, Barath et al. were the first to utilize the CD4+CD25^{high}FOXP3+ immunophenotype for Tregs characterization [112]. They found these cells in significantly lower levels as compared to healthy controls, whereas the inducible CD4+IL-10+ Tregs did not display any significant quantitative differences. At the tissue level, CD4+CD25+FOXP3+ Tregs were found in decreased numbers in the skin lesions of active cutaneous lupus as compared to other inflammatory skin diseases, such as psoriasis, atopic dermatitis, and lichen planus [119].

In 2008, a new subpopulation was described, namely the CD4+CD25–FOXP3+ T cells [50]. These cells were found in increased numbers in newly diagnosed SLE patients and were associated with other indices of disease activity, such as low complement C3 and C4 [51]. Their function was primarily regulatory as they were able to suppress the effector T cell proliferation but not IFN-γ production [51]. Other investigators opposed these findings by performing the measurements in untreated lupus patients, reaching the conclusion that not all FOXP3 expressing T cells are Tregs [120].

The association of Tregs with SLE disease activity was tested in several studies with a small number of patients. Most of them reported a strongly inverse correlation [14, 113], whereas others found insignificant correlations [109, 112].

In the first large-scale (n = 100 patients), longitudinal (mean follow up of 5 years) study of CD4+CD25^{high}FOXP3+ Tregs as a biomarker of disease activity, we found that these cells are gradually decreased from healthy controls to patients with inactive, mild, or severe disease [113]. Moreover, we observed inverse alterations in cases of changing disease activity; these cells were reduced during disease flare and increased upon remission, while numbers remained stable during stable disease activity. Their sensitivity and specificity to assess a clinically significant change in global disease activity was 88 and 74%, respectively. Their positive and negative predictive values were 85 and 79%, respectively. In the same study, we reported decreased Tregs numbers in active lupus nephritis and active neuropsychiatric involvement, whereas no differences were observed in patients with active antiphospholipid syndrome (APS). The ability of CD4+CD25^{high}FOXP3+ Tregs to predict disease flares was low (positive predictive value 17%).

Concerning the influence of certain therapeutic approaches, we prospectively showed that Tregs' numerical restoration after treatment is independent of the occasional medication administered [121]. In that study, patients achieved remission after administration of various immunomodulatory agents, including glucocorticoids (oral and intravenous), cyclophosphamide, intravenous immuno globulins, azathioprine and hydroxy chloroquxine. In all cases, a significant increase of CD4+CD25^{high}FOXP3+ Tregs was observed. That restoration was faster with the intravenous regimens as compared to oral therapies. Cyclophosphamide pulse therapy, in particular, led to a significant increase of Tregs after the fourth pulse in patients with active lupus nephritis and/or neuropsychiatric involvement [122]. Of note, an even faster response (shortly after the first infusion) was documented after treatment with intravenous tocilizumab in patients with rheumatoid arthritis [123].

4.2. Novel theories for Tregs in the pro-inflammatory environment of SLE

As mentioned above, most studies on Tregs have been conducted *in vitro*; thus, their reliability and accuracy pertaining to the actual function of these cells *in vivo* are questionable. After the discovery that a fully demethylated TSDR is required for intense and sustained expression of FOXP3, the hallmark of regulatory function, many beliefs have been revised [39]. In this context, Helios+FOXP3+ T cells, with a fully demethylated TSDR, were found in increased numbers in active lupus patients; their function was intact [124]. It is not yet known if Helios represents a unique marker for Tregs; however, the epigenetic change is believed to differentiate between natural and inducible Tregs. Nevertheless, there is disequilibrium between Tregs and effector cells that is more prominent in the pro-inflammatory environment of SLE.

Several studies have reported on altered ratios between Tregs and T effectors in lupus patients [125]. The most striking feature, among other findings, was that there is plasticity between

Tregs and Th17 populations, and the latter may derive from the former under certain circumstances [126]. In this regard, the presence of TGF-β alone will drive naive CD4+ T cells towards Tregs differentiation, while the simultaneous presence of IL-6 will lead to Th17 proliferation [127]. Other transitions have also been described between Th1 and Th17 cells, based on the presence of IL-12 receptors on the surface of Th17 cells; upon activation with IL-12, these cells are capable of producing IFN-γ [125, 127]. Of note, it has been documented that some Tregs down-regulate FOXP3 expression and act as effectors, promoting inflammation through the secretion of IL-17 and IFN-α [39]. These cells are called ex Tregs and believed to derive from the Tregs lineage prior to natural Tregs commitment. They acquire pro-inflammatory characteristics in the periphery, probably in the context of a generalized immune response.

The concept of Tregs/Th17 imbalance, in particular, seems of paramount importance in SLE. It has been demonstrated that disease relapses may occur as a consequence of an impaired Tregs/Th17 ratio, in favour of the latter, in animal models [128]. Those findings were later confirmed in lupus patients, in whom the altered Tregs/Th17 ratio was documented even in clinically quiescent disease; this may represent a hallmark of SLE [129, 130]. In this context, it is believed that the sole targeting of the Th17 arm of the immune response will not render meaningful results; approaches aiming at the restoration of the Tregs/Th17 balance will be more likely to exert beneficial effects [125, 131].

The disturbed balance between T effectors (Th1, Th2, Th17) and Tregs is driven by a relative IL-2 deficiency in SLE [132]. Treatment with low doses of IL-2 re-established the equilibrium between Tregs and T effectors in animal models of the disease; accordingly, IL-2 neutralization or CD25 depletion accelerated disease onset [39]. Studies in lupus patients showed that FOXP3+Helios+ Tregs were capable of proliferating despite the reduced IL-2 levels; however, the integrity of their suppressive function has not been confirmed [124]. Apart from IL-2, other cytokines, such as IL-6, IL-21 and IFN-α may inhibit the Tregs function and/or render T effectors resistant to regulation. All these cytokines are found in abundance in SLE and are positively correlated to disease activity. On the other hand, the main regulatory cytokine, TGF-β, is lower in active disease, generating hypotheses that the cytokine disequilibrium drives the imbalance of Tregs and T effectors. The exact mechanisms by which these cytokines increase the T effectors' resistance to Tregs suppression have not been elucidated yet [39].

4.3. Epigenetics and Tregs

Latest studies revealed that certain epigenetic mechanisms, such as methylation, histone modification and miRNAs, play a significant role in Tregs biology [38]. In this regard, the methylation status of the TSDR is of paramount importance for the sustained expression of FOXP3 and, hence, the intensity of Treg suppressive function. Histone modification is another mechanism involved in Tregs functional differentiation. The acetylation of histones H3 and H4 has been shown to reliably differentiate Tregs than FOXP3+ effectors [133]. Modification of the FOXP3 promoter by other genes influenced dramatically the rate of differentiation of iTregs in the periphery [38]. Finally, miRNA-155 is associated with less Tregs, though functionally intact, in mice, while miRNA-126 up-regulates Tregs and enhances their function [134].

Epigenetic regulation of the FOXP3 gene has been reported in lupus patients. In this context, decreased peripheral Tregs were associated with hypermethylation of the promoter of the FOXP3 gene [135]. Genome-wide studies have shown that virtually all immune cells in SLE, including Tregs, had severe hypomethylation in interferon-type I-related genes [38]. Treatment with a histone modification inhibitor the enhanced Tregs number and function in lupus-prone mice [136]; the same results were reached with an inhibitor of the protein kinase IV [137]. It is believed that these approaches will soon be tested in lupus patients [38].

5. Tregs-based therapeutic approaches in SLE

5.1. Adoptive transfer of *ex vivo* expanded Tregs

Based on the aforementioned data, Tregs may represent a promising target in SLE therapeutics. Several groups have tried to manipulate this cellular subpopulation in order to restore the defective immune tolerance that is a crucial component of disease pathophysiology [138]. Early experiments in mice models showed that adoptive transfer of *ex vivo* expanded Tregs was capable of ameliorating the disease [139, 140]. In the first experiment, T cells treated with IL-2 and TGF-β lost their ability to induce a graft-versus-host disease and prevented other effector T cells from activating B cells [139]. In addition, when transferred to animals with high titers of anti-dsDNA antibodies, they led to a significant reduction of their titers and doubled survival. In New Zealand black/New Zealand white mice, a well-studied lupus model, transfer of thymic Tregs (CD4+CD25+CD62L^{high}) decreased the rate of glomerulonephritis, the severity of proteinuria and improved survival [140]. The precise mechanism by which these Tregs suppress the autoimmune response has not been elucidated; however, it was demonstrated that the induction of tolerogenic DCs plays a critical role [141]. These DCs were also able to expand the recipient's CD4+FOXP3+ Tregs (infectious tolerance).

Studies in humans also showed that *in vitro* expanded Tregs, both polyclonal [142] and antigen-specific [143] may display enhanced regulatory activity. These encouraging results led to the implementation of this strategy in phase I and II clinical trials in other autoimmune diseases. Seminal studies in type 1 diabetes (T1D) proved the feasibility of generating purified iTregs for therapeutic purposes [144, 145]. Bluestone et al. demonstrated that Tregs could survive for more than 1 year after infusion in 14 patients with T1D; although there were no significant reactions to infusion, from an efficacy standpoint there was no significant improvement in C-peptide levels and HbA1c [144]. In another study of 12 children with T1D, adoptive transfer of Tregs led to significant reduction in exogenous insulin needs and improvement in C-peptide levels. Of note, two children were insulin independent after 12 months [145]. In chronic graft-versus-host disease (GVHD), adoptive transfer of Tregs ameliorated symptoms in two out of five patients, while the remaining patients did not show any deterioration after 21 months of follow-up [146]. In another study, where umbilical cord-derived Tregs were used in 11 patients, there was a significant reduction in the rate of severe acute GVHD, whereas chronic GVHD at 1 year was 0% in Treg-treated patients and 14% in patients who received the conventional therapy with immunosuppressives (sirolimus and mycophenolate mofetil)

[147]. All the aforementioned studies reported a purity of approximately 90%, demonstrating that this approach is feasible; on the other hand, survival of Tregs *in vivo* (after infusion) was limited with a dramatic decline after 14 days from infusion. There are several currently ongoing clinical trials based on adoptive Treg transfer mainly in solid organ transplantation [147]. Such therapeutic approaches have not been published yet in lupus patients; one phase I clinical trial aiming to assess Treg efficacy in cutaneous lupus started in 2015 [148].

5.2. Hematopoietic and mesenchymal stem cell transplantation

Hematopoietic and mesenchymal stem cell transplantation (HSCT and MSCT, respectively) aim at immune reconstitution after intensive chemotherapy and have been implemented in cases with refractory autoimmune diseases.

In the context of SLE, HSCT has been shown to induce long-term remission for approximately 5 years in half patients, whereas relapse was usually mild [149, 150]. On the other hand, MSCT exerts potent immunosuppressive capacity since mesenchymal stem cells do not require MHC (major histocompatibility complex) restriction for their function [151]. The effects of these therapeutic approaches on Tregs numbers and function have a critical role with respect to their efficacy. Zhang et al. showed that CD4+CD25^{high}FOXP3+ Tregs were reconstituted in levels comparable to those of normal individuals after autologous HSCT in 15 SLE patients [152]. In addition, a novel Tregs subset (CD8+LAPhighCD103^{high}) was induced and capable of maintaining remission through TGF-β mediated suppression. On the contrary, Szodoray et al. did not find any significant differences in Tregs numbers (pre- and post-transplant) in 12 patients with various systemic autoimmune diseases; only three lupus patients were enrolled in that study [153].

Concerning MSCT, a report on nine patients with refractory SLE showed good safety profile after 6 years; unfortunately, Tregs were not assessed in this study [154]. Limited case reports demonstrated a significant increase of peripheral Tregs in three lupus patients; however, clinical remission was not achieved [155, 156]. Of note, mesenchymal stem cells were shown to increase Tregs in 30 active lupus patients, in a dose-dependent fashion, even after 1 week after transplantation, and this was sustained for 1 and 3 months after transplant [157]. In the same study, Th17 cells were accordingly reduced after 3 months.

5.3. IL-2-based approaches

Extensive research on IL-2 and IL-2 receptor (IL-2R) biology has shed light on its critical importance for the maintenance of immune tolerance by influencing Tregs number and function [132]. Administration of low doses of IL-2 led to remission and decreased glucocorticoid dose in lupus patients [158], while it was shown that Tregs expansion (CD4+CD25^{high}CD127low) and a decrease in T effectors/Tregs ratio were the primary mechanism [159]. The same results were observed in other diseases, such as GVHD and HCV-related vasculitis [160]. Interestingly, IL-2/anti-IL-2 immunocomplexes were capable of reducing the severity of renal inflammation in NZB/W F1 mice by inducing CD4+CD25+FOXP3+ Tregs. With regard to proteinuria, this approach was superior to the combination of glucocorticoids and mycophenolate mofetil, the current standard of care for LN [161].

5.4. All-trans retinoic acid (atRA)

This approach has been used in various autoimmune diseases with inconsistent and contradictory results, possibly due to the small sample sizes [162]. Limited data in lupus patients showed that Tregs could be induced by atRA [163]; however, these results were not confirmed [164]. In a more recent study, retinoic acid increased Treg numbers (and decreased Th17 cells) in lupus patients with low levels of vitamin A [165].

5.5. Tolerogenic peptides

The rationale behind the use of tolerogenic peptides in SLE therapeutics is that a dysregulated immune system can be modified by inducing tolerance against a specific antigen. This is a crucial component of this approach since non-specific tolerance may lead to generalized immune suppression and secondary immunodeficiency. In this context, such different molecules (hCDR1, pCons, P140, etc.) have been administered in lupus prone mice with subsequent expansion of Tregs and suppression of effector cells and pro-inflammatory cytokines [166, 167]. These encouraging results led to the first peptide-based randomized controlled trial in SLE with 149 patients [168]. Although the effect on Tregs was not assessed, approximately 62% of the peptide-treated patients achieved the primary clinical end-point as compared to 38.6% of the placebo arm (all patients received standard of care therapy).

5.6. Effect of other medications on Tregs

Apart from the aforementioned approaches that implicate Tregs in their mechanism of action, medications commonly used in SLE patients have been demonstrated to increase their numbers and/or restore their function. Several studies have demonstrated a significant Tregs expansion after treatment with glucocorticoids [121, 122, 169–171]. Moreover, intravenous methylprednisolone pulses led to a dramatic and sustained increase in CD4+CD25^{high}FOXP3+ Tregs numbers, regardless of the initial clinical indication [121]; this was noted even from the first few days after the pulses [172]. The mechanism by which these medications lead to Treg proliferation is yet unknown; however, a steroid-mediated up-regulation of FOXP3 has been described [171].

Immunosuppressive drugs have also been shown to affect Tregs in active SLE. Cyclophosphamide pulse therapy led to a significant increase in Tregs numbers after the 4th month of administration, which reflected clinical remission [121], although the effect of concomitant glucocorticoid treatment may have a role. Similar results were obtained with azathioprine and hydroxychloroquine [121]. Of note, polyclonal intravenous immunoglobulins (IVIGs) also led to Tregs increase, possibly through up-regulation of FOX3 and intracellular IL-10 and TGF-β [173]. Rituximab was demonstrated to enhance the Tregs numbers and function in lupus patients whereas the increased and sustained FOXP3 mRNA expression was associated with favourable outcome [174]. In general, *in vivo* expansion of Tregs after treatment might be the result of a change of Th1/Th17 to Th2 balance, which could lead to disease remission and not a direct drug-specific reaction [121].

Other medications that are increasingly used in lupus patients and may affect Tregs include statins. These drugs display multiple beneficial effects in atherosclerosis through different mechanisms among which immune modulation is critical [175]. Several experiments in animal models showed that statins increase the numbers and suppressive capacity of Tregs as well as their accumulation in the atherosclerotic plaque [176]. Atorvastatin, in particular, exerted similar results in human Tregs [177].

All the pre-mentioned therapeutic interventions are summarized in **Table 1**.

5.7. Barriers in Tregs-based therapeutic approaches

Although the above-mentioned data are encouraging for SLE patients, several challenges still exist. The multiple phenotypes that have been used to characterize Tregs in the different studies have demonstrated that all Tregs are not functionally capable of suppressing autoimmune responses [160]. In the chronic inflammatory environment of SLE, it cannot be predicted which regulatory cells are likely to function more beneficially; furthermore, effector cells are more capable of escaping regulatory mechanisms under these circumstances [106]. Furthermore, tissue distribution of Tregs, after infusion, is unknown, while their survival and maintenance of regulatory capacity have not been precisely defined in the context of SLE. Other considerations include technical aspects, such as the purity and cost-effectiveness of these approaches.

Therapy	Mechanism	Approach	Efficacy	Notes
Adoptive transfer of *ex vivo* expanded Tregs	Increase of Tregs pool	Experimental and clinical trials in other immune-mediated diseases	Moderate	High purification rates, low Tregs survival
HSCT/MSCT	Immune system reconstitution	Limited clinical trials	Moderate	Inconsistent clinical results
IL-2	Enhanced survival and function of Tregs	Limited clinical trials	Moderate	IL-2/anti-IL-2 complexes provided favourable results in LN
Retinoids	Induction of Tregs	Limited clinical trials	Inconsistent	Mainly in patients with low vitamin A
Tolerogenic peptides	Induction of Tregs	Experimental studies and one RCT	Moderate	Ongoing phase III clinical trials
Glucocorticoids	Up-regulation of FOXP3	Limited observational trials	Good	Rapid induction of Tregs
Immunomodulating agents	Induction of Tregs	Limited observational trials	Good	Regardless of the agent used, probably an epiphenomenon to disease remission
Statins	Enhanced numbers and function of Tregs	Experimental and limited observational trials	Good	Accumulation of Tregs in the atherosclerotic plaques

Table 1. Therapeutic approaches targeting Tregs in SLE.

6. Conclusion

Most well-designed studies have concluded that Tregs are significantly depleted from the periphery of active lupus SLE patients and this reduction is in accordance with disease activity. Moreover, Tregs follow alterations in disease activity (with inverse changes) quite reliably; numeric increase is not drug specific but characterizes disease remission. Their value as an activity biomarker has been demonstrated and may be helpful in assessing disease status in controversial circumstances. Their potential to be used for therapeutic purposes, either by direct adoptive transfer or by approaches aiming to increase their numbers, is quite promising in the field of SLE.

Author details

Konstantinos Tselios[1], Alexandros Sarantopoulos[2], Ioannis Gkougkourelas[2] and Panagiota Boura[2]*

*Address all correspondence to: boura@med.auth.gr

1 Centre for Prognosis Studies in the Rheumatic Diseases, Toronto Western Hospital, University of Toronto Lupus Clinic, Toronto, ON, Canada

2 Clinical Immunology Unit, 2nd Department of Internal Medicine, Hippokration General Hospital, Aristotle University of Thessaloniki, Thessaloniki, Greece

References

[1] Tsokos GC. Systemic lupus erythematosus. The New England Journal Medicine. 2011;**365**:2110–2121. DOI: 10.1056/NEJMra1100359

[2] Scheinecker C, Bonelli M, Smolen JS. Pathogenetic aspects of systemic lupus erythematosus with an emphasis on regulatory T cells. Journal of Autoimmunity. 2010;**35**:269–275. DOI: 10.1016/j.jaut.2010.06.018

[3] Gershon RK. A disquisition on suppressor T cells. Transplantation Reviews. 1975;**26**:170

[4] Sakaguchi S, Fukuma K, Kuribayashi K, Masuda T. Organ-specific autoimmune diseases induced in mice by elimination of a T cell subset. Evidence for the active participation of T cells in natural self-tolerance; deficit of a T cell subset as a possible cause of autoimmune disease. Journal of Experimental Medicine. 1985;**161**:72–87. DOI: 10.1084/jem.161.1.72

[5] Gershon RK, Kondo K. Infectious immunological tolerance. Immunology. 1971;**21**:903–914

[6] Germain RN. Special regulatory T-cell review. A rose by any other name: From suppressor T cells to Tregs, approbation to unbridled enthusiasm. Immunology. 2008;**123**:20–27. DOI: 10.1111/j.1365-2567.2007.02779.x

[7] Kapp JA. Special regulatory T-cell review: Suppressors regulated but unsuppressed. Immunology. 2008;**123**:28–32. DOI: 10.1111/j.1365-2567.2007.02773.x

[8] Sakaguchi S, Sakaguchi N, Asano M, Itoh M, Toda M. Immunologic self-tolerance maintained by activated T cells expressing IL-2 receptor alpha-chain (CD25). Breakdown of a single mechanism of self-tolerance causes various autoimmune diseases. Journal of Immunology. 1995;**155**:1151–1164

[9] Sakaguchi S, Wing K, Miyara M. Regulatory T cells- a brief history and perspective. European Journal of Immunology. 2007;**37**:S116–123. DOI: 10.1002/eji.200737593

[10] Thornton A, Shevach EM. CD4+CD25+ immunoregulatory T cells suppress polyclonal T cell activation in vitro by inhibiting interleukin-2 production. Journal of Experimental Medicine. 1998;**188**:287–296. DOI: 10.1084/jem.188.2.287

[11] Jonuleit H, Schmitt E, Stassen M, Tuettenberg A, Knop J, Enk AH. Identification and functional characterization of human CD4+CD25+ T cells with regulatory properties isolated from peripheral blood. Journal of Experimental Medicine. 2001;**193**:1285–1294. DOI: 10.1084/jem.193.11.1285

[12] Liston A, Rudensky AY. Thymic development and peripheral homeostasis of regulatory T cells. Current Opinion in Immunology. 2007;**19**:176–185. DOI: 10.1016/j.coi.2007.02.005

[13] Shevach EM. From vanilla to 28 flavours: Multiple varieties of T regulatory cells. Immunity. 2006;**25**:195–201. DOI: 10.1016/j.immuni.2006.08.003

[14] Miyara M, Amoura Z, Parizot C, Badoual C, Dorgham K, Trad S, et al. Global natural regulatory T cell depletion in active systemic lupus erythematosus. Journal of Immunology. 2005;**175**:8392–8400. DOI: https://doi.org/10.4049/jimmunol.175.12.8392

[15] Brunkow ME, Jeffery EW, Hjierrild KA, Paeper B, Clark LB, Yasayko SA, et al. Disruption of a new forkhead/winged-helix protein, scurfin, results in the fatal lymphoproliferative disorder of the scurfy mouse. Nature Genetics. 2001;**27**:68–73. DOI: 10.1038/83784

[16] Chatila TA, Blaeser F, Ho N, Lederman HM, Voulgaropoulos C, Helms C, et al. JM2, encoding a fork head-related protein, is mutated in X-linked autoimmunity-allergic dysregulation syndrome. The Journal of Clinical Investigation. 2000;**106**:R75–R81. DOI: 10.1172/JCI11679

[17] Wildin RS, Ramsdell F, Peake J, Faravelli F, Casanova JL, Buist N, et al. X-linked neonatal diabetes mellitus, enteropathy and endocrinopathy syndrome is the human equivalent of mouse scurfy. Nature Genetics. 2001;**27**:18–20. DOI: 10.1038/83707

[18] Bennett CL, Christie J, Ramsdell F, Brunkow ME, Ferguson PJ, Whitesell L, et al. The immune dysregulation, polyendocrinopathy, enteropathy, X-linked syndrome (IPEX) is caused by mutations of Foxp3. Nature Genetics. 2001;**27**:20–21. DOI: 10.1038/83713

[19] Hori S, Nomura T, Sakaguchi S. Control of regulatory T cell development by the transcription factor FoxP3. Science. 2003;**299**:1057–1061. DOI: 10.1126/science.1079490

[20] Marson A, Kretschmer K, Frampton GM, Jacobsen ES, Polansky JK, MacIsaac KD, et al. Foxp3 occupancy and regulation of key target genes during T-cell stimulation. Nature. 2007;**445**:931. DOI: 10.1038/nature05478

[21] Zheng Y, Josefowicz SZ, Kas A, Chu TT, Gavin MA, Rudensky AY. Genome-wide analysis of Foxp3 target genes in developing and mature regulatory T cells. Nature. 2007;**445**:936. DOI: 10.1038/nature05563

[22] Roncarolo MG, Gregori S. Is FOXP3 a bonafide marker for human regulatory T cells? European Journal of Immunology. 2008;**38**:925–927. DOI: 10.1002/eji.200838168

[23] Shevach EM. Certified professionals: CD4+CD25+ suppressor T cells. The Journal of Experimental Medicine. 2001;**193**:F41–F45. DOI: 10.1084/jem.193.11.F41

[24] Walker LSK. CD4+CD25+ Treg: Divide and rule? Immunology. 2004;**111**:129–137. DOI: 10.1111/j.0019-2805.2003.01788.x

[25] Coutinho A, Caramalho I, Seixas E, Demengeot J. Thymic commitment of regulatory T cells is a pathway of TCR-dependent selection that isolates repertoires undergoing positive or negative selection. Current Topics in Microbiology and Immunology. 2005;**293**:43–71

[26] Maggi E, Cosmi L, Liotta F, Romagnani P, Romagnani S, Annunziato F. Thymic regulatory T cells. Autoimmunity Reviews. 2005;**4**:579–586. DOI: 10.1016/j.autrev.2005.04.010

[27] Raimondi G, Turner MS, Thomson AW, Morel PA. Naturally occurring regulatory T cells: Recent insights in health and disease. Critical Reviews in Immunology. 2007;**27**:61–95. DOI: 10.1615/CritRevImmunol.v27.i1.50

[28] Griesemer AD, Sorenson EC, Hardy MA. The role of the thymus in tolerance. Transplantation. 2010;**90**:465–474. DOI: 10.1097/TP.0b013e3181e7e54f

[29] Bour-Jordan H, Bluestone JA. Regulating the regulators: Costimulatory signals control the homeostasis and function of regulatory T cells. Immunological Reviews. 2009;**229**:41–66. DOI: 10.1111/j.1600-065X.2009.00775.x

[30] Yi H, Zhen Y, Jiang L, Zheng J, Zhao Y. The phenotypic characterization of naturally occurring regulatory CD4+CD25+ T cells. Cellular & Molecular Immunology. 2006;**3**:189–195

[31] Wysocki CA, Jiang Q, Panoskaltsis-Mortari A, Taylor PA, McKinnon KP, Su L, et al. Critical role for CCR5 in the function of donor CD4+CD25+ regulatory T cells during acute graft-versus-host disease. Blood. 2005;**106**:3300–3307. DOI: 10.1182/blood-2005-04-1632

[32] Nakamura K, Kitami A, Strober W. Cell contact-dependent immunosuppression by CD4+CD25+ regulatory T cells is mediated by cell surface-bound transforming growth factor β. Journal of Experimental Medicine. 2001;**194**:629–644. DOI: 10.1084/jem.194.5.629

[33] Bruder D, Probst-Kepper M, Westendorf AM, Geffers R, Beissert S, Loser K, et al. Neuropilin-1: A surface marker of regulatory T cells. European Journal of Immunology. 2004;**34**:623–630. DOI: 10.1002/eji.200324799

[34] Workman CJ, Vignali DA. Negative regulation of T cell homeostasis by lymphocyte activation gene-3 (CD223). Journal of Immunology. 2005;**174**:688–695. DOI: https://doi.org/10.4049/jimmunol.174.2.688

[35] Yamaguchi T, Hirota K, Nagahama K, Ohkawa K, Takahashi T, Nomura T, et al. Control of immune responses by antigen-specific regulatory T cells expressing the folate receptor. Immunity. 2007;**27**:145–159. DOI: 10.1016/j.immuni.2007.04.017

[36] Tran DQ, Glass DD, Uzel G, Darnell DA, Spalding C, Holland SM, et al. Analysis of adhesion molecules, target cells and role of IL-2 in human FOXP3+ regulatory T cell suppressor function. Journal of Immunology. 2008;**182**:2929–2938. DOI: 10.4049/jimmunol.0803827

[37] Zabransky DJ, Nirschl CJ, Durham NM, Park BV, Ceccato CM, Bruno TC, et al. Phenotypic and functional properties of Helios+regulatory T cells. PLoS One. 2012;7:e34547. DOI: 10.1371/journal.pone.0034547

[38] Shu Y, Hu Q, Long H, Chang C, Lu Q, Xiao R. Epigenetic variability of CD4+CD25+ Tregs contributes to the pathogenesis of autoimmune diseases. Clinical Reviews in Allergy & Immunology. 29 September 2016 [Epub ahead of print]. DOI: 10.1007/s12016-016-8590-3

[39] Ohl K, Tenbrock K. Regulatory T cells in systemic lupus erythematosus. European Journal of Immunology. 2015;**45**:344–355. DOI: 10.1002/eji.201344280

[40] Chatenoud L, Bach JF. Adaptive human regulatory T cells: Myth or reality? The Journal of Clinical Investigation. 2006;**116**:2325–2327. DOI: 10.1172/JCI29748

[41] Barrat FJ, Cua DJ, Boonstra A, Richards DF, Crain C, Savelkoul HF, et al. In vitro generation of interleukin 10-producing regulatory CD4 (+) T cells is induced by immunosuppressive drugs and inhibited by T helper type 1 (Th1) - and Th2-inducing cytokines. Journal of Experimental Medicine. 2002;**195**:603–616. DOI: 10.1084/jem.20011629

[42] Kemper C, Chan AC, Green JM, Brett KA, Murphy KM, Atkinson JP. Activation of human CD4+ cells with CD3 and CD46 induces a T-regulatory cell 1 phenotype. Nature. 2003;**421**:388–392. DOI: 10.1038/nature01315

[43] Levings M, Gregori S, Tresoldi E, Cazzaniga S, Bonini C, Roncarolo MG. Differentiation of Tr1 cells by immature dendritic cells requires IL-10 but no CD25+CD4+ Tr cells. Blood. 2004;**105**:1162–1169. DOI: 10.1182/blood-2004-03-1211

[44] Vieira PL, Christensen JR, Minaee S, O'Neill EJ, Barrat FJ, Boonstra A, et al. IL-10-secreting regulatory T cells do not express Foxp3 but have comparable regulatory function to naturally occurring CD4+CD25+ regulatory T cells. Journal of Immunology. 2004;**172**:5986–5993. DOI: https://doi.org/10.4049/jimmunol.172.10.5986.

[45] Langier S, Sade K, Kivity S. Regulatory T cells in allergic asthma. The Israel Medical Association Journal. 2012;**14**:180–183

[46] Cerwenka A, Swain SL. TGF-β1: Immunosuppressant and viability factor for T lymphocytes. Microbes and Infection. 1999;**1**:1291–1296. DOI: http://dx.doi.org/10.1016/S1286-4579(99)00255-5

[47] Tang Q, Boden EK, Henriksen KJ, Bour-Jordan H, Bi M, Bluestone JA. Distinct roles of CTLA-4 and TGF-β in CD4+CD25+ regulatory T cell function. European Journal of Immunology. 2004;**34**:2996–3005. DOI: 10.1002/eji.200425143

[48] Zheng SG, Gray JD, Ohtsuka K, Yamagiwa S, Horwitz DA. Generation ex vivo of TGF-beta- producing regulatory T cells from CD4+CD25− precursors. Journal of Immunology. 2002;**169**:4183–4189. DOI: https://doi.org/10.4049/jimmunol.169.8.4183

[49] Carrier Y, Yuan J, Kuchroo VK, Weiner HL. Th3 cells in peripheral tolerance. I. Induction of Foxp3-positive regulatory T cells by Th3 cells derived from TGF-β T cell-transgenic mice. Journal of Immunology. 2007;**178**:179–185. DOI: https://doi.org/10.4049/jimmunol.178.1.179

[50] Zhang B, Zhang X, Tang FL, Zhu LP, Liu Y, Lipsky PE. Clinical significance of increased CD4+CD25-FOXP3+ T cells in patients with new-onset systemic lupus erythematosus. Annals of the Rheumatic Diseases. 2008;**67**:1037–1040. DOI: 10.1136/ard.2007.083543

[51] Bonelli M, Savitskaya A, Steiner CW, Rath E, Smolen JS, Scheinecker C. Phenotypic and functional analysis of CD4+CD25-FOXP3+ T cells in patients with systemic lupus erythematosus. Journal of Immunology. 2009;**182**:1689–1695. DOI: https://doi.org/10.4049/jimmunol.182.3.1689

[52] Miyara M, Yoshioka Y, Kitoh A, Shima T, Wing K, Niwa A, et al. Functional delineation and differentiation dynamics of human CD4+ T cells expressing the FOXP3 transcription factor. Immunity. 2009;**30**:899–911. DOI: 10.1016/j.immuni.2009.03.019

[53] Afzali B, Mitchell PJ, Edozie FC, Povoleri GA, Dowson SE, Demandt L, et al. CD161 expression characterizes a subpopulation of human regulatory T cells that produces IL-17 in a STAT-3 dependent manner. European Journal of Immunology. 2013;**43**:2043–2054. DOI: 10.1002/eji.201243296

[54] Ma L, Zhao P, Jiang Z, Shan Y, Jiang Y. Imbalance of different types of CD4+ forkhead box protein 3 (FOXP3)+ T cells in patients with new-onset systemic lupus erythematosus. Clinical and Experimental Immunology. 2013;**174**:345–355. DOI: 10.1111/cei.12189

[55] Peterson RA. Regulatory T-cells: Diverse phenotypes integral to immune homeostasis and suppression. Toxicologic Pathology. 2012;**40**:186–204. DOI: 10.1177/0192623311430693

[56] Corthay A. How do regulatory T cells work? Scandinavian Journal of Immunology. 2009;**70**:326–336. DOI: 10.1111/j.1365-3083.2009.02308.x

[57] Sakaguchi S, Wing K, Onishi Y, Prieto-Martin P, Yamaguchi T. Regulatory T cells: How do they suppress immune responses? International Immunology. 2009;**21**:1105–1111. DOI: 10.1093/intimm/dxp095

[58] Tang Q, Bluestone JA. The Foxp3+ regulatory T cell: A jack-of-all-trades, master of regulation. Nature Immunology. 2008;**9**:239–244. DOI: 10.1038/ni1572

[59] Sojka DK, Huang YH, Fowell DJ. Mechanisms of regulatory T-cell suppression-a diverse arsenal for a moving target. Immunology. 2008;**124**:13–22. DOI: 10.1111/j.1365- 2567.2008.02813.x

[60] Tselios K, Boura P, Kountouras J. T regulatory cells in Helicobacter pylori-associated diseases. Immunogastroenterology. 2013;**2**:38–46. DOI: 10.7178/ig.27

[61] Furtado GC, Curotto de Lafaille MA, Kutchukhidze N, Lafaille JJ. Interleukin 2 signalling is required for CD4 (+) regulatory T cell function. Journal of Experimental Medicine. 2002;**196**:851–857. DOI: 10.1084/jem.20020190

[62] De la Rosa M, Rutz S, Dorninger H, Scheffold A. Interleukin-2 is essential for CD4+CD25+ regulatory T cell function. European Journal of Immunology. 2004;**34**:2480–2488. DOI: 10.1002/eji.200425274

[63] Pandiyan P, Zheng L, Ishihara S, Reed J, Lenardo MJ. CD4+CD25+Foxp3+ regulatory T cells induce cytokine deprivation-mediated apoptosis of effector CD4+ T cells. Nature Immunology. 2007;**8**:1353–1362. DOI: 10.1038/ni1536

[64] Barthlott T, Moncrieffe H, Veldhoen M, Atkins CJ, Christensen J, O' Garra A, et al. CD25+CD4+ T cells compete with naive CD4+ T cells for IL-2 and exploit it for the induction of IL-10. International Immunology. 2005;**17**:279–288. DOI: 10.1093/intimm/dxh207

[65] Takahashi T, Tagami T, Yamazaki S, Uede T, Shimizu J, Sakaguchi N, et al. Immunologic self-tolerance maintained by CD4+CD25+ regulatory T cells constitutively expressing cytotoxic T lymphocyte-associated antigen 4. Journal of Experimental Medicine. 2000;**192**:303–310. DOI: 10.1084/jem.192.2.303

[66] Read S, Malmstrom V, Powrie F. Cytotoxic T lymphocyte-associated antigen 4 plays an essential role in the function of CD25+CD4+ regulatory cells that control intestinal inflammation. Journal of Experimental Medicine. 2000;**192**:295–302. DOI: 10.1084/jem.192.2.295

[67] Marie JC, Letterio JJ, Gavin M, Rudensky AY. TGF-β1 maintains suppressor function and Foxp3 expression in CD4+CD25+ regulatory T cells. Journal of Experimental Medicine. 2005;**201**:1061–1067. DOI: 10.1084/jem.20042276

[68] Wan YY, Flavell RA. Regulatory T cells, transforming growth factor-β, and immune suppression. Proceedings of the American Thoracic Society. 2007;**4**:271–276. DOI: 10.1513/pats.200701-020AW

[69] Liang B, Workman C, Lee J, Chew C, Dale BM, Colonna L, et al. Regulatory T cells inhibit dendritic cells by LAG-3 engagement of MHC class II. Journal of Immunology. 2008;**180**:5916–5926. DOI: https://doi.org/10.4049/jimmunol.180.9.5916

[70] Kanamaru F, Youngnak P, Hashiguchi M, Nishioka T, Takahashi T, Sakaguchi S, et al. Costimulation via glucocorticoid-induced TNF receptor in both conventional and CD15+ regulatory CD4+ T cells. Journal of Immunology. 2004;**172**:7306–7314. DOI: https://doi.org/10.4049/jimmunol.172.12.7306

[71] Shevach EM, Stephens GL. The GITR-GITRL interaction: Co-stimulation or contra-suppression of regulatory activity? Nature Reviews Immunology. 2006;**6**:613–618. DOI: 10.1038/nri1867

[72] Fife BT, Pauken KE, Eagar TN, Obu T, Wu J, Tang Q, et al. Interactions between programmed death ligand-1 promote tolerance by blocking the T cell receptor-induced stop signal. Nature Immunology. 2009;**10**:1185–1192. DOI: 10.1038/ni.1790

[73] Gondek DC, Lu LF, Quezada SA, Sakaguchi S, Noelle RJ. Cutting edge: Contact-mediated suppression by CD4+CD25+ regulatory cells involves a granzyme B-dependent, perforin-independent mechanism. Journal of Immunology. 2005;**174**:1783–1786. DOI: https://doi.org/10.4049/jimmunol.174.4.1783

[74] Gondek DC, Devries V, Nowak EC, et al. Transplantation survival is maintained by granzyme B+ regulatory cells and adaptive regulatory T cells. Journal of Immunology. 2008;**181**:4752–4760. DOI: https://doi.org/10.4049/jimmunol.181.7.4752

[75] Bodor J, Fehervari Z, Diamond B, Sakaguchi S. Regulatory T-cell mediated suppression: Potential role of ICER. Journal of Leukocyte Biology. 2007;**81**:161–167. DOI: 10.1189/jlb.0706474

[76] Chen W, Jin W, Hardegen N, Lei KJ, Marinos N, McGrady, G, et al. Conversion of peripheral CD4+CD25- naove T cells to CD4+CD25+ regulatory T cells by TGF-β induction of transcription factor Foxp3. Journal of Experimental Medicine. 2003;**198**:1875–1886. DOI: 10.1084/jem.20030152

[77] Davidson TS, DiPaolo RJ, Andersson J, Shevach EM. Cutting edge: IL-2 is essential for TGF-beta-mediated induction of Foxp3 T regulatory cells. Journal of Immunology. 2007;**178**:4022–4026. DOI: https://doi.org/10.4049/jimmunol.178.7.4022

[78] Moore KW, de Waal Malefyt R, Coffman RL, et al. Interleukin-10 and the interleukin-10 receptor. Annual Review of Immunology. 2001;**19**:683–765. DOI: 10.1146/annurev.immunol.19.1.683

[79] Rubtsov YP, Rasmussen JP, Chi EY, Fontenot J, Castelli L, Ye X, et al. Regulatory T cell-derived interleukin-10 limits inflammation at environmental interfaces. Immunity. 2008;**28**:546–558. DOI: 10.1016/j.immuni.2008.02.017

[80] Collison LW, Workman CJ, Kuo TT, Boyd K, Wang Y, Vignali KM, et al. The inhibitory cytokine IL-35 contributes to regulatory T-cell function. Nature. 2007;**450**:566–569. DOI: 10.1038/nature06306

[81] Bettini M, Vignalli DA. Regulatory T cells and inhibitory cytokines in autoimmunity. Current Opinion in Immunology. 2009;**21**:612–618. DOI: 10.1016/j.coi.2009.09.011

[82] Banchereau J, Pascual V, O'Garra A. From IL-2 to IL-37: The expanding spectrum of anti-inflammatory cytokines. Nature Immunology. 2012;**13**:925–931. DOI: 10.1038/ni.2406

[83] Bopp T, Becker C, Klein M, Klein-Hessling S, Palmetshofer A, Serfling E, et al. Cyclic adenosine monophosphate is a key component of regulatory T cell-mediated suppression. Journal of Experimental Medicine. 2007;**204**:1303–1310. DOI: 10.1084/jem.20062129

[84] Deaglio S, Dwyer KM, Gao W, Friedman D, Usheva A, Erat A, et al. Adenosine generation catalysed by CD39 and CD73 expressed on regulatory T cells mediates immune suppression. Journal of Experimental Medicine. 2007;**204**:1257–1265. DOI: 10.1084/jem.20062512

[85] Zarek PE, Huang CT, Lutz ER, Kowalski J, Horton MR, Linden J, et al. A2A receptor signalling promotes peripheral tolerance by inducing T-cell anergy and the generation of adaptive regulatory T cells. Blood. 2008;**111**:251–259. DOI: 10.1182/blood-2007-03-081646

[86] Ernst PB, Garrison JC, Thompson LF. Much ado about adenosine: Adenosine synthesis and function in regulatory T cell biology. Journal of Immunology. 2010;**185**:1993–1998. DOI: 10.4049/jimmunol.1000108

[87] Tadokoro CE, Shakhar G, Shen S, Ding Y, Lino AC, Maraver A, et al. Regulatory T cells inhibit stable contacts between CD4+ T cells and dendritic cells in vivo. Journal of Experimental Medicine. 2006;**203**:505–511. DOI: 10.1084/jem.20050783

[88] Houot R, Perrot I, Garcia E, Durand I, Lebecque S. Human CD4+CD25high regulatory T cells modulate myeloid but not plasmacytoid dendritic cells activation. Journal of Immunology. 2006;**176**:5293–5298. DOI: https://doi.org/10.4049/jimmunol.176.9.5293

[89] Cederbom L, Hall H, Ivars F. CD4+CD25+ regulatory T cells down-regulate co-stimulatory molecules on antigen-presenting cells. European Journal of Immunology. 2000;**30**:1538–1543. DOI: 10.1002/1521- 4141(200006)30:6<1538::AID-IMMU1538>3.0.CO;2-X

[90] Oderup C, Cederbom L, Makowska A, Cilio CM, Ivars F. Cytotoxic T lymphocyte antigen-4-dependent down-modulation of costimulatory molecules on dendritic cells in CD4+CD25+ regulatory T-cell-mediated suppression. Immunology. 2006;**118**:240–249. DOI: 10.1111/j.1365- 2567.2006.02362.x

[91] Kornete M, Piccirillo CA. Functional crosstalk between dendritic cells and Foxp3(+) regulatory T cells in the maintenance of immune tolerance. Frontiers in Immunology. 2012;**3**:165. DOI: 10.3389/fimmu.2012.00165

[92] Liu X, Nurieva RI, Dong C. Transcriptional regulation of follicular T-helper (Tfh) cells. Immunological Reviews. 2013;**252**:139–145. DOI: 10.1111/imr.12040

[93] Burchill MA, Yang J, Vogtenhuber C, Blazar BR, Farrar MA. IL-2 receptor beta-dependent STAT5 activation is required for the development of Foxp3+ regulatory T cells. Journal of Immunology. 2007;**178**:280–290. DOI: https://doi.org/10.4049/jimmunol.178.1.280

[94] Campbell DJ, Koch MA. Phenotypical and functional specialization of FOXP3+ regulatory T cells. Nature Reviews Immunology. 2011;**11**:119–130. DOI: 10.1038/nri2916

[95] Chauhdry A, Rudra D, Treuting P, Samstein RM, Liang Y, Kas A, et al. CD4+ regulatory T cells control Th17 responses in a STAT3-dependent manner. Science. 2009;**326**:986–991. DOI: 10.1126/science.1172702

[96] Wan YY. Regulatory T cells: Immune suppression and beyond. Cellular & Molecular Immunology. 2010;**7**:204–210. DOI: 10.1038/cmi.2010.20

[97] McClymont SA, Putnam AL, Lee MR, Esensten JH, Liu W, Hulme MA, et al. Plasticity of human regulatory T cells in healthy subjects and patients with type 1 diabetes. Journal of Immunology. 2011;**186**:3918–3926. DOI: 10.4049/jimmunol.1003099

[98] Suri-Prayer E, Amar AZ, McHugh R, Natarajan K, Marqulies DH, Shevach EM. Post-thymectomy autoimmune gastritis, fine specificity and pathogenicity of anti-H/K APTase-reactive T cells. European Journal of Immunology. 1999;**29**:669–677. DOI: 10.1002/(SICI)1521-4141(199902)29:02<669::AID-IMMU669>3.0.CO;2-J

[99] Horwitz DA, Zheng SG, Gray JD. The role of the combination of IL-2 and TGF-β or IL-10 in the generation and function of CD4+ CD25+ and CD8+ regulatory T cell subsets. Journal of Leukocyte Biology. 2003;**74**:471–478. DOI: 10.1189/jlb.0503228

[100] Zou L, Barnett B, Safah H, Larussa VF, Evdemon-Hogan M, Mottram P, et al. Bone marrow is a reservoir for CD4+CD25+ regulatory T cells that traffic through CXCL12/CXCR4 signals. Cancer Research. 2004;**64**:8451–8455. DOI: 10.1158/0008-5472.CAN-04-1987

[101] Mailloux AW, Young MR. Regulatory T cell trafficking: From thymic development to tumour-induced immune suppression. Critical Reviews in Immunology. 2010;**30**:435–447

[102] Lim HW, Hillsamer P, Kim CH. Regulatory T cells can migrate to follicles upon T cell activation and suppress GC-Th cells and GC-Th cell-driven B responses. The Journal of Clinical Investigation. 2004;**114**:1640–1649. DOI: 10.1172/JCI22325

[103] Walker LS. Regulatory T cells overtuned: The effectors fight back. Immunology. 2009;**126**:466–474. DOI: 10.1111/j.1365-2567.2009.03053.x

[104] Liu G, Zhao Y. Toll-like receptors and immune regulation: Their direct and indirect modulation on regulatory CD4+CD25+ T cells. Immunology. 2007;**122**:149–156. DOI: 10.1111/j.1365-2567.2007.02651.x

[105] King C, Ilic A, Koelsch K, Sarvetnick N. Homeostatic expansion of T cells during immune insufficiency generates autoimmunity. Cell. 2004;**117**:265–277. DOI: http://dx.doi.org/10.1016/S0092-8674(04)00335-6

[106] Pasare C, Medzhitov R. Toll pathway-dependent blockade of CD4+CD25+ T cell-mediated suppression by dendritic cells. Science. 2003;**299**:1033–1036. DOI: 10.1126/science.1078231

[107] Crispin JC, Martinez A, Alcocer-Varela J. Quantification of regulatory T cells in patients with systemic lupus erythematosus. Journal of Autoimmunity. 2003;**21**:273–276. DOI: http://dx.doi.org/10.1016/S0896-8411(03)00121-5

[108] Liu MF, Wang CR, Fung LL, Wu CR. Decreased CD4+CD25+ T cells in peripheral blood of patients with systemic lupus erythematosus. Scandinavian Journal of Immunology. 2004;**59**:198–202. DOI: 10.1111/j.0300-9475.2004.01370.x

[109] Fathy A, Mohamed RW, Tawfik GA, Omar AS. Diminished CD4+CD25+ T-lymphocytes in peripheral blood of patients with systemic lupus erythematosus. The Egyptian Journal of Immunology. 2005;**12**:25–31

[110] Valencia X, Yarboro C, Illei G, Lipsky PE. Deficient CD4+CD25high T regulatory cell function in patients with active systemic lupus erythematosus. Journal of Immunology. 2007;**178**:2579–2588. DOI: https://doi.org/10.4049/jimmunol.178.4.2579

[111] Lyssouk EY, Torgashina AV, Soloviev SK, Nassonov EL, Bykovskaia SN. Reduced number and function of CD4+CD25highFOXP3+ regulatory T cells in patients with systemic lupus erythematosus. Advances in Experimental Medicine and Biology. 2007;**601**:113–119. DOI: 10.1007/978-0-387-72005-0_12

[112] Barath S, Aleksza M, Tarr T, Sinka S, Szegedi G, Kiss E. Measurement of natural (CD4+CD25high) and inducible (CD4+IL-10+) regulatory T cells in patients with systemic lupus erythematosus. Lupus. 2007;**16**:488–496. DOI: 10.1177/0961203307080226

[113] Tselios K, Sarantopoulos A, Gkougkourelas I, Boura P. CD4+CD25highFOXP3+ T regulatory cells as a biomarker of disease activity in systemic lupus erythematosus: A prospective study. Clinical and Experimental Rheumatology. 2014;**32**:630–639

[114] Yates J, Whittington A, Mitchell P, Lechler RI, Lightstone L, Lombardi G. Natural regulatory T cells: Number and function are normal in the majority of patients with systemic lupus erythematosus. Clinical and Experimental Immunology. 2008;**153**:44–55. DOI: 10.1111/j.1365-2249.2008.03665.x

[115] Alvarado-Sanchez B, Hernandez-Castro B, Portales-Perez D, Baranda L, Layseca-Espinosa E, Abud-Mendoza C, et al. Regulatory T cells in patients with systemic lupus erythematosus. Journal of Autoimmunity. 2006;**27**:110–118. DOI: 10.1016/j.jaut.2006.06.005

[116] Lin SC, Chen KH, Lin CH, Kuo CC, Ling QD, Chan CH. The quantitative analysis of peripheral blood FOXP3-expressing T cells in systemic lupus erythematosus and rheumatoid arthritis patients. European Journal of Clinical Investigation. 2007;**37**:987–996. DOI: 10.1111/j.1365-2362.2007.01882.x

[117] Venigalla RK, Tretter T, Krienke S, Max R, Eckstein V, Blank N, et al. Reduced CD4+CD25- T cell sensitivity to the suppressive function of CD4+CD25highCD127low regulatory T cells in patients with active systemic lupus erythematosus. Arthritis and Rheumatism. 2008;**58**:2120–2130. DOI: 10.1002/art.23556

[118] Zhang B, Zhang X, Tang F, Zhu L, Liu Y. Reduction of forkhead box P3 levels in CD4+CD25high T cells in patients with new-onset systemic lupus erythematosus. Clinical and Experimental Immunology. 2008;**153**:182–187. DOI: 10.1111/j.1365-2249.2008.03686.x

[119] Kuhn A, Beissert S, Krammer PH. CD4+CD25+ regulatory T cells in systemic lupus erythematosus. Archives of Dermatological Research. 2009;**301**:71–81. DOI: 10.1007/s00403-008-0891-9

[120] Yang HX, Zhang W, Zhao LD, Li Y, Zhang FC, Tang FL, et al. Are CD4+CD25-FOXP3+ cells in untreated new-onset lupus patients regulatory T cells? Arthritis Research & Therapy. 2009;**11**:R153. DOI: 10.1186/ar2829

[121] Tselios K, Sarantopoulos A, Gkougkourelas I, Boura P. The influence of therapy on CD4+CD25highFOXP3+ regulatory T cells in systemic lupus erythematosus patients: A prospective study. Scandinavian Journal of Rheumatology. 2015;**44**:29–35. DOI: 10.3109/03009742.2014.922214

[122] Tselios K, Sarantopoulos A, Gkougkourelas I, Papagianni A, Boura P. Increase of peripheral T regulatory cells during remission induction with cyclophosphamide in active systemic lupus erythematosus. International Journal of Rheumatic Diseases. 2014;**17**:790–795. DOI:10.1111/1756-185X.12500

[123] Sarantopoulos A, Tselios K, Gkougkourelas I, Pantoura M, Georgiadou AM, Boura P. Tocilizumab treatment leads to a rapid and sustained increase in Treg cell levels in rheumatoid arthritis patients: Comment on the article of Thiolat et al. Arthritis Rheumatology. 2014;**66**:2638. DOI: 10.1002/art.38714

[124] Alexander T, Sattler A, Templin L, Kohler S, Gross C, Meisel A, et al. Foxp3+Helios+ regulatory T cells are expanded in active systemic lupus erythematosus. Annals of the Rheumatic Diseases. 2013;**72**:1549–1558. DOI: 10.1136/annrheumdis-2012-202216

[125] Alunno A, Bartoloni E, Bistoni O, Nocentini G, Ronchetti S, Caterbi S, et al. Balance between regulatory T and Th17 cells in systemic lupus erythematosus: The old and the new. Clinical & Developmental Immunology. 2012;**2012**:823085. DOI: 10.1155/2012/823085

[126] Valmori D, Raffin C, Raimbaud I, Ayyoub M. Human RORγt+ TH17 cells preferentially differentiate from naive FOXP3+ Tregs in the presence of lineage-specific polarizing factors. Proceedings of the National Academy of Sciences. 2010;**107**:19402–19407. DOI: 10.1073/pnas.1008247107

[127] Lee YK, Mukasa R, Hatton RD, Weaver CT. Developmental plasticity of Th17 and Treg cells. Current Opinion in Immunology. 2009;**21**:274–280. DOI: 10.1016/j.coi.2009.05.021

[128] Yang J, Chu Y, Yang X, Gao D, Zhu L, Yang X, et al. Th17 and natural Treg cell population dynamics in systemic lupus erythematosus. Arthritis and Rheumatism. 2009;**60**:1472–1483. DOI: 10.1002/art.24499

[129] Ma J, Yu J, Tao X, Cai L, Wang J, Zheng SG. The imbalance between regulatory and IL-17-secreting CD4+ T cells in lupus patients. Clinical Rheumatology. 2010;**29**:1251–1258. DOI: 10.1007/s10067-010-1510-7

[130] Dolff S, Bijl M, Huitema MG, Limburg PC, Kallenberg CG, Abdulahad WH. Disturbed Th1, Th2, Th17 and Treg balance in patients with systemic lupus erythematosus. Clinical Immunology. 2011;**141**:197–204. DOI: 10.1016/j.clim.2011.08.005

[131] Yang J, Yang X, Zou H, Chu Y, Li M. Recovery of the immune balance between Th17 and regulatory T cells as a treatment for systemic lupus erythematosus. Rheumatology (Oxford). 2011;**50**:1366–1372. DOI: 10.1093/rheumatology/ker116

[132] Mizui M, Tsokos GC. Low-dose IL-2 in the treatment of lupus. Current Rheumatology Reports. 2016;**18**:68

[133] Zhang B, Dou Y, Xu X, Wang X, Xu B, Du J, et al. Endogenous FOXP3 inhibits cell proliferation, migration and invasion in glioma cells. International Journal of Clinical and Experimental Medicine. 2015;8:1792–1802

[134] Qin A, Wen Z, Zhou Y, Li Y, Li Y, Luo J, et al. MicroRNA-126 regulates the induction and function of CD4+FOXP3+ regulatory T cells through PI3K/AKT pathway. Journal of Cellular and Molecular Medicine. 2013;**17**:252–264. DOI: 10.1111/jcmm.12003

[135] Zhao M, Liang GP, Tang MN, Luo SY, Zhang J, Cheng WJ, et al. Total glucosides of paeony induces regulatory CD4+CD25+ T cells by increasing FOXP3 demethylation in lupus CD4+ T cells. Clinical Immunology. 2012;**143**:180–187. DOI: 10.1016/j.clim.2012.02.002

[136] Regna NL, Chafin CB, Hammond SE, Puthiyaveetil AG, Caudell DL, Reilly CM. Class I and II histone deacetylase inhibition by ITF2357 reduces SLE pathogenesis in vivo. Clinical Immunology. 2014;**151**:29–42. DOI: 10.1016/j.clim.2014.01.002

[137] Koga T, Mizui M, Yoshida N, Otomo K, Lieberman LA, Crispin JC, et al. KN-93, an inhibitor of calcium/calmodulin-dependent protein kinase IV promotes generation and function of FOXP3+ regulatory T cells in MRL/lpr MICE. Autoimmunity. 2014;**47**:445–450. DOI: 10.3109/08916934.2014.915954

[138] Stohl W. Future prospects in biologic therapy for systemic lupus erythematosus. Nature Reviews Rheumatology. 2013;**9**:705–720. DOI: 10.1038/nrrheum.2013.136

[139] Zheng SG, Wang JH, Koss MN, Quismorio Jr. F, Gray JD, Horwitz DA. CD4+ and CD8+ regulatory T cells generated ex vivo with IL-2 and TGF-beta suppress a stimulatory graft-versus-host disease with a lupus-like syndrome. Journal of Immunology 2004;**172**:1531–1539. DOI: https://doi.org/10.4049/jimmunol.172.3.1531

[140] Scalapino KJ, Tang Q, Bluestone JA, Bonyhadi ML, Daikh DI. Suppression of disease in New Zealand black/New Zealand white lupus-prone mice by adoptive transfer of ex vivo expanded regulatory T cells. Journal of Immunology. 2006;**177**:1451–1459. DOI: https://doi.org/10.4049/jimmunol.177.3.1451

[141] Lan Q, Zhou X, Fan H, Chen M, Wang J, Ryffel B, et al. Polyclonal CD4+Foxp3+ Treg cells induce TGFβ-dependent tolerogenic dendritic cells that suppress the murine lupus-like syndrome. The Journal of Molecular Cell Biology. 2012;**4**:409–419. DOI: 10.1093/jmcb/mjs040

[142] Cao T, Wenzel SE, Faubion WA, Harriman G, Li L. Enhanced suppressive function of regulatory T cells from patients with immune-mediated diseases following successful ex vivo expansion. Clinical Immunology. 2010;**136**:329–337. DOI: 10.1016/j.clim.2010.04.014

[143] Hahn BH, Anderson M, Le E, La Cava A. Anti-DNA Ig peptides promote Treg cell activity in systemic lupus erythematosus patients. Arthritis and Rheumatism. 2008;**58**:2488–2497. DOI: 10.1002/art.23609

[144] Bluestone JA, Buckner JH, Fitch M, Gitelman SE, Gupta S, Hellerstein MK, et al. Type 1 diabetes immunotherapy using polyclonal regulatory T cells. Science Translational Medicine. 2015;**7**:315ra189. DOI: 10.1126/scitranslmed.aad4134

[145] Marek-Trzonkowska N, Mysliwiec M, Dobyszuk A, Grabowska M, Derkowska I, Juscinska J, et al. Therapy of type 1 diabetes with CD4+CD25highCD127- regulatory

T cells prolongs survival of pancreatic islets- results of one year follow-up. Clinical Immunology. 2014;**153**:23–30. DOI: 10.1016/j.clim.2014.03.016

[146] Theil A, Tuve S, Oelschlagel U, Maiwald A, Dohler D, Obmann D, et al. Adoptive transfer of allogeneic regulatory T cells into patients with chronic graft-versus-host disease. Cytotherapy. 2015;**17**:473–486. DOI: 10.1016/j.jcyt.2014.11.005

[147] Brunstein CG, Miller JS, McKenna DH, Hippen KL, DeFor TE, Sumstad D, et al. Umbilical cord blood-derived T regulatory cells to prevent GVHD: Kinetics, toxicity profile and clinical effect. Blood. 2016;**127**:1044–1051. DOI: 10.1182/blood-2015-06-653667

[148] Jeffery HC, Braitch MK, Brown S, Oo YH. Clinical potential of regulatory T cell therapy in liver diseases: An overview and current perspectives. Frontiers in Immunology. 2016;**7**:334. DOI: 10.3389/fimmu.2016.00334

[149] Hugle T, Daikeler T. Stem cell transplantation for autoimmune diseases. Haematologica. 2010;**95**:185–188. DOI: 10.3324/haematol.2009.017038

[150] Burt RK, Traynor A, Statkute L, Barr WG, Rosa R, Schroeder J, et al. Nonmyeloablative hematopoietic stem cell transplantation for systemic lupus erythematosus. Journal of the American Medical Association. 2006;**295**:527–535. DOI: 10.1001/jama.295.5.527

[151] Figueroa FE, Cuenca Moreno J, La Cava A. Novel approaches to lupus drug discovery using stem cell therapy. Role of mesenchymal-stem-cell-secreted factors. Expert Opinion on Drug Discovery. 2014;**9**:555–566. DOI: 10.1517/17460441.2014.897692

[152] Zhang L, Bertucci AM, Ramsey-Goldman R, Burt RK, Datta SK. Regulatory T cell (Treg) subsets return in patients with refractory lupus following stem cell transplantation and TGF-beta-producing CD8+ Treg cells are associated with immunological remission of lupus. Journal of Immunology. 2009;**183**:6346–6358. DOI: 10.4049/jimmunol.0901773

[153] Szodoray P, Varoczy L, Papp G, Barath S, Nakken B, Szegedi G, et al. Immunological reconstitution after autologous stem cell transplantation in patients with refractory systemic autoimmune diseases. Scandinavian Journal of Rheumatology. 2012;**41**:110–5. DOI: 10.3109/03009742.2011.606788

[154] Wang D, Niu L, Feng X, Yuan X, Zhao S, Zhang H, et al. Long-term safety of umbilical cord mesenchymal stem cells transplantation for systemic lupus erythematosus: A 6-year follow-up study. Clinical and Experimental Medicine. 7 June 2016 [Epub ahead of print]. DOI: 10.1007/s10238-016-0427-0

[155] Carrion F, Nova E, Ruiz C, Diaz F, Inostroza C, Rojo D, et al. Autologous mesenchymal stem cell treatment increased T regulatory cells with no effect on disease activity in two systemic lupus erythematosus patients. Lupus. 2010;**19**:317–322. DOI: 10.1177/0961203309348983

[156] Wang Q, Qian S, Li J, Che N, Gu L, Wang Q, et al. Combined transplantation of autologous hematopoietic stem cells and allogenic mesenchymal stem cells increases T regulatory cells in systemic lupus erythematosus with refractory lupus nephritis and leukopenia. Lupus. 2015;**24**:1221–1226. DOI: 10.1177/0961203315583541

[157] Wang D, Huang S, Yuan X, Liang J, Xu R, Yao G, et al. The regulation of the Treg/Th17 balance by mesenchymal stem cells in human systemic lupus erythematosus. Cellular & Molecular Immunology 5 October 2015 [Epub ahead of print]. DOI: 10.1038/cmi.2015.89

[158] He J, Zhang X, Wei Y, Sun X, Chen Y, Deng J, et al. Low-dose interleukin-2 treatment selectively modulated CD4+ T cell subsets in patients with systemic lupus erythematosus. Nature Medicine. 2016;**22**:991–993. DOI: 10.1038/nm.4148

[159] Von Spee-Mayer C, Siegert E, Abdirama D, Rose A, Klaus A, Alexander T, et al. Low-dose interleukin-2 selectively corrects regulatory T cell defects in patients with systemic lupus erythematosus. Annals of the Rheumatic Diseases. 2016;**75**:1407–1415. DOI: 10.1136/annrheumdis-2015-207776

[160] Giang S, La Cava A. Regulatory T cells in SLE: Biology and use in treatment. Current Rheumatology Reports. 2016;**18**:67. DOI: 10.1007/s11926-016-0616-6

[161] Yan JJ, Lee JG, Jang JY, Koo TY, Ahn C, Yang J. IL-2/anti-IL-2 complexes ameliorates lupus nephritis by expansion of CD4+CD25+FOXP3+ regulatory T cells. Kidney International. 30 November 2016 [Epub ahead of print]. DOI: 10.1016/j.kint.2016.09.022

[162] Miyabe Y, Miyabe C, Nanki T. Could retinoids be a potential treatment for rheumatic diseases? Rheumatology International. 2015;**35**:35–41. DOI: 10.1007/s00296-014-3067-2

[163] Lu L, Ma J, Li Z, Lan Q, Chen M, Liu Y, et al. All-trans retinoic acid promotes TGF-β-induced Tregs via histone modification but not DNA demethylation on Foxp3 gene locus. PLoS One. 2011;**6**:e24590. DOI: 10.1371/journal.pone.0024590

[164] Sobel ES, Brusko TM, Butfiloski EJ, Hou W, Li S, Cuda CM, et al. Defective response of CD4+ T cells to retinoic acid and TGFβ in systemic lupus erythematosus. Arthritis Research & Therapy. 2011;**13**:R106. DOI: 10.1186/ar3387

[165] Handono K, Firdausi SN, Pratama MZ, Endharti AT, Kalim H. Vitamin A improves Th17 and Treg regulation in systemic lupus erythematosus. Clinical Rheumatology. 2016;**35**:631–638. DOI: 10.1007/s10067-016-3197-x

[166] Sharabi A, Mozes E. The suppression of murine lupus by a tolerogenic peptide involves Foxp3-expressing CD8+ cells that are required for the optimal induction and function of Foxp3-expressing CD4 cells. Journal of Immunology. 2008;**181**:3243–3251. DOI: https://doi.org/10.4049/jimmunol.181.5.3243

[167] Singh RP, La Cava A, Hahn B. pConsensus peptide induces tolerogenic CD8+ T cells in lupus-prone (NXBxNZW) F1 mice by differentially regulating Foxp3 and PD1 molecules. Journal of Immunology. 2008;**180**:2069–2080. DOI: https://doi.org/10.4049/jimmunol.180.4.2069

[168] Zimmer R, Scherbarth HR, Rillo OL, Gomez-Reino JJ, Muller S. Lupuzor/P140 peptide in patients with systemic lupus erythematosus: A randomized, double-blind, placebo-controlled phase IIb clinical trial. Annals of the Rheumatic Diseases. 2013;**72**:1830–1835. DOI: 10.1136/annrheumdis-2012-202460

[169] Suarez A, Lopez P, Gomez J, Gutierrez C. Enrichment of CD4+CD25high T cell population in patients with systemic lupus erythematosus treated with glucocorticoids. Annals of the Rheumatic Diseases. 2006;**65**:1512–1517. DOI: 10.1136/ard.2005.049924

[170] Azab NA, Bassyouni IH, Emad Y, Abd El-Wahab GA, Hamdy G, Mashahit MA. CD4+CD25+ regulatory T cells (TREG) in systemic lupus erythematosus (SLE) patients: The possible influence of treatment with corticosteroids. Clinical Immunology. 2008;**127**:151–157. DOI: 10.1016/j.clim.2007.12.010

[171] Prado C, Gomez J, Lopez P, De Paz B, Gutierrez C, Suarez A. Dexamethasone upregulates FOXP3 expression without increasing regulatory activity. Immunobiology. 2011;**216**:386–392. DOI: 10.1016/j.imbio.2010.06.013

[172] Mathian A, Jouenne R, Chader D, Cohen-Aubart F, Haroche J, Fadlallah J, et al. Regulatory T cell responses to high-dose methylprednisolone in active systemic lupus erythematosus. PLoS One. 2015;**10**:e0143689. DOI: 10.1371/journal.pone.0143689

[173] Kessel A, Ammuri H, Peri R, Pavlotzky ER, Blank M, Shoenfeld Y, et al. Intravenous immunoglobulin therapy affects T regulatory cells by increasing their suppressive function. Journal of Immunology. 2007;**179**:5571–5575. DOI: https://doi.org/10.4049/jimmunol.179.8.5571

[174] Sfikakis PP, Souliotis VL, Fragiadaki KG, Moutsopoulos HM, Boletis JN, Theofilopoulos AN. Increased expression of the FoxP3 functional marker of regulatory T cells following B cell depletion with rituximab in patients with lupus nephritis. Clinical Immunology. 2007;**123**:66–73. DOI: 10.1016/j.clim.2006.12.006

[175] Ulivieri C, Baldari CT. Statins: From cholesterol-lowering drugs to novel immunomodulators for the treatment of Th17-mediated autoimmune diseases. Pharmacological Research. 2014;**88**:41–52. DOI: 10.1016/j.phrs.2014.03.001

[176] Tselios K, Sarantopoulos A, Gkougkourelas I, Boura P. T regulatory cells: A promising new target in atherosclerosis. Critical Reviews in Immunology. 2014;**34**:389–397

[177] Mausner-Fainberg K, Luboshits G, Mor A, Maysel-Auslender S, Rubinstein A, Keren G, et al. The effect of HMG-CoA reductase inhibitors on naturally occurring CD4+CD25+ T cells. Atherosclerosis. 2008;**197**:829–839. DOI: 10.1016/j.atherosclerosis.2007.07.031

Section 3

Additional Complications in Lupus

Chapter 6

Accelerated Atherosclerosis in Patients with Systemic Lupus Erythematosus and the Role of Selected Adipocytokines in This Process

Eugeniusz Hrycek, Iwona Banasiewicz-Szkróbka, Aleksander Żurakowski, Paweł Buszman and Antoni Hrycek

Additional information is available at the end of the chapter

http://dx.doi.org/10.5772/68016

Abstract

Systemic lupus erythematosus (SLE) can affect various systems and organs. The most severe forms of the disease affect the kidneys, the central nervous system, and the heart. Cardiac and cardiovascular system diseases are inter alia caused by atherosclerosis, vasculitis, and thromboembolic events. Patients with SLE are at a higher risk of developing accelerated atherosclerosis. This process in SLE patients cannot be explained solely based on classical risk factors. Recently, some adipocytokines/adipokines have been indicated in the development of atherosclerosis, inflammation, and immune processes. It has also been postulated that adipokines might regulate the immune response and hence the atherogenic process. In this work, the factors contributing to accelerated atherosclerosis in SLE patients with special respect to vasculitis/vascular injury are presented, and selected adipocytokines, that is leptin, resistin, and adiponectin, with their relation to atherosclerosis and SLE, are under discussion.

Keywords: systemic lupus erythematosus, pathogenesis, atherosclerosis, adipocytokines, associations

1. Introduction

Systemic lupus erythematosus (SLE) is an organ-nonspecific autoimmune disease, more prevalent in young women than in men. It is characterized by periods of varying activity, sometimes even spontaneous remission. However, there can also be life-threatening disease flares, especially in those patients who undergo incorrect treatment.

The pathogenesis of SLE involves different factors and generally speaking, complex gene-environment interactions [1, 2]. More specifically, abnormal lymphocyte count (T-helper/T-suppressor cell quotient) and defects in T- and B-lymphocyte functions should be emphasized. Ineffective clearance of apoptotic cells [3, 4] and of immune complexes containing host auto-antigens and autoantibodies may also play a role in the development of SLE. Host lipids may contribute to the formation of immune complexes leading to the production of anticardiolipin antibodies [5]. Extracellular DNA molecules generated from apoptotic cells may also contribute to SLE as they promote the origin of anti-DNA autoantibodies, which are characteristic of the disease [6–8]. It should be noted though that the cause of SLE is not fully known.

As already mentioned, SLE is an organ-non-specific autoimmune disease that can affect almost any organ or system; the most severe forms affect the kidneys, the central nervous system, and the heart. Cardiac and cardiovascular system involvement may result from atherosclerosis, vasculitis, and thromboembolic lesions that are known to be interrelated processes [9, 10].

Although SLE patients constitute a small proportion of the population dying from cardiovascular events, they tend to suffer from cardiovascular complications at a young age [11]. Previous studies on SLE-related mortality revealed that early deaths were associated with disease activity and infections, whereas late deaths frequently resulted from atherosclerotic disease [12, 13]. It is noteworthy that these patients often suffer from accelerated atherosclerosis, which is associated inter alia with lipid disturbances, vasculitis, and vascular injury. The latter result from the activity of autoantibodies and immune complexes, which, via the activation of the complement system, lead to autoimmune inflammation of the vascular wall. Long-term side effects of lupus medications may also contribute to the development of cardiovascular disease (CVD) [4, 7, 11, 14, 15].

2. Factors contributing to accelerated atherosclerosis in patients with SLE with special respect to vasculitis/vascular injury

Patients in early stages of SLE rarely exhibit cardiac manifestations. Nevertheless, in over 50% of severe cases, the heart is affected, and the patients suffer from pericarditis, myocarditis, Libman-Sacks endocarditis, pulmonary hypertension, and coronary artery disease (CAD)—the development of which is related to autoimmune processes characteristic of SLE [16].

Among CVD diagnosed in SLE patients, particular attention should be paid to angiopathy, which is due to a chronic inflammatory process within the vascular wall and underlies premature atherosclerosis [17–20]. Atherosclerosis is a progressive disease resulting from a multitude of factors, including altered composition of the extracellular matrix and activation of vascular smooth muscle cells in the arterial walls, which leads to atherosclerotic plaque formation.

Due to modern immunosuppressive therapy, prognosis in SLE patients has markedly improved. However, arterial disease (including CAD) and strokes still account for a large proportion of SLE-related morbidity and mortality, while their pathogenesis has not been fully elucidated [21]. It has been estimated that the incidence of acute coronary syndromes is 50-fold higher in patients with SLE compared to the control [19, 22–25], while the CAD mortality rate ranges from 3.5 to 15.7% [26]. It should be noted that diagnostic imaging revealed subclinical atherosclerosis in 30–52% of SLE patients [24, 25, 27, 28].

The mechanisms of accelerated atherosclerosis in SLE patients are not fully understood and remain controversial. Its development cannot be accounted for based on traditional risk factors such as age, male sex, arterial hypertension, abnormalities in serum lipids, smoking, diabetes mellitus, obesity, and abnormal results of laboratory tests including high levels of C-reactive protein (CPR), fibrinogen, and homocysteine [4, 11, 29–34]. Other causative factors that might promote accelerated atherosclerosis should also be considered [35].

It has been suggested that atherosclerosis could be caused by an immune reaction against autoantigens at the endothelial level, which include oxidized low-density lipoprotein (LDL) and heat shock proteins (HSP) 60/65. Endothelial dysfunction plays a key role. It has also been speculated that immune mechanisms might be responsible for conversion of stable to instable plaque with resultant rupture [36].

Thus, it is not surprising that several autoimmune diseases, for example, SLE and antiphospholipid syndrome, are considered to raise the risk of CAD [37]; nevertheless, the precise mechanism is yet to be defined [38]. Multiple researchers believe that atherosclerosis is associated with immune responses [37, 39, 40]; it should be emphasized though that considering atherosclerosis as a solely autoimmune condition would be an oversimplification since metabolic disorders and hemodynamic factors are also involved in its development [41].

Although there is a lot of evidence that inflammation plays a central role in atherosclerosis, its pathogenesis is also associated with other risk factors often connected with SLE, that is arterial hypertension (especially renal hypertension), prolonged exposure to high doses of glucocorticoids (which, apart from having a beneficial anti-inflammatory action, also influence blood pressure and glucose metabolism), lupus-associated antiphospholipid syndrome, diabetes mellitus, and hypercholesterolemia [23, 25]. It should be noted that a regimen of ≤ 10 mg prednisone daily is considered safe in this respect [25]; however, the problem of metabolic disorders seen in SLE patients and its relation to glucocorticoid doses has not been satisfactorily elucidated. Contrary to steroids, antimalarial drugs used in SLE patients have a beneficial effect on their lipid profile.

Patients with SLE also exhibit other metabolic disturbances that may promote accelerated atherosclerosis and accelerated CAD. These include hypertriglyceridemia, high homocysteine levels, and early menopause [25].

The multifactorial etiology of atherosclerosis makes it difficult to unambiguously determine why SLE patients develop atherosclerotic lesions earlier in life and more frequently than the general population. Researchers are often confronted with inconsistent results [23, 42]; hence, it has been suggested SLE might be considered an independent risk factor for atherosclerosis including CAD [24, 43–45] and CVD [23].

The factors underlying the atherosclerotic process undoubtedly comprise pro-inflammatory cytokines, antiphospholipid antibodies, antiendothelial cell antibodies (AECAs), and antineutrophil cytoplasmic antibodies (ANCAs), all acting directly on blood vessels or forming deposits of immune complexes. Monocyte chemotactic protein-1 (MCP-1) [7] is also involved; its higher concentrations were revealed in the blood of our study participants with mild-to-moderate SLE [46]. Other researchers investigated the relationships between atherosclerotic plaques in the carotid arteries, antiphospholipid antibodies, and peripheral blood leukocyte count, an established indicator of inflammation [25]. There is also a spectrum of vascular abnormalities in SLE, resulting from adverse effects of several drugs or induced by infections, etc. [15].

It is important to note that vascular injury may develop not only due to an inflammatory condition but also as a result of non-inflammatory factors including environmental influences (toxicity, medication, or micro-organisms), neoplastic process, etc. [14]. Vascular disease in SLE patients can occur due to a combination of different pathological processes, for example, atherosclerosis, clotting disorders, and systemic vasculitis associated with vascular wall injury (especially endothelial dysfunction), caused by an autoimmune process [24, 28].

SLE patients most typically exhibit cutaneous vasculitis; systemic vasculitis develops in 10–18% of these patients and, as a life-threatening condition, may require aggressive therapy [14, 15].

Recently, it has been suggested that adipokines might play a causative role in the development of atherosclerosis, inflammatory, and immune processes [47]. These factors, secreted by the white adipose tissue, have autocrine-like actions, locally affecting adipocyte biology. They also act as endocrine factors that regulate systemic processes, for example, food intake, insulin sensitivity, bone growth and energy homeostasis, and affect development of obesity and metabolic syndrome [40, 48]. Adipokines have been indicated in the link between immune response and atherosclerotic process [49].

Since patients with SLE develop metabolic syndrome, insulin resistance, dyslipidemia, or hypertension more frequently than the general population [50–54], the interest in the adipose tissue is justified in the group of rheumatic diseases [55, 56]. Identification of mechanisms common to inflammation and CVD might be of considerable interest especially in the context SLE, which is, potentially, a model disease for gaining a deeper insight into such mechanisms [13]. Generally, the relationship of adipokines to inflammation and coronary atherosclerosis in patients with SLE has not been fully elucidated [57]; for example, it has not been determined whether adiponectin concentrations in SLE result from metabolic disorders or inflammatory processes and nor has it been determined whether adipokine abnormalities associated with connective tissue diseases contribute to disease development or are caused by inflammation induced by other pro-inflammatory factors [58].

3. Adipocytokines and their relation to atherosclerosis and systemic lupus erythematosus

White adipose tissue is a loose connective tissue composed of adipocytes and also containing adipocyte precursors, immune system cells fibroblasts, and other cell types [59]. Previously, this tissue had been considered an energy store (triglycerides) but now it is known to produce a number of biologically active substances that act at autocrine, paracrine, and endocrine levels. They regulate homeostasis through regulation of food intake, energy balance, lipid,

http://dx.doi.org/10.5772/68016

and carbohydrate metabolism. They also modulate the insulin effects, angiogenesis, and vascular remodeling, regulate arterial pressure, affect inflammatory processes as well as associated immune response, and have metabolic effects including an impact on the development of atherosclerosis [47, 50, 57, 59–63]. Since the structure of these substances resembles that of the cytokine family, they have been referred to as adipocytokines or adipokines [60]. Their multifunctionality underlies the relationship between white adipose tissue, metabolic disorders, and autoimmune diseases [59]. Actions of selected adipokines are summarized in **Table 1**.

The role of adipokines in atherosclerosis deserves particular attention as they modulate inflammatory processes and initiate its development [60]. Adipokines may constitute a link between impaired insulin sensitivity, obesity, chronic inflammation, and atherosclerosis in patients with SLE [57, 64]. It has been speculated that altered serum/plasma levels of adipokines in SLE might be related to coronary atherosclerosis, insulin resistance, and the inflammatory process [57]; however, these correlations need to be further explored and documented [65]. A deep insight into the mechanisms of adipokine actions would help develop new therapies—also for autoimmune disorders [58, 66].

It is assumed that resistin or leptin have pro-inflammatory and proatherosclerotic effects; they have also been implicated in insulin resistance [57, 67]. Conversely, adiponectin has an inverse association with inflammatory states, atherosclerosis, and insulin resistance [68]; hence, independent of traditional risk factors, low level of adiponectin might also contribute to the development of the abovementioned diseases [57, 69]. However, other studies did not confirm these causative associations [69–71] with respect to total adiponectin levels but only to some adiponectin isoforms determined in the serum [69]. The reported research results are therefore inconsistent.

Resistin plays an important role in the inflammatory process, but its amount in adipocytes is quite small. Greater resistin concentrations have been found in adipose tissue monocytes and macrophages and peripheral blood monocytes [72, 73]. It is also present in neutrophils and is capable of inducing the production of IL-6 and TNFα [42, 74–76]. These facts may indicate pro-inflammatory properties of resistin [73]. Patients with severe inflammatory disease exhibit significant increases in plasma resistin [77]. It is also noteworthy that endothelial cells exhibit sensitivity to resistin.

Resistin	Adiponectin	Leptin
Obesity	Obesity	Insulin resistance
Type 2 diabetes mellitus	Rheumatoid arthritis	Rheumatoid arthritis
Sleep apnea	Degenerative joint disease	Degenerative joint disease
Chronic kidney disease	Diabetes mellitus	Hepatitis
Atherosclerosis	Liver damage	Inflammatory bowel disease
Arthritis	Cardiovascular disease	Sepsis
Nonalcoholic fatty liver disease		Encephalomyelitis
Cardiovascular disease		

Table 1. Relationships between selected adipokines and disease processes in humans.

Although the role of resistin in SLE has not been fully determined [57, 58], its concentrations in the peripheral blood of SLE patients are elevated and have been found to correlate with inflammatory markers, glomerular filtration rate, and glucocorticoid therapy [75, 78]. However, other studies did not reveal significant differences in serum resistin between patients with SLE and control participants [78]. Hence, reports on resistin levels in SLE patients are not consistent and its role remains to be elucidated.

It has been argued that resistin concentrations might be predictive of coronary atherosclerosis, acute coronary events, and associated mortality [74, 78, 79]. It has been hypothesized that resistin secreted from macrophages in atheromas could affect vascular cell function and promote atherosclerosis [80]. Furthermore, it has been suggested that the levels of serum resistin might help determine the severity of myocardial ischemia [81], and its reduction could possibly reduce the risk for CVD [47]. It has also been speculated that this adipokine is more related to the inflammatory process and atherosclerosis than to obesity and insulin resistance [47].

Plasma leptin is known to be proportional to the total amount of adipose tissue, and therefore it is directly related to obesity and associated CVDs including atherosclerosis. Leptin exerts its atherogenic effects via induction of endothelial dysfunction, stimulation of inflammatory response, oxidative stress, platelet aggregation, migration, hypertrophy, and proliferation of vascular smooth muscle cells [82]. It regulates blood pressure and this is probably independent of body adiposity [83]. Plasma leptin concentration correlates with markers of subclinical atherosclerosis such as extracranial carotid intima-media thickness and coronary artery calcification. Beltowski [82] speculates that inhibition of leptin activity might slow down the progression of atherosclerosis in obese individuals with hyperleptinemia.

There are also data on the involvement of leptin in the immune response [77] and its modulatory effect on monocytes/macrophages, neutrophils, basophils, eosinophils, natural killer cells (NK), and dendritic cells [63, 84]. It has also been indicated in lymphocyte reactivity [85]. As already mentioned, leptin is considered a pro-inflammatory adipokine; therefore, changes in its plasma levels observed in SLE patients are not surprising. Leptin modulates the cardiovascular risk in these patients [86], and several authors have suggested that the adipokine might act as an independent risk factor for CVD [68].

Patients with SLE had higher plasma leptin compared to the control [49, 57, 87, 88], but clinical relevance of leptin level changes in autoimmune disorders remains unclear [87]. Several researchers believe that leptin is involved in the pathogenesis thereof [88, 89]. The evaluation of leptin concentrations in SLE patients with correction for BMI (body mass index) also revealed higher levels in the study group [42]. However, other authors concluded that leptin levels in SLE patients were lower or comparable to those found in healthy controls [90, 91].

Adiponectin, the major product of adipocytes, functions as an autocrine/paracrine factor within the adipose tissue and exerts endocrine effects on distant tissues thus influencing whole-body metabolism [92].

http://dx.doi.org/10.5772/68016

The role of adiponectin in SLE remains controversial. Several researchers observed an increase in adiponectin concentration in SLE patients [57, 91], while others did not find differences compared to the control [50, 58]. However, plasma adiponectin levels tend to be higher in patients with renal SLE in comparison to healthy controls and patients with nonrenal SLE [93].

Although the role of adiponectin in SLE pathogenesis has not been fully elucidated [86], higher local and/or systemic concentrations of this adipokine have been noted in chronic inflammatory conditions including SLE [94]. Nevertheless, processes leading to adiponectin levels elevation in chronic inflammatory/autoimmune diseases are still to be clarified [94].

The significance of adiponectin in atherosclerosis also needs clarification [72]. It was postulated that the anti-inflammatory effects of adiponectin were associated with the inhibition of pro-inflammatory cytokines, decreased leukocyte adhesion, and enhanced production of anti-inflammatory cytokines [95]. Adiponectin mediates inhibition of macrophage phagocytosis and decreases the production of IL-6 and TNF. It strongly inhibits B-lymphopoiesis, reduces T-lymphocyte response, and induces the production of anti-inflammatory agents (e.g., IL-10) in human monocytes, macrophages, and dendritic cells [62, 63]. Adiponectin also suppresses monocyte adhesion to endothelial cells as well as migration and proliferation of smooth muscle cells [30]. Hence, it may exert a beneficial effect in the metabolic syndrome and coronary heart disease. Low adiponectin concentrations have been found to enhance insulin resistance and the risk for coronary heart disease. It is noteworthy, though, that, contrary to its protective role with respect to obesity and vascular disease, adiponectin seems to have pro-inflammatory effects in joint diseases [58, 62, 63].

Summing up, it should be noted that metabolic disorders frequently seen in patients with SLE might result from the disease itself or genetic influences/long-term treatment. Patients with SLE also tend to more frequently develop a classic metabolic disease, that is obesity, which is associated with chronic, although not severe, inflammatory conditions. The latter has an impact on insulin resistance-related type 2 diabetes as well as on atherosclerosis and ischemic heart disease.

Author details

Eugeniusz Hrycek[1*], Iwona Banasiewicz-Szkróbka[1], Aleksander Żurakowski[1], Paweł Buszman[1,2] and Antoni Hrycek[2]

*Address all correspondence to: ehrycek@gmail.com

1 American Heart of Poland, Chrzanów, Poland

2 Department of Internal, Autoimmune and Metabolic Diseases, Medical University of Silesia, Katowice, Poland

References

[1] Hrycek A, Siekiera U, Cieślik P, Szkróbka W. HLA-DRB1 and DQB1 alleles and gene polymorphisms of selected cytokines in systemic lupus erythematosus. Rheumatol Int 2005: 26; 1–6.

[2] Hrycek A, Olszanecka-Glinianowicz M. Pylica płuc z towarzyszącym toczniem rumieniowatym układowym – opis przypadku. Pol Merk Lek 2008: 24; 18–19.

[3] Jasiuk B, Reich A. Znaczenie apoptozy w patogenezie tocznia rumieniowatego układowego. Dermatol Klin 2005: 7; 97–100.

[4] Wade NS, Major AS. The problem of accelerated atherosclerosis in systemic lupus erythematosus: insights into a complex co-morbidity. Thromb Haemost 2011: 106; 849–857.

[5] Jovanović V, Aziz NA, Lim YT, Poh ANA, Chan SJH, Pei EHX, Lew FCH, Shui G, Jenner AM, Bowen L, McKinney EF, Lyons PA, Kemeny MD, Smith KGC, Wenk MR, MacAry PA. Lipid anti-lipid antibody responses correlate with disease activity in systemic lupus erythematosus. PloS One 2013: 8; e55639.

[6] Su K-Y, Pisetsky DS. The role of extracellular DNA in autoimmunity in SLE. Scand J Immunol 2009: 70; 175–183.

[7] Narshi CB, Giles IP, Rahman A. The endothelium: an interface between autoimmunity and atherosclerosis in systemic lupus erythematosus? Lupus 2011: 20; 5–13.

[8] Hrycek A, Cieślik P. Annexin A5 and anti-annexin antibodies in patients with systemic lupus erythematosus. Rheumatol Int 2012: 32; 1335–1342.

[9] Irzyk K, Ciurzyński M. Zmiany naczyniowe w chorobach układowych tkanki łącznej. Pol Przegl Kardiol 2011: 13; 171–176.

[10] Gęsikowska K, Kandera-Anasz Z, Mielczarek-Palacz A, Sikora J, Machaj I, Smycz M. Toczeń rumieniowaty układowy – ciągle aktualny problem kliniczny i diagnostyczny. Pol Merk Lek 2012: 32; 111–115.

[11] Swacha M, Więsik-Szewczyk E, Olesińska M. Ocena ryzyka sercowo-naczyniowego u chorych na toczeń rumieniowaty układowy – aspekty praktyczne. Reumatologia 2011: 49; 419–425.

[12] Urowitz MB, Bookman AA, Koehler BE, Gordon DA, Smythe HA, Ogryzlo MA. The bimodal mortality pattern of systemic lupus erythematosus. Am J Med 1976: 60; 221–225.

[13] Bruce IN. Atherogenesis and autoimmune disease: the model of lupus. Lupus 2005: 14; 687–690.

[14] Cieślik P, Hrycek A, Kłuciński P. Vasculopathy and vasculitis in systemic lupus erythematosus. Pol Arch Med Wewn 2008: 118; 57–63.

[15] Radic M, Kaliterna DM, Radic J. Vascular manifestations of systemic lupus erythematosus. Neth J Med 2013: 71; 10–16.

[16] de Godoy MF, de Oliveira CM, Fabri VA, de Abreu LC, Valenti VE, Pires AC, Raimundo RD, Figueiredo JL, Bertazzi GRL. Long-term cardiac changes in patients with systemic lupus erythematosus. BMI Res Notes 2013: 6; 171–177.

[17] Escárcega RO, Carrasco MG, Alexandro SF, Jara LJ, Rodriguez JR, Linares LEE, Cervera R. Insulin resistance, chronic inflammatory state and the link with systemic lupus erythematosus related coronary disease. Autoim Rev 2006: 6; 48053.

[18] Płazak W, Gryga K, Dziedzic H, Tomkiewicz-Pająk L, Konieczyńska M, Podolec P, Musiał J. Influence of atorvastatin on coronary calcifications and myocardial perfusion defects in systemic lupus erythematosus patients: prospective, randomized, double-masked, placebo-controled study. Arthritis Res Ther 2011: 13; R117.

[19] Kotlarczyk A, Konarski ł, Matuszczyk A, Misztal K. Wybrane zagadnienia dotyczące układu sercowo-naczyniowego u chorych na toczeń rumieniowaty układowy. Ann Acad Med Siles 2013: 67; 137–141.

[20] Dahl TB, Yndestad A, Skjelland M, Øie E, Dahl A, Michelsen A, Damås JK, Tunheim SH, Ueland T, Smith C, Bendz B, Tonstad S, Gullestad L, Frøland SS, Krohg-Sørensen K, Russell D, Aukrust P, Halvorsen B. Increased expression of visfatin in macrophages of human unstable carotid and coronary atherosclerosis. Possible role in inflammation and plaque destabilization. Circulation 2007: 115; 972–980.

[21] Sada K-E, Yamasaki Y, Maruyama M, Sugiyama H, Yamamura M, Maeshima Y, Makino H. Altered levels of adipocytokines in association with insulin resistance in patients with systemic lupus erythematosus. J Rheumatol 2006: 33; 1545–1552.

[22] Manzi S, Meilahan EN, Rairie JE, Conte CG, Medsger TA Jr, Jansen-McWilliams L, D'Agostino RB, Kuller LH. Age-specific incidence rates of myocardial infarction and angina in women with systemic lupus erythematosu: comparison with the Framingham Study. Am J Epidemiol 1997: 145; 408–415.

[23] Zeller CB, Appenzeller S. Cardiovascular disease in systemic lupus erythematosus: the role of traditional and lupus related risk factors. Curr Cardiol Rev 2008: 4; 116–122.

[24] Pyrpasopoulou A, Chatzimichailidou S, Aslanidis S. Vascular disease in systemic lupus erythematosus. Autoimmune Dis 2012: Article ID 876456, 4 p.

[25] Bruce IN. "Not only...but also": factors that contribute to accelerated atherosclerosis and premature coronary heart disease in systemic lupus erythematosus. Rheumatology 2005: 44; 1492–1502.

[26] Matsumoto Y, Wakabayashi H, Otsuka F, Inoue K, Takano M, Sada KE, Makino H. Systemic lupus erythematosus complicated with acute myocardial infarction and ischemic colitis. Intern Med 2011: 50; 2669–2673.

[27] Doria A, Shoenfeld Y, Wu R, Gambari PF, Puato M, Ghirardello A, Gilburd B, Carbanese S, Patniak M, Zampieri S, Peter JB, Favaretto E, Laccarino L, Sherer Y, Todesco S, Pauletto P. Risk factors for subclinical atherosclerosis in a prospective cohort of patients with systemic lupus erythematosus. Ann Rheum Dis 2003: 62; 1071–1077.

[28] Croca SA, Rahman A. Imaging assessment of cardiovascular disease in systemic lupus erythematosus. Clin Develop Immunol 2012, Article ID 694143, 7 p.

[29] De Leeuw K, Freire B, Smit AJ, Bootsoma H, Kallenberg CG, Bijl M. Traditional and non-traditional risk factors contribute to the development of accelerated atherosclerosis in patients with systemic lupus erythematosus. Lupus 2006: 15; 675–682.

[30] Kahlenberg JM, Kaplan MJ. The interplay of inflammation and cardiovascular disease in systemic lupus erythematosus. Arth Res Ther 2011: 13; 203–213.

[31] Funakubo Asanuma Y. Accelerated atherosclerosis and inflammation in systemic lupus erythematosus. Nihon Rhinsho Meneki Gakkai Kaishi 2012: 35; 470–480.

[32] Skaggs BJ, Hahn BH, McMahon M. The role of the immune system in atherosclerosis: molecules, mechanisms an implications for management of cardiovascular risk and disease in patients with rheumatic diseases. Nat Rev Rheumatol 2012: 8; 214–223.

[33] Vadacca M, Zardi EM, Margiotta D, Rigon A, Cacciapaglia F, Arcarese L, Buzzulini F, Amoroso A, Afeltra A. Leptin, adiponectin and vascular stiffness parameters in women with systemic lupus erythematosus. Intern Emerg Med 2013: 8; 705–712.

[34] Parker B, Urowitz MB, Gladman DD, Lunt M, Bae S-CH et al. Clinical associations of the metabolic syndrome in systemic lupus erythematosus: data from an international inception cohort. Ann Rheum Dis 2013: 72; 1308–1314.

[35] McMahon M, Hahn BH, Skaggs BJ. Systemic lupus erythematosus and cardiovascular disease: prediction and potential for therapeutic intervention. Expert Rev Clin Immunol 2011: 7; 227–241.

[36] Blasi C. The autoimmune origin of atherosclerosis. Atherosclerosis 2008: 201; 17–32

[37] Shoenfeld Y, Gerli R, Doria A, Matsuura E, Cerinic MM, Ronda N, Jara LJ, Abu-Shakra M, Meroni PL, Sherer Y. Accelerated atherosclerosis in autoimmune rheumatic diseases. Circulation 2005: 112; 3337–3347.

[38] Haque S, Gordon C, Isenberg D, Rahman A, Lanyon P et al. Risk fctors for clinical coronary heart disease in systemic lupus erythematosus: the lupus and atherosclerosis evaluation of risk [LASER] study. J Rheumatol 2010: 37; 322–329.

[39] Shoenfeld Y, Sherer Y, Harats D. Atherosclerosis as an infectious, inflammatory and autoimmune disease. Trends Immunol 2001: 22; 293–295.

[40] Gonzalez-Gay MA, Vazquez-Rodriguez TR, Garcia-Unzueta MT, Berja A, Miranda-Filloy JA, de Matias JM, Gonzalez-Juanatey C, Liorca J. Visfatin is not associated with inflammation or metabolic syndrome in patients with severe rheumatoid arthritis undergoing anti-TNF-α therapy. Clin Exp Rheumatol 2010: 28; 56–62.

[41] Sherer Y, Zinger H, Shoenfeld Y. Atherosclerosis in systemic lupus erythematosus. Autoimmunity 2010: 43; 98–102.

[42] Scotece M, Conde J, Gómez R, López V, Pino J, González A, Lago F, Gómez-Reino JJ, Gualillo O. Role of adipokines in atherosclerosis: interference with cardiovascular complications in rheumatic diseases. Mediators Inflamm 2012: Article ID125458.

[43] Romero-Diaz J, Vargas-Vóracková F, Kimura-Hayama E, Cortázar-Benitez E, Gijón-Mitre R, Criales S, Cabiedes-Contreras J, Ińiguez-Rodriguez Mdel R, Lora-Garcia EA, Núńez-Alvarez C, Liorente L, Aguilar-Salinas C, Sánocha-Guerreo J. Systemic lupus erythematosus risk factors for coronary artery calcifications. Rheumatology 2012: 51; 110–119.

[44] Roman MJ, Shanker B-A, Davis A, Lockshin MD, Sammaritano L, Simantov R, Crow MK, Schwartz JE, Paget SA, Devereux RB, Salmon JE. Prevalence and correlates of accelerated atherosclerosis in systemic lupus erythematosus. N Eng J Med 2003: 349; 2399–2406.

[45] Zinger H, Sherer Y, Shoenfeld Y. Atherosclerosis in autoimmune rheumatic diseases-mechanisms and clinical findings. Clin Rev Allerg Immunol 2009: 37; 20–28.

[46] Hrycek E, Franek A, Błaszczak E, Dworak J, Hrycek A. Serum levels of selected chemokines in systemic lupus erythematosus patients. Rheumatol Int 2013: 33; 242–247.

[47] Baran A, Flisiak I, Chodynicka B. Znaczenie wybranych adipokin w łuszczycy. Przegl Dermatol 2011: 98; 422–428.

[48] Bozaoglu K, Segal D, Shields KA, Cummings N, Curran JE, Comuzzie AG, Mahaney C, Rainwater DL, VandeBerg JL, MacCluer JW, Collier G, Blangero J, Walder K, Jowett JBM. Chemerin is associated with metabolic syndrome phenotypes in a Mexican-American population. J Clin Endocrinol Metab 2009: 94; 3085–3088.

[49] McMahon M, Skaggs B, Sahakian L, Grossman J, FritzGerald J, Ragavendra N,Charles-Schoeman CH, Chernishof M, Gorn A, Witztum JL, Wong WK, Weisman M, Wallace DJ, La Cava A, Hahn BH. High plasma leptin levels confer increased risk of atherosclerosis in women with systemic lupus erythematosus, and are associated with inflammatory oxidized lipids. Ann Rheum Dis 2011: 70; 1619–1624.

[50] Vadacca M, Margiotta D, Rigon A, Cacciapaglia F, Coppolino G, Amoroso A, Afeltra A. Adipokines and systemic lupus erythematosus: relationships with metabolic syndrome and cardiovascular disease risk factors. J Rheumatol 2009: 36; 295–297.

[51] Chung CP, Avales I, Oeser A, Gebretsodik T, Shintani A, Raggi P, Stein CM. High prevalence of the metabolic syndrome in patients with systemic lupus erythematosus: association with disease characteristics and cardiovascular risk factors. Ann Rheum Dis 2007: 66; 208–214.

[52] Bultink IEM, Turkstra F, Diamant M, Dijkmans BAC, Voskuyl AE. Prevalence of and risk factors for the metabolic syndrome in women with systemic lupus erythematosus. Clin Exp Rheumatol 2008: 26; 32–38.

[53] Tellels R, Lanna C, Ferreira G, Ribeiro A. Metabolic syndrome in patients with systemic lupus erythematosus: association with traditional risk factors for coronary heart disease and lupus characteristics. Lupus 2010: 19; 803–809.

[54] dos Santos FMM, Borges MC, Telles RW, Correia MITD, Lanna CCD. Excess weight and associated risk factors in patients with systemic lupus erythematosus. Rheumatol Int 2013: 33; 681–688.

[55] Gómez R, Conde J, Scotece M, Gómez-Reino J, Lago F, Gualillo O. What's new in our understanding of the role of adipokines in rheumatic diseases? Nat Rev Rheumatol 2011: 7; 528–536.

[56] Barbosa VS, Rêgo J, da Silva NA. Possible role of adipokines in systemic lupus erythematosus and rheumatoid arthritis. Rev Bras Rheumatol 2012: 52; 271–287.

[57] Chung CP, Long AG, Solus JF, Rho YH, Oeser A, Raggi P, Stein M. Adipocytokines in systemic lupus erythematosus: relationships to inflammation, insulin resistance and coronary atherosclerosis. Lupus 2009: 18; 799–806.

[58] Krysiak R, Handzlik-Orlik G, Okopień B. The role of adipokines in connective tissue diseases. Eur J Nutr 2012: 51; 513–528.

[59] Olewicz-Gawlik A, Dańczak-Pazdrowska A, Klama K, Mackiewicz S, Silny W, Hrycaj P. Rola adipokin w patogenezie twardziny układowej – badania własne i przegląd literatury. Reumatologia 2009: 47; 329–331.

[60] Szadkowska A. Adipokiny w Miażdżyca u Dzieci i Młodzieży. Redakcja Mirosława Urban. Wydawca Cornetis 2007r.

[61] Juge-Aubry CHE, Henrichot E, Meier CHA. Adipose tissue: a regulator of inflammation. Best Pract Res Clin Endocrinol Metab 2005: 19; 547–566.

[62] Lago F, Dieguez C, Gómez-Reino J, Gualillo O. The emerging role of adipokines as mediators of inflammation and immune responses. Cytokine Growth Factor Rev 2007: 18; 313–325.

[63] Lago F, Dieguez C, Gómez-Reino J, Gualillo O. Adipokines as emerging mediators of immune response and inflammation. Nature Publishing Group. Nat Clin Pract Rheumatol 2007: 3; 716–724.

[64] Niedzwiedzka-Rystwej P, Deptuła W. Tkanka tłuszczowa a układ odpornościowy. Allergia Astma Immunol 2009: 15; 101–105.

[65] Al M, Ng L, Tyrrell P, Bargman J, Bradley T, Silverman E. Adipokines as novel biomarkers to pediatric systemic lupus erythematosus. Rheumatology 2009: 48; 497–501.

[66] Tilg H, Moschen AR. Adipocytokines: mediators linking adipose tissue, inflammation and immunity. Nature Publishing Group. Nat Rev Immunol 2006: 6; 773–783.

[67] Guzik TJ, Mangalat D, Korbut R. Adipokines – novel link between inflammation and vascular function? J Physiol Pharmacol 2006: 57; 505–528.

[68] Wu Z, Zhao S. Adipocyte: a potential target for the treatment of atherosclerosis. Med Hypoth 2006: 67; 82–86.

[69] Baessler A, Schlossbauer S, Stark K, Strack CH, Riegger G, Schunkert H, Hengstenberg C, Fischer M. Adiponectin multimetric forms but not total adiponectin levels are associated with myocardial infarction in non-diabetic men. J Atheroscler Thromb 2011: 18; 616–627.

[70] Lawlor DA, Davey Smith G, Ebrahim S, Thompson S, Sattor N. Plasma adiponectin levels are associated with insulin resistance, but do not predict future risk of coronary heart disease in women. J Clin Endocrinol Metab 2005: 90; 5677–5683.

[71] Khalili P, Flyvbjerg A, Frystyk J, Lundin F, Jundle J, Engstrom, Nilsson PM. Total adiponectins does not predict cardiovascular events in middle-aged men in a prospective long-term follow-up study. Diab Metab 2010: 31; 137–143.

[72] Miranda-Filloy JA, López-Mejias R, Genre F, Carnero-López B, Ochoa R, Diaz de Terán T, González-Juanatey C, Blanco R, González-Gay MA. Adiponectin and resistin serum levels in non-diabetic ankylosing spondylitis patients undergoing TNF-α antagonist therapy. Clin Exp Rheumatol 2013: 31; 365–371.

[73] Bokarewa M, Nagaev I, Dahlberg L, Smith U, Tarkowski A. Resistin an adipokine with potent proinflammatory properties. J Immunol 2005: 174; 5789–5795.

[74] Reilly MP, Lehrke M, Wolfe ML, Rohatgi A, Lazar MA, Rader DJ. Resistin is an inflammatory marker of atherosclerosis in humans. Circulation 2005: 111; 932–939.

[75] Almehed K, d'Elia HF, Bokarewa M, Carlsten H. Role of resistin as a marker of inflammation in systemic lupus erythematosus. Ann Res Ther 2008: 10; 1–9.

[76] Johnston A, Arnadottir S, Gudjonsson JE, Aphale A, Sigmarsdottir AA, Gunnarsson SJ, Steinsson JT, Elder JT, Valdimarsson H. Obesity in psoriasis; leptin and resistin as mediators of cutaneous inflammation. Br J Dermatol 2008: 159; 342–350.

[77] Kumor-Kisielewska A, Kierszniewska-Stępień D, Pietras T, Kroczyńska-Bednarek J, Kurmanowska Z, Antczak A, Górski P. Assessment of leptin and resistin levels in patients with chronic obstructive pulmonary disease. Pol Arch Med Wewn 2013: 123; 215–220.

[78] Baker JF, Morales M, Qatanani M, Cucchira A, Nackos E, Lazar MA, Teff K, von Feldt JM. Resistin levels in lupus and association with disease-specific measures, insulin resistance, and coronary calcification. J Rheumatol 2011: 38; 2369–2375.

[79] Fiková M, Haluzik M, Gay S, Šenolt L. The role of resistin as a reulator of inflammation: implications for various human pathologies. Clin Immunol 2009: 133; 157–170.

[80] Jung HS, Park KH, Cho YM, Chung SS, Cho HJ, Cho SY, Kim SJ, Kim SY, Lee HK, Park KS. Resistin is secreted from macrophages in atheromas and promotes atherosclerosis. Cardiovasc Res 2006: 69: 76–85.

[81] Zheng H, Xu H, Xie N, Huang J, Fang H, Luo M. Association of serum resistin with peripheral arterial disease. Pol Arch Med Wewn 2013: 123; 680–685.

[82] Beltowski J. Leptin and atherosclerosis. Atherosclerosis 2006: 189; 47–60.

[83] Beltowski J. Role of leptin in blood pressure regulation and arterial hypertension. J Hypertens 2006: 24; 789–801.

[84] Matarese G, Maschos S, Mantzoros CS. Leptin in immunology. J Immunol 2005: 174; 3137–3142.

[85] Lord GM, Matarese G, Howard JK, Baker RJ, Blooms SR, Lechler RI. Leptin modulates the T-cell immune response and reverses starvation-induced immunosuppression. Nature 1998: 394; 897–901.

[86] Scotece M, Conde J, Gómez R, López V, Lago F, Gómez-Reino J, Gualillo O. Beyond fat mass: exploring the role of adipokines in rheumatic diseases. Sci World J 2011: 11; 1932–1947.

[87] Garcia-Gonzalez A, Gonzalez-Lopez L, Valera-Gonzalez IC, Gardona-Muñoz EG, Salazar-Parmo M, González-Ortiz M, Martinez-Abundis E, Gamez-Nawa JI. Serum leptin levels in women with systemic lupus erythematosus. Rheumatol Int 2002: 22; 138–141.

[88] Xu W-D, Zhang M, Zhang Y-J, Liu S-S, Pan H-F, Ye DQ. Association between leptin and systemic lupus erythematosus. Rheumatol Int 2014: 34; 559–563.

[89] Otero M, Lago R, Gomez R, Dieguez C, Lago F, Gómez-Reino J, Gualillo O. Towards a pro-inflammatory and immunomodulatory emergin role of leptin. Rheumatology 2006: 45; 944–950.

[90] De Sanctis JB, Zabaleta M, Bianco NE, Garmendia JV, Rivas L. Serum adipokine levels in patients with systemic lupus erythematosus. Autoimmunity 2009: 42; 272–274.

[91] Wisłowska M, Rok M, Stępień K, Kuklo-Kowalska A. Serum leptin in systemic lupus erythematosus. Rheumatol Int 2008: 28; 467–473.

[92] Lara-Castro C, Fu Y, Chung BH, Garvey WT. Adiponectin and metabolic syndrome: mechanisms mediating risk for metabolic and cardiovascular diseases. Curr Opin Lipidol 2007: 18; 263–270.

[93] Rovin BH, Song H, Herbert LA, Nadasdy T, Nadasdy G, Birmingham DJ, Yu CY, Nagaraja HN. Plasma, urine and renal expression of adiponectin in human systemic lupus erythematosus. Kidney Intern 2005: 68; 1825–1833.

[94] Fantuzzi G. Adiponectin and inflammation: consensus and controversy. J Allergy Clin Immunol 2008: 121; 326–330.

[95] Song H, Chan J, Rovin BH. Induction of chemokine expression by adiponectin in vitro is isoform dependent. Transl Res 2009: 54; 18–26.

Chapter 7

Idiopathic Osteonecrosis and Atypical Femoral Fracture in Systemic Lupus Erythematosus

Takeshi Kuroda and Hiroe Sato

Additional information is available at the end of the chapter

http://dx.doi.org/10.5772/intechopen.68143

Abstract

Osteonecrosis and osteoporosis are frequent adverse effects of glucocorticoid therapy of systemic lupus erythematosus (SLE). Idiopathic osteonecrosis (ION) of the femoral head occurs in 3–40% of patients receiving glucocorticoid, and can also develop in other bones. Higher doses of glucocorticoid and steroid pulse therapy are considered to be risk factors for ION of the femoral head. To analyze these risk factors, it seems important to detect early changes in the femoral head by magnetic resonance imaging and to monitor early clinical events attributable to steroid therapy. Prophylaxis with statins and warfarin remains debatable. The use of glucocorticoid is increase the risk of bone fractures. Bisphosphonate (BP) is used for its prevention and treatment of osteoporosis. Atypical femoral fracture (AFF) has been recently recognized as a complication associated with BP use. AFF is considered to be a form of stress fracture; localized periosteal thickening of the lateral cortex is often present at the fracture site. The thickening has been recently recognized as a complication associated with the use of antiresorptive agents such as BP and denosumab. As long-term BP/glucocorticoid use is a risk factor for beaking in patients with SLE , temporary withdrawal of BP administration should be considered.

Keywords: systemic lupus erythematosus, glucocorticoid, osteonecrosis, bisphosphonate, atypical femoral fracture

1. Introduction

Systemic lupus erythematosus (SLE) is a chronic, inflammatory, systemic autoimmune disease of unknown etiology characterized by production of antinuclear autoantibodies. It mainly affects young women and shows a broad spectrum of manifestations such as general fatigue, skin rash, fever, and arthritis and disorders involving the kidney, heart, and central nervous system. These organ involvements occur in patients with severer disease status and indicate a poor prognosis. Glucocorticoid has been used as a first-line therapy for SLE. Glucocorticoid exerts strong anti-inflammatory effects and is widely used for the treatment of uncontrolled disease activity in patients with SLE, such as central nervous system lupus (CNS), severe lupus nephritis, and other life-threatening conditions [1]. Glucocorticoid therapy is successful in most cases when high doses are employed, and as a result the prognosis of the SLE has improved remarkably. On the other hand, as glucocorticoid has adverse side effects on many organ systems, only the minimum effective dose is used for treatment. For example, skin thinning and purpura are commonly observed, and the risk of both cataracts and glaucoma is increased. Glucocorticoid use is associated with an increased risk of ischemic heart disease and heart failure, and also an increased risk of gastritis, gastric ulcer, and gastrointestinal bleeding. In the musculoskeletal system, osteoporosis is one of the more serious adverse effects of glucocorticoid [2], and osteonecrosis is also a significant problem [3]. Bisphosphonate (BP) is a key drug used for prevention and treatment of osteoporosis. The risk of osteonecrosis caused by glucocorticoid is higher in patients with SLE. Glucocorticoid causes a dose-dependent, mild increase in the fasting glucose level and a greater increase in postprandial hyperglycemia in patients without preexisting diabetes mellitus (DM), whereas it worsens control of the blood glucose level in patients with DM. The adverse effect of glucocorticoid on atherosclerotic vascular disease is thought to be mediated in part by elevated levels of nonfunctional lipoprotein. In patients with SLE, the adverse effects of glucocorticoid on lipid profiles are dose-dependent, occurring only at prednisone doses exceeding 10 mg/day. Systemic glucocorticoid also has many effects on both innate and acquired immunity, resulting in a dose-dependent increase in the risk of infection, especially with common bacterial, viral, and fungal pathogens [4]. Conventional immunosuppressive agents such as mycophenolate mofetil, azathioprine, and cyclophosphamide are also widely used in the management of SLE, and current treatment regimens optimize the use of these agents while minimizing their potential toxicity [5]. Tacrolimus may be particularly useful as adjunctive therapy in patients with persistent proteinuria despite other therapies, and in the management of lupus nephritis in pregnancy. The advent of biological agents has advanced the treatment of SLE, particularly in patients with refractory disease. The CD20 monoclonal antibody rituximab and the anti-BLyS agent belimumab are widely used in clinical practice. The prognosis of SLE has improved markedly, and long-term survival has increased. Prior to 1955, fewer than 50% of patients survived 5 years after diagnosis whereas now, 10-year survival exceeds 90% [6]. Our recent data have also confirmed that the 5-year survival rates of patients diagnosed as having SLE before 1970, between 1970 and 1979, between 1980 and 1989, between 1990 and 1999, and after 2000 were 71.4, 83.1, 94.5, 93.4, and 96.4%, respectively. Previously, the causes of death in patients with SLE were mainly infection and renal disease, but recently atherosclerotic cardiovascular disease emerging in the long term has become a focus of concern. Musculoskeletal conditions that impair the quality of life have also become problematic, including osteonecrosis and atypical femoral fracture (AFF). Here we discuss osteonecrosis and AFF in patients with SLE.

2. Incidence, etiology, and pathogenesis

Idiopathic osteonecrosis (ION) of the femoral head occurs frequently (3–40%) in patients receiving glucocorticoid for underlying conditions such as nephrotic syndrome and renal transplantation [7–10]. It is also known to occur as one of the serious complications of glucocorticoid treatment *of* SLE. Among several factors *related to* ION, glucocorticoid therapy is considered to be one of *essential* importance [3]. There have been *a lot of* reports of ION onset in SLE patients to date, but the *exact* incidence of ION in this group is unknown. The etiology or pathogenesis of this disorder has not been fully clarified, and no prophylaxis has been established to date. The risk of ION in SLE patients is considered to be due to both the SLE itself and the concomitant use of glucocorticoid because, in occasional cases, ION has been noted in the absence of glucocorticoid therapy [3]. In addition, the risk of developing ION has been linked to numerous factors such as glucocorticoid use, alcohol consumption, cigarette smoking, and several rheumatic diseases including SLE. Although the pathogenesis remains unclear, involvement of lipid metabolism abnormality [11], hypercoagulability [12], oxidative stress [13], and vascular endothelial dysfunction [14] has been suggested from basic and clinical research. Several studies investigating the association of ION with steroid treatment have yielded conflicting results with regard to the cumulative dosage, maximum dose, route of administration, and duration of treatment. Glucocorticoid dose and duration seem to be important factors related to ION, but there is considerable controversy about this issue [3, 15–20]. ION may develop in patients who have received high-dose, short-term, or long-term steroid. However, in the early phase, the relationship between steroid and ION has yet been not fully investigated. In our present study, the patients were treated with steroid for the first time, and our observation period was short. Additionally, the initial dose of prednisolone (PSL) for treatment of SLE has sometimes been determined according to the patient's weight or body surface area (BSA) [21]. Therefore, we investigated the relationship of body mass index (BMI) [22] and BSA with the initial dose of PSL. We found that the initial dose of PSL, steroid pulse therapy, BMI, and BSA were not correlated with asymptomatic ION, similar to the results obtained by Sekiya et al. [23]. Also, we failed to identify any relationship between BMI, BSA, the initial dose of PSL per unit BW, the initial dose of PSL relative to BMI, or the initial dose of PSL relative to BSA. None of the factors evaluated were associated with asymptomatic ION. Recent meta-analysis data have shown that the likelihood of ION developing in patients receiving glucocorticoid at more than 20 mg/day is significantly higher than in patients receiving less than 20 mg/day. In the early phase, corticosteroid at over 20 mg/day may trigger ION. In addition, it has been revealed that increasing the steroid dose at the time of SLE recurrence is a risk factor for development of new ION [24].

3. Timing of osteonecrosis-related ischemia in patients with SLE

Radiographically, at the earliest stage of ION, plain radiographs show normal features, whereas axial and coronal T1- and T2-weighted MR images show low-density signals in the femoral head (**Figure 1**).

From this viewpoint, osteonecrosis associated with renal transplantation can provide important information. The band patterns on MRI correspond to repair tissue located between necrotic and intact areas [25, 26]. Thus, there is a time lag between the occurrence of ischemia and the appearance of the band pattern. It has been reported that 1 month after internal fixation of a femoral neck fracture, MRI can reveal band patterns in the femoral head away

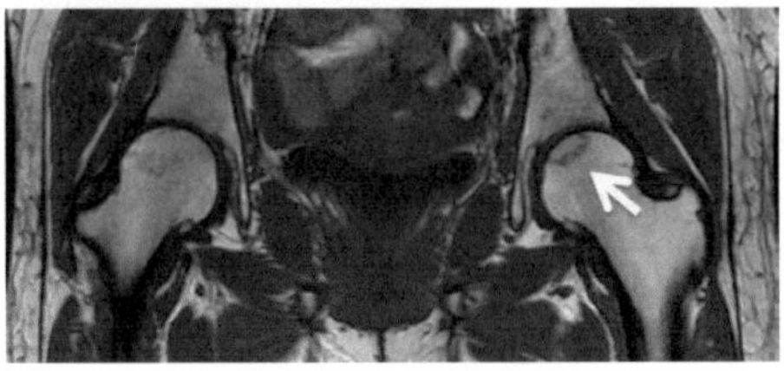

Figure 1. A T1-weighted image demonstrates a ring-like subchondral area of osteonecrosis (white arrow) present in the femoral head.

from the fracture line [27]. In patients who develop ION after renal transplantation, it is presumed that intraosseous ischemia occurs earlier than 6–12 weeks postoperatively [28, 29] when band patterns are observed on T1-weighted MRI. In experimental animal models of osteonecrosis, it has been shown that intraosseous ischemia occurs quite soon after administration of large doses of steroid, that is, on the fifth and third day, respectively. The total dose of steroid administered in the first 2 weeks after renal transplantation is related to ION development [30]. This suggests the occurrence of an event in the bone that may lead to the development of ION at a very early stage after steroid administration. The widespread use of MRI now makes it possible to detect osteonecrotic change in SLE patients soon after administration of glucocorticoid, thus facilitating early diagnosis. Nagasawa et al. reported that 33% of patients developed ION within 3 months after the start of glucocorticoid treatment and that symptomatic ION became apparent at 2 years and beyond [31]. Radiographically, a subchondral radiolucency known as the crescent sign appeared at a late stage in ION, indicating subchondral fracture. However, that study was a multicenter one, and several strategies were selected for treatment of SLE according to the clinical conditions of the patients, resulting in slight differences among the participating hospitals. Several strategies have been selected for treatment of SLE *in conformity with* the clinical conditions of the affected patients, and there are *many* differences among hospitals, such as the indications for immunosuppressants. However, for any study performed at a single institution, the strategy *of treatment*, the steroid *selection*, the initial dose of steroid, and concomitant drugs would be more uniform. In addition, the speed of steroid tapering would also be quite uniform. This would allow better clarification of the background factors associated with ION. On the basis of this concept, we investigated the early development of ION in a cohort of strictly selected SLE patients using MRI and the early changes in laboratory parameters associated with steroid therapy [32].

4. Classification of osteonecrosis

Diagnosis of ION of the femoral head relies on the combination of clinical symptoms and radiographs and/or magnetic resonance imaging (MRI) *changes*. To evaluate the evolution of ION of the femoral head, the Ficat (**Table 1**) [33] and the Association Research Circulation Osseous (ARCO) classification (**Table 2**) [34] are *generally* used to *evaluate* both imaging modalities. For comparative purposes, these classifications need to be reliable and *uniform definition* to provide sufficient therapy options for the patient.

Stage	Radiographic signs	Clinical features
0	Inconspicuous/normal findings	0 ("silent hip")
I	Inconspicuous findings or minor changes (slight patchy osteoporosis, blurring of trabecular pattern, subtle loss of clarity)	+
II A	Diffuse/focal radiological changes (osteoporosis, sclerosis, cysts)	+
II B	Subchondral fracture ("crescent sign") segmental flattening of femoral head ("out-of-round appearance")	+
III	Broken contour of femoral head, bone sequestrum, joint space normal	++
IV	Flattened contour of femoral head, decreased joint space collapse of femoral head, acetabular osteoarthritic changes	+++

Table 1. Scheme of Ficat classification (1985).

Stage	Radiological findings	Subclassification	
0	Positive: histology negative/normal: radiograph/CT/MRI/scintigraphy	–	
I	Positive: MRI and/or bone scintigraphy negative/normal: radiograph/CT	+	(a)
II	Radiograph: sclerotic, cystic or osteoporotic changes of femoral head	+	(a)
III	Radiograph: subchondral fracture ("crescent sign")	+	(a)
IV	Radiograph: flattening of femoral head	++	(b)
V	Radiograph: flattening of femoral head and osteoarthritic changes: decreased joint space and acetabular changes	+++	(b)
VI	Complete joint destruction	–	

Note: (a) Location of femoral head necrosis: (1) medial third, (2) median third, and (3) lateral third. Size of femoral head necrosis: (A) <15%, (B) 15–30%, (C) >30%.

(b) Intrusion degree of femoral head contour: (A) <2 mm, (B) 2–4 mm, and (C) >4 mm.

Table 2. Scheme of ARCO classification system (1992).

5. Early changes in MRI features and laboratory parameters of SLE patients

In previous multicenter studies, several strategies were selected for treatment of SLE according to the clinical conditions of the patients, resulting in slight differences among the participating hospitals. This allowed us to investigate the very early development of ION at 3 months after the start of steroid therapy using MRI imaging to clarify the background factors associated with ION. We found that the prevalence of asymptomatic ION among our patients was 26.9%, similar to that described previously [23]. We found no differences in the clinical characteristics of the patients, such as sex, age, height, and body weight and clinical features. The Systemic Lupus Erythematosus Disease Activity Index (SLEDAI) *is shown to be a valid and reliable measure of disease activity of SLE patients* [35]. The SLEDAI score *is assessed using a combination of clinical history, physical examination, organ-specific function test and serological test.* Almost all of our patients showed high or very high disease activity at the time of steroid initiation. However, the SLEDAI score was not correlated with asymptomatic ION [32]. In SLE, as is the case for antiphospholipid syndrome (APS), about 30–40% of patients have detectable antiphospholipid antibodies [36] and a positive lupus anticoagulant test and anticardiolipin antibody are detected in approximately 10–30% and 20–40% of patients, respectively. The prevalence of a so-called clinically significant anticardiolipin profile is considered to be about 30–40% [37]. APS antibodies as a prothrombotic factor might predispose to ION by causing microvascular thrombosis. However, the link between APS antibodies and ION is controversial [38–41]. In our study, there was no significant association between APS antibody and ION [32]. A Japanese nationwide study revealed that cigarette smoking was an independent risk factor for ION [42]. However, in our present study, cigarette smoking was not correlated with ION in SLE patients [32].

6. Serological parameters and ION

Serological activity of SLE was determined on the basis of decreased CH50 and increased anti-DNA antibodies. We also investigated serological parameters such as C3, C4, CH50, and anti-ds DNA antibody, as well as renal function parameters such as the serum creatinine level, estimated glomerular filtration rate, and *proteinuria*. However, these factors were *not* correlated with ION. Thus, both *initial* serological *disease* activity and *initial* renal function, as the most common forms of organ involvement, did not appear to be correlated with ION [32]. Similar results were obtained in a previous single-center study [23].

7. Lipid levels, statins, and ION

Several studies of ION have indicated the association of lipid. Nagasawa et al. [31] investigated the rate of increase in serum total cholesterol (TC) levels 1 month after glucocorticoid administration in patients with new-onset SLE, and found that they were significantly high in the ION group. It was also found that lipid levels, and the rates of increase in almost all the TC and triglyceride (TG) parameters, were higher in the group that developed ION. TC levels tended to be higher than that in the non-ION group, and the maximum levels and *increasing rates* were significantly higher, suggesting that a rapid rise in serum lipids soon after an increase in glucocorticoid dose might affect the onset of ION [23]. Our data *suggested* that the level of TG both before and after the *initiation* of steroid *therapy* was higher in patients with ION [32]. *The TG level before PSL therapy was associated future risk of asymptomatic ION.* As the *association* between TG before PSL therapy and the initial dose of PSL was not significant, the effect of *TG* before PSL therapy on asymptomatic ION would not have been modified by the initial dose of subsequent PSL. Several studies have *shown* that a high TG level is a strong risk factor for *stroke and ischemic heart disease* [43–45]. ION is caused by partial or total *interruption* of blood flow to the femoral head, and SLE patients *thought to* develop asymptomatic ION through a similar mechanism. *Additionally*, it is well known that steroid *therapy* induces iatrogenic metabolic syndrome, and *from this point of view*, a high TG level is considered to be an important risk factor for asymptomatic ION. Furthermore, *the TC level* after steroid *therapy* tended to be higher in patients with asymptomatic ION. *However*, the levels of high-density lipoprotein cholesterol (HDL-C) and low-density lipoprotein cholesterol (LDL-C) were not correlated with asymptomatic ION. As described previously, the TC level after 1 month of steroid treatment was significantly higher in patients with asymptomatic ION. Our data are similar to those reported previously [46]. In the early phase, lipids—especially TG—play an important role in the development of ION in patients with SLE. HMG-CoA reductase inhibitors (statins) have been widely used for the treatment of dyslipidemia as well as for prevention of *ischemic heart* disease. *According to* a chicken model, Wang et al. suggested that lovastatin prevented steroid-induced ION [47], and a study by Nishida et al. using a rabbit model also *revealed* that pitavastatin had a similar effect [48]. In humans, it has been reported that the incidence of osteonecrosis was decreased by 1% by administration of statins in a study of 284 patients with various disorders (excluding SLE) who received glucocorticoid treatment [49]. We used pravastatin, pitavastatin, lovastatin, and atorvastatin for prevention of ION, but no such preventive effect was observed [32]. Until now, no randomized controlled trial has been reported to successfully prevent steroid-induced ION. In patients with SLE, treatment with statins alone is insufficient for prevention of ION.

8. Prevention of osteonecrosis

In patients at risk of osteonecrosis, several factors are controllable, and thus prevention is the best approach. Hyperlipidemia and DM should be managed appropriately and alcohol consumption minimized [42]. Smoking should also be avoided, if possible [50]. The dosage of glucocorticoid should be minimized as far as possible, as described previously. Statins may help to protect against osteonecrosis. One database review found that only 1% of 284 patients developed ION after treatment with statins before glucocorticoid use. In renal transplant recipients, among 338 patients who were treated with statins, 15 (4.4%) developed ION and among 2543 patients who were not treated with statins, 180 (7%) patients developed ION [49]. Antioxidant agents have been shown to inhibit osteonecrosis in animal models [51]. Further accumulation of similar studies is needed to clarify the preventive effect of statins against SLE-associated ION.

9. Treatment of ION

The management of ION is usually determined by the degree of femoral head involvement. If the subchondral shell remains intact, there is still a possibility of healing, but if collapse occurs, healing is impossible. If the necrotic area is small and there are no symptoms, ION should be followed up because some cases may spontaneously progress over time. If femoral head ION is diagnosed early, core depression is a commonly used form of prophylactic surgery to prevent the development of arthritis. One study has demonstrated long-term spontaneous repair of osteonecrotic lesions during low-dose glucocorticoid therapy [52]. Conservative treatment of ION involves limiting the degree of weight-bearing on the hip joint in conjunction with analgesia. In general, simple observation may be considered for asymptomatic lesions. Symptomatic lesions will likely progress to collapse, and if observation is chosen, the next joint-preserving procedure should be considered. Various forms of medication have been tried. BP is regularly used for prevention of insufficiency fractures, and several studies have shown that alendronate can reduce pain and slow the progression of collapse [53–55]. Treatment with BP is effective before subchondral collapse, but after subchondral collapse, the effects of treatment for inhibiting destruction of the femoral head are limited. Lipid-lowering agents, especially statins, are hypothesized to have a protective effect against ON. The prevalence of a clinically significant antiphospholipid profile is approximately 20% in SLE patients, and these antiphospholipid antibodies are believed to contribute to ION though hypercoagulation. Accordingly, anticoagulation therapy has been tried for prevention of ION in SLE patients, and warfarin has been modestly beneficial in this respect. One study of 60 SLE patients receiving prednisolone at more than 40 mg/day found that treatment with warfarin significantly reduced the onset of ION [31]. Among various physical modalities, extracorporeal shockwave therapy, hyperbaric oxygen, and pulsed electromagnetic therapy have yielded encouraging results, but further large prospective studies will be necessary to confirm these effects. Surgical treatments to prevent joint destruction include hip arthroplasty, core decompression, osteotomy, and vascularized bone grafting. Core decompression is commonly performed as prophylactic surgery for pre-collapse osteonecrosis of the femoral head. This decreases intramedullary pressure within the femoral head and neck, and has been postulated to improve blood circulation to the femoral head. Core decompression is often combined with bone grafting to help regenerate healthy bone and support cartilage at the hip joint. Bone grafting involves transplantation of healthy bone tissue to an area of the body where it is needed. Another option that has had some degree of success is harvesting and *in vitro* culture of autologous mesenchymal stem cells and their re-implantation into the core decompression site [56–58]. Long-term studies to confirm the success of this approach are still underway. Hip arthroplasty is the most commonly performed procedure for postcollapse lesions of the femoral head. Recent mid- and long-term studies have yielded satisfactory results [59]. Transtrochanteric anterior rotational osteotomy moves the symptomatic portion of the antero-superior femoral head out of the weight-bearing dome, enabling the normal posterior aspect of the head to bear weight, thus helping to preserve the joint [60]. These procedures have yielded favorable success rates, but are associated with a moderate risk of nonunion. Vascularized fibular grafting is a more complex procedure in which a segment of bone is taken from the fibula of the patient, along with the arterial and venous blood supply. This is then transplanted into a hole created in the femoral neck and head. Vascularized fibular grafting has yielded successful outcomes in patients with precollapse lesions and moderate success in those with postcollapse lesions [61]. Additionally, use of autogenic or allogeneic cortical bone grafts and cancellous bone grafts has yielded good results for the treatment of precollapse and/or early precollapse osteonecrotic lesions of the femoral head.

10. Atypical femoral fracture

Glucocorticoid-induced osteoporosis (GIO) is an important problem in patients with SLE. BP is a key drug used for prevention and treatment of GIO. Patients with SLE often need to continue glucocorticoid and BP therapy for a long time, even if they are young. AFF has recently been recognized as a complication of long-term BP use [62, 63]. AFF is defined as a fracture located along the femoral diaphysis from just distal to the lesser trochanter to just proximal to the supracondylar flare, as distinguished from typical femoral fracture which occurs at the femoral neck or intertrochanteric area and is related to osteoporosis [63]. Diagnosis of AFF requires the presence of four of five major features (**Table 3**).

Beaking is one of these features, and is defined as localized periosteal or endosteal thickening of the lateral cortex at the fracture site. Since cortical thickening at the fracture site characterizes stress fracture, the mechanism of AFF is considered to involve stress [63]. The age-standardized incidence rates of AFF have been reported to be 16 per 100,000 person-years for patients treated with BPs over 5 years and 133 for those treated with BPs over 10 years [62], and AFF occurs much less frequently than osteoporosis-related fractures. However, once it occurs, it takes much time to heal [64, 65], and the daily life activities of the patient are often impaired. Risk factors for AFF other than long-term BP use include glucocorticoid therapy [66, 67], complicating connective tissue disease [67], lateral bowing of the femur [68, 69], a low level of serum 25-hydroxyvitamin D [66], and female gender [70]. Glucocorticoid therapy has been reported to have an important impact on AFF [66, 67], although no significant

To satisfy the case definition of AFF, the fracture must be located along the femoral diaphysis from just distal to the lesser trochanter to just proximal to the supracondylar flare. In addition, at least four of the five major features must be present. None of the minor features is required but have sometimes been associated with these fractures.
Major features
The fracture is associated with minimal or no trauma, as in a fall from a standing height or less
The fracture line originates at the lateral cortex and is substantially transverse in its orientation, although it may become oblique as it progresses medially across the femur
Complete fractures extend through both cortices and may be associated with a medial spike; incomplete fractures involve only the lateral cortex
The fracture is noncomminuted or minimally comminuted
Localized periosteal or endosteal thickening of the lateral cortex is present at the fracture site ("beaking" or "flaring")
Minor features
Generalized increase in cortical thickness of the femoral diaphyses
Unilateral or bilateral prodromal symptoms such as dull or aching pain in the groin or thigh
Bilateral incomplete or complete femoral diaphysis fractures
Delayed fracture healing

Table 3. ASBMR Task Force 2013 Revised Case Definition of AFFs [63].

association has yet been proved in several studies [71, 72]. Girgis et al. reviewed 152 femoral shaft fractures and classified 20 of them as AFF; they concluded that the use of glucocorticoid therapy for more than 6 months was significantly associated with AFF [66]. In a fracture location-, age-, and gender-matched case-control study, Saita et al. reviewed 2238 hip and femoral shaft fractures and diagnosed 10 of them as AFF, concluding that glucocorticoid therapy and complicating connective tissue disease were significant risk factors for AFF [67]. We recently evaluated the incidence of latent femoral beaking (**Figure 2**), which may precede AFF, in 125 patients with autoimmune diseases [65 (52%) with SLE] taking BP and glucocorticoid [73].

Our data revealed that the incidence of beaking was 8% and increased to 10% over 2 years. A case of complete AFF from the tip of the beaking occurred in one patient. The risk factors for beaking were BP therapy for a period of >4 years, age 40–60 years, and presence of diabetes mellitus [73]. Although few studies have investigated AFF in patients with SLE, the frequency of beaking in our study was thought to be higher than in conventional reports of AFF, possibly because all of the patients were taking BP (mean therapy duration 5.1 ± 2.7 years) and glucocorticoid (mean dose 10.0 ± 3.8 mg). Both BP and prolonged glucocorticoid therapy reduce bone remodeling [64, 74], thus, impairing the healing of microdamage occurring during normal daily life activities. BP also changes bone plasticity [75], and glucocorticoid therapy leads to a deterioration of bone quality [76]. Thus, a combination of BP and glucocorticoid therapies enhances microdamage accumulation, producing conditions in which beaking can easily occur. Generally, lateral bowing of the femur is considered to be a risk factor for AFF. Hyodo et al. indicated that

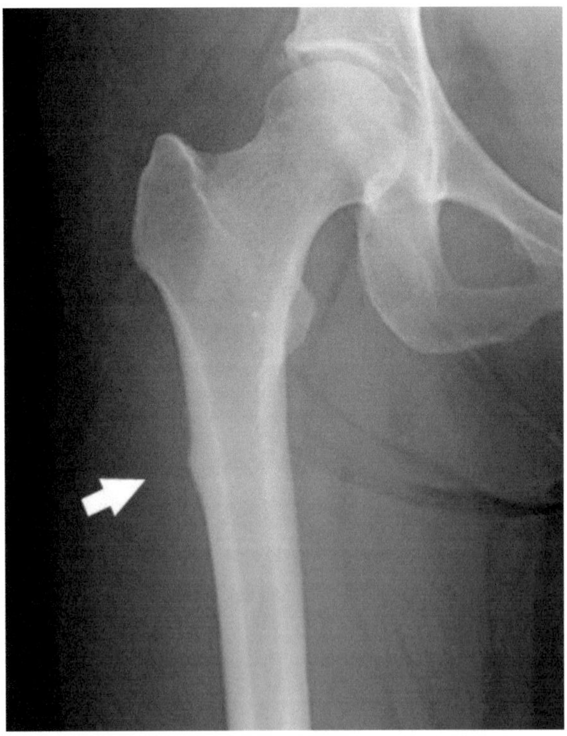

Figure 2. X-ray of the hip joint showing beaking (white arrow).

AFF located in the mid femur was significantly related to femoral bowing, whereas AFF in the proximal femur was related to glucocorticoid use [68]. In our previous study of patients with autoimmune diseases taking BP and glucocorticoid, the femoral beaking was mostly located at the subtrochanter, and was not related to lateral bowing of the femur [73]. Therefore, AFF and beaking in patients taking BP and glucocorticoid may generally occur irrespective of lateral femoral bowing. In order to properly benefit from BP and to minimize the risk of AFF, a BP "drug holiday" has been proposed. Postmenopausal women treated orally with BP for over 5 years can be considered for such a break in drug therapy if they have no osteoporotic fractures, their hip T score is >–2.5 and their fracture risk is not high [62]. For patients with GIO, few studies have investigated the safety and effectiveness of temporary drug withdrawal, and further studies are required. Because of the high frequency of beaking in patients taking BP and glucocorticoid [73], regular femoral X-ray screening for beaking is strongly recommended for AFF prevention, and once beaking is detected, a BP drug holiday should be considered.

11. Conclusion

SLE is a chronic inflammatory autoimmune disease mainly affecting young women; the mortality has recently been improved by treatments including glucocorticoid therapy. However, several adverse effects of glucocorticoid may decrease the quality of life. Even though some of these adverse effects have been overcome recently, AFF and ION are still persistent problems, and further work needs to be done to alleviate them.

Acknowledgements

This study was supported by a research grant from the Research Committee on Idiopathic Osteonecrosis of the Femoral Head of the Ministry of Health, Labour, and Welfare of Japan.

Author details

Takeshi Kuroda* and Hiroe Sato

*Address all correspondence to: kurodat@med.niigata-u.ac.jp

Niigata University Health Administration Center, Nishi-ku, Niigata City, Japan

References

[1] Boumpas DT, Chrousos GP, Wilder RL, Cupps TR, Balow JE. (1993). Glucocorticoid therapy for immune-mediated diseases: basic and clinical correlates. Ann Intern Med. 15;119(12): 1198–1208.

[2] Zonana-Nacach A, Barr SG, Magder LS, Petri M. (2000). Damage in systemic lupus erythematosus and its association with corticosteroids. Arthritis Rheum. 43(8): 1801–1808.

[3] Calvo-Alén J, McGwin G, Toloza S, Fernández M, Roseman JM, Bastian HM, Cepeda EJ, González EB, Baethge BA, Fessler BJ, Vilá LM, Reveille JD, Alarcón GS; LUMINA Study Group. Systemic lupus erythematosus in a multiethnic US cohort (LUMINA): XXIV. (2006). Cytotoxic treatment is an additional risk factor for the development of symptomatic osteonecrosis in lupus patients: results of a nested matched case-control study. Ann Rheum Dis. 65(6): 785–790.

[4] Kirou KA, Boumpus DT. Dubois' lupus erytheamtosus and related syndrome. Wallace DJ, Haln BH (Eds.) Saunders-Elsevier, Philadelphia. 2012. p. 597

[5] Kalunian KC, Kim M, Xie X, Baskaran A, Daly RP, Merrill JT. (2016). Impact of standard of care treatments and disease variables on outcomes in systemic lupus erythematosus trials: analysis from the Lupus Foundation of America Collective Data Analysis Initiative. Eur J Rheumatol. 3(1): 13–19.

[6] Moroni G, Quaglini S, Gallelli B, Banfi G, Messa P, Ponticelli C. (2007). The long-term outcome of 93 patients with proliferative lupus nephritis. Nephrol Dial Transplant. 22(9): 2531–2539.

[7] Abeles M, Urman JD, Rothfield NF. (1987). Aseptic necrosis of bone in systemic lupus erythematosus. Relationship to corticosteroid therapy. Arch Intern Med. 138(5): 750–754.

[8] Koo KH, Kim R. (1995). Quantifying the extent of osteonecrosis of the femoral head. A new method using MRI. J Bone Joint Surg Br. 77(6): 875–880.

[9] Landmann J, Renner N, Gächter A, Thiel G, Harder F. (1978). Cyclosporin a and osteonecrosis of the femoral head. J Bone Joint Surg Am. 69(8): 1226–1228.

[10] Mont MA, Hungerford DS. (1995). Non-traumatic avascular necrosis of the femoral head. J Bone Joint Surg Am 77(3): 459–474.

[11] Moskal JT, Topping RE, Franklin LL. (1997). Hypercholesterolemia: an association with osteonecrosis of the femoral head. Am J Orthop. 26(9): 609–612.

[12] Oinuma K, Harada Y, Nawata Y, Kobayashi K, Abe I, Kamikawa K, Moriya H. (2000). Sustained hemostatic abnormality in patients with steroid-induced osteonecrosis in the early period after high dose corticosteroid therapy. J Orthop Sci. 5(4): 374–379.

[13] Ichiseki T, Matsumoto T, Nishino M, Kaneuji A, Katsuda S. (2004). Oxidative stress and vascular permeability in steroid-induced osteonecrosis model. J Orthop Sci. 9(5): 509–515.

[14] Iuchi T, Akaike M, Mitsui T, Ohshima Y, Shintani Y, Azuma H, Matsumoto T. (2003). Glucocorticoid excess induces superoxide production in vascular endothelial cells and elicits vascular endothelial dysfunction. Circ Res. 92(1): 81–87.

[15] Abeles M, Urman JD, Rothfield NF. (1978). Aseptic necrosis of bone in systemic lupus erythematosus. Relationship to corticosteroid therapy. Arch Intern Med. 138(5): 750–754.

[16] Dimant J, Ginzler EM, Diamond HS, Schlesinger M, Marino CT, Weiner M, Kaplan D. (1978). Computer analysis of factors influencing the appearance of aseptic necrosis in patients with SLE. J Rheumatol. 5(2): 136–141.

[17] Nagasawa K, Tsukamoto H, Tada Y, Mayumi T, Satoh H, Onitsuka H, Kuwabara Y, Niho Y. (1994). Imaging study on the mode of development and changes in avascular necrosis of the femoral head in systemic lupus erythematosus: long-term observations. Br J Rheumatol. 33(4): 343–347.

[18] Weiner ES, Abeles M. (1989). Aseptic necrosis and glucocorticosteroids in systemic lupus erythematosus: a reevaluation. J Rheumatol. 16(5): 604–608.

[19] Massardo L, Jacobelli S, Leissner M, González M, Villarroel L, Rivero S. (1992). High-dose intravenous methylprednisolone therapy associated with osteonecrosis in patients with systemic lupus erythematosus. Lupus. 1(6): 401–405.

[20] Gladman DD, Urowitz MB, Chaudhry-Ahluwalia V, Hallet DC, Cook RJ. (2001). Predictive factors for symptomatic osteonecrosis in patients with systemic lupus erythematosus. J Rheumatol. 28(4): 761–765.

[21] DuBois D, DuBois EF. (1989). A formula to estimate the approximate surface area if height and weight be known. 1916. Nutrition. 5(5): 303–311; discussion 312–313.

[22] Garrow JS, Webster J. (1985). Quetelet's index (W/H2) as a measure of fatness. Int J Obes. 9(2): 147–153.

[23] Sekiya F, Yamaji K, Yang K, Tsuda H, Takasaki Y. (2010). Investigation of occurrence of osteonecrosis of the femoral head after increasing corticosteroids in patients with recurring systemic lupus erythematosus. Rheumatol Int. 30(12): 1587–1593.

[24] Mont MA, Pivec R, Banerjee S, Issa K, Elmallah RK, Jones LC. (2015). High-dose corticosteroid use and risk of hip osteonecrosis: meta-analysis and systematic literature review. J Arthroplasty. 30(9): 1506–1512.

[25] Hauzeur JP, Sintzoff S Jr., Appelboom T, De Maertelaer V, Bentin J, Pasteels JL. (1992). Relationship between magnetic resonance imaging and histologic find-ings by bone biopsy in nontraumatic osteonecrosis of the femoral head. J Rheumatol. 19 (3): 385–392.

[26] Kubo T, Yamamoto T, Inoue S, Horii M, Ueshima K, Iwamoto Y, Hirasawa Y. (2000). Histological findings of bone marrow edema pattern on MRI in osteonecrosis of the femoral head. J Orthop Sci. 5(5): 520–523.

[27] Sugano N, Masuhara K, Nakamura N, Ochi T, Hirooka A, Hayami Y. (1996). MRI of early osteonecrosis of the femoral head after transcervical fracture. J Bone Joint Surg (Br). 78(2): 253–257.

[28] Kubo T, Yamazoe S, Sugano N, Fujioka M, Naruse S, Yoshimura N, Oka T, Hirasawa Y. (1997). Initial MRI findings of non-traumatic osteonecrosis of the femoral head in renal allograft recipients. Magn Reson Imaging. 15(9): 1017–1023.

[29] Fujioka M, Kubo T, Nakamura F, Shibatani M, Ueshima K, Hamaguchi H, Inoue S, Sugano N, Sakai T, Torii Y, Hasegawa Y, Hirasawa Y. (2001). Initial changes of non-traumatic osteonecrosis of femoral head in fat suppression images: bone marrow edema was not found before the appearance of band patterns. Magn Reson Imaging. 19 (7): 985–991.

[30] Saito M, Ueshima K, Fujioka M, Ishida M, Goto T, Arai Y, Ikoma K, Fujiwara H, Fukushima W, Kubo T. (2014). Corticosteroid administration within 2 weeks after renal-transplantation affects the incidence of femoral head osteonecrosis. Acta Orthop. 85(3): 266–270.

[31] Nagasawa K, Tada Y, Koarada S, Tsukamoto H, Horiuchi T, Yoshizawa S, Murai K, Ueda A, Haruta Y, Ohta A. (2006). Prevention of steroid-induced osteonecrosis of femoral head in systemic lupus erythematosus by anti-coagulant. Lupus. 15(6): 354–357.

[32] Kuroda T, Tanabe N, Wakamatsu A, Takai C, Sato H, Nakatsue T, Wada Y, Nakano M, Narita I. (2015). High triglyceride is a risk factor for silent osteonecrosis of the femoral head in systemic lupus erythematosus. Clin Rheumatol. 34(12): 2071–2077.

[33] Ficat RP. (1985). Idiopathic bone necrosis of the femoral head. Early diagnosis and treatment. J Bone Joint Surg Br. 67(1): 3–9.

[34] Gardeniers JW (1992). A new international classification of osteonecrosis of the ARCO Committee on terminology and classification. J Jpn Orthop Assoc 66(1): 18–20.

[35] Bombardier C, Gladman DD, Urowitz MB, Carton D, Chang CH. (1992). Derivation of the SLEDAI. A disease activity index for lupus patients. The committee on prognosis studies in SLE. Arthritis Rheum. 35(6): 630–640.

[36] Galli M, Luciani D, Bertolini G, Barbui T. (2003). Lupus anticoagulants are stronger risk factors for thrombosis than anticardiolipin antibodies in the antiphospholipid syndrome:a systemtic review of the literature. Blood. 101(5): 1827–1832.

[37] Taraborelli M, Leuenberger L, Lazzaroni MG, Martinazzi N, Zhang W, Franceschini F, Salmon J, Tincani A, Erkan D. (2016). The contribution of antiphospholipid antibodies to organ damage in systemic lupus erythematosus. Lupus. 25(12): 1365–1368.

[38] Asherson RA, Lioté F, Page B, Meyer O, Buchanan N, Khamashta MA, Jungers P, Hughes GR. (1993). Avascular necrosis of bone and antiphospholipid antibodies in systemic lupus erythematosus. J Rheumatol. 20(2): 284–288.

[39] Mont MA, Glueck CJ, Pacheco IH, Wang P, Hungerford DS, Petri M. (1997). Risk factors for osteonecrosis in systemic lupus erythematosus. J Rheumatol. 24(4): 654–662.

[40] Faezi ST, Hoseinian AS, Paragomi P, Akbarian M, Esfahanian F, Gharibdoost F, Akhlaghi M, Nadji A, Jamshidi AR, Shahram F, Nejadhosseinian M, Davatchi F. (2015). Non-corticosteroid risk factors of symptomatic avascular necrosis of bone in

systemic lupus erythematosus: a retrospective case-control study. Mod Rheumatol. 25(4): 590–594.

[41] Mok MY, Farewell VT, Isenberg DA. (2000). Risk factors for avascular necrosis of bone in patients with systemic lupus erythematosus: is there a role for antiphospholipid antibodies? Ann Rheum Dis. 59(6): 462–467.

[42] Sakaguchi M, Tanaka T, Fukushima W, Kubo T, Hirota Y. (2010). Idiopathic ONF multicenter case-control study group. Impact of oral corticosteroid use for idiopathic osteonecrosis of the femoral head: a nationwide multicenter case-control study in Japan. J Orthop Sci. 15(2): 185–191.

[43] Noda H, Iso H, Saito I, Konishi M, Inoue M, Tsugane S, JPHC Study Group. (2009). The impact of the metabolic syndrome and its components on the incidence of ischemic heart disease and stroke: the Japan public health center-based study. Hypertens Res. 32(4): 289–298.

[44] Patel A, Barzi F, Jamrozik K, Lam TH, Ueshima H, Whitlock G, Woodward M, Asia Pacific Cohort Studies Collaboration. (2004). Serum triglycerides as a risk factor for cardiovascular diseases in the Asia-Pacific region. Circulation. 110(17): 2678–2686.

[45] Sarwar N, Danesh J, Eiriksdottir G, Sigurdsson G, Wareham N, Bingham S, Boekholdt SM, Khaw KT, Gudnason V. (2007). Triglycerides and the risk of coronary heart disease: 10,158 incident cases among 262,525 participants in 29 Western prospective studies. Circulation. 115(4): 450–458.

[46] Nagasawa K, Tada Y, Koarada S, Horiuchi T, Tsukamoto H, Murai K, Ueda A, Yoshizawa S, Ohta A. (2005). Very early development of steroid-associated osteonecrosis of femoral head in systemic lupus erythematosus: prospective study by MRI. Lupus. 14(5): 385–390.

[47] Wang GJ, Sweet DE, Reger SI, Thompson RC. (1977). Fat-cell changes as a mechanism of avascular necrosis of the femoral head in cortisone-treated rabbits. J Bone Joint Surg Am. 59(6): 729–735.

[48] Nishida K, Yamamoto T, Motomura G, Jingushi S, Iwamoto Y. (2008). Pitavastatin may reduce risk of steroid-induced osteonecrosis in rabbits: a preliminary histological study. Clin Orthop Relat Res. 466(5): 1054–1058.

[49] Pritchett JW. (2001). Statin therapy decreases the risk of osteonecrosis in patients receiving steroids. Clin Orthop Relat Res. 386: 173–178.

[50] Takahashi S, Fukushima W, Kubo T, Iwamoto Y, Hirota Y, Nakamura H. (2012). Pronounced risk of nontraumatic osteonecrosis of the femoral head among cigarette smokers who have never used oral corticosteroids: a multicenter case-control study in Japan. J Orthop Sci. 17(6): 730–736.

[51] Mikami T, Ichiseki T, Kaneuji A, Ueda Y, Sugimori T, Fukui K, Matsumoto T. (2010). Prevention of steroid-induced osteonecrosis by intravenous administration of vitamin E in a rabbit model. J Orthop Sci. 15(5): 674–677.

[52] Shigemura T, Nakamura J, Kishida S, Harada Y, Ohtori S, Kamikawa K, Ochiai N, Takahashi K. (2011). Incidence of osteonecrosis associated with corticosteroid therapy among different underlying diseases: prospective MRI study. Rheumatology (Oxford). 50(11): 2023–2028.

[53] Agarwala S, Shah S, Joshi VR. (2009). The use of alendronate in the treatment of avascular necrosis of the femoral head: follow-up to eight years. J Bone Joint Surg Br. 91(8): 1013–1018.

[54] Lai KA1, Shen WJ, Yang CY, Shao CJ, Hsu JT, Lin RM. (2005). The use of alendronate to prevent early collapse of the femoral head in patients with nontraumatic osteonecrosis. A randomized clinical study. J Bone Joint Surg Am. 87(10): 2155–2159.

[55] Nishii T, Sugano N, Miki H, Hashimoto J, Yoshikawa H. (2006). Does alendronate prevent collapse in osteonecrosis of the femoral head? Clin Orthop Relat Res. 443: 273–279.

[56] Gangji V, Toungouz M, Hauzeur JP. (2005). Stem cell therapy for osteonecrosis of the femoral head. Expert Opin Biol Ther. 5(4): 437–442.

[57] Hernigou P, Beaujean F. (2002). Treatment of osteonecrosis with autologous bone marrow grafting. Clin Orthop Relat Res. 405: 14–23.

[58] Hauzeur JP, Gangji V. (2010). Phases 1–3 clinical trials using adult stem cells in osteonecrosis and nonunion fractures. Stem Cells Int. 2010: 410170.

[59] Woo MS, Kang JS, Moon KH. (2014). Outcome of total hip arthroplasty for avascular necrosis of the femoral head in systemic lupus erythematosus. J Arthroplasty. 29(12): 2267–2270.

[60] Atsumi T, Muraki M, Yoshihara S, Kajihara T. (1999). Posterior rotational osteotomy for the treatment of femoral head osteonecrosis. Arch Orthop Trauma Surg. 119(7–8): 388–393.

[61] Malizos KN, Quarles LD, Seaber AV, Rizk WS, Urbaniak JR. (1993). An experimental canine model of osteonecrosis: characterization of the repair process. J Orthop Res. 11(3): 350–357.

[62] Adler RA, El-Hajj Fuleihan G, Bauer DC, Camacho PM, Clarke BL, Clines GA, Compston JE, Drake MT, Edwards BJ, Favus MJ, Greenspan SL, McKinney R Jr., Pignolo RJ, Sellmeyer DE. (2016). Managing osteoporosis in patients on long-term bisphosphonate treatment: report of a task force of the American society for bone and mineral research. J Bone Miner Res. 31(1): 16–35.

[63] Shane E, Burr D, Abrahamsen B, Adler RA, Brown TD, Cheung AM, Cosman F, Curtis JR, Dell R, Dempster DW, Ebeling PR, Einhorn TA, Genant HK, Geusens P, Klaushofer K, Lane JM, McKiernan F, McKinney R, Ng A, Nieves J, O'Keefe R, Papapoulos S, Howe TS, van der Meulen MC, Weinstein RS, Whyte MP. (2014). Atypical subtrochanteric and

diaphyseal femoral fractures: second report of a task force of the American society for bone and mineral research. J Bone Miner Res. 29(1): 1–23.

[64] Odvina CV, Zerwekh JE, Rao DS, Maalouf N, Gottschalk FA, Pak CY. (2005). Severely suppressed bone turnover: a potential complication of alendronate therapy. J Clin Endocrinol Metab. 90(3): 1294–1301.

[65] Kondo N, Yoda T, Fujisawa J, Arai K, Sakuma M, Ninomiya H, Sano H, Endo N. (2015). Bilateral atypical femoral subtrochanteric fractures in a premenopausal patient receiving prolonged bisphosphonate therapy: evidence of severely suppressed bone turnover. Clin Cases Miner Bone Metab. 12(3): 273–277.

[66] Girgis CM, Sher D, Seibel MJ. (2010). Atypical femoral fractures and bisphosphonate use. N Engl J Med. 362(19): 1848–1849.

[67] Saita Y, Ishijima M, Mogami A, Kubota M, Baba T, Kaketa T, Nagao M, Sakamoto Y, Sakai K, Homma Y, Kato R, Nagura N, Miyagawa K, Wada T, Liu L, Matsuoka J, Obayashi O, Shitoto K, Nozawa M, Kajihara H, Gen H, Kaneko K. (2015). The incidence of and risk factors for developing atypical femoral fractures in Japan. J Bone Miner Metab. 33(3): 311–318.

[68] Hyodo K, Nishino T, Kamada H, Nozawa D, Mishima H, Yamazaki M. (2017). Location of fractures and the characteristics of patients with atypical femoral fractures: analyses of 38 Japanese cases. J Bone Miner Metab. 35(2):209–214.

[69] Saita Y, Ishijima M, Mogami A, Kubota M, Baba T, Kaketa T, Nagao M, Sakamoto Y, Sakai K, Kato R, Nagura N, Miyagawa K, Wada T, Liu L, Obayashi O, Shitoto K, Nozawa M, Kajihara H, Gen H, Kaneko K. (2014). The fracture sites of atypical femoral fractures are associated with the weight-bearing lower limb alignment. Bone. 66: 105–110.

[70] Beaudouin-Bazire C, Dalmas N, Bourgeois J, Babinet A, Anract P, Chantelot C, Farizon F, Chopin F, Briot K, Roux C, Cortet B, Thomas T. (2013). Real frequency of ordinary and atypical sub-trochanteric and diaphyseal fractures in France based on X-rays and medical file analysis. Joint Bone Spine. 80(2): 201–205.

[71] Giusti A, Hamdy NA, Dekkers OM, Ramautar SR, Dijkstra S, Papapoulos SE. (2011). Atypical fractures and bisphosphonate therapy: a cohort study of patients with femoral fracture with radiographic adjudication of fracture site and features. Bone. 48(5): 966–971.

[72] Warren C, Gilchrist N, Coates M, Frampton C, Helmore J, McKie J, Hooper G. (2012). Atypical subtrochanteric fractures, bisphosphonates, blinded radiological review. ANZ J Surg. 82(12): 908–912.

[73] Sato H, Kondo N, Wada Y, Nakatsue T, Iguchi S, Fujisawa J, Kazama JJ, Kuroda T, Nakano M, Endo N, Narita I. (2016). The cumulative incidence of and risk factors for latent beaking in patients with autoimmune diseases taking long-term glucocorticoids and bisphosphonates. Osteoporos Int. 27(3): 1217–1225.

[74] Teitelbaum SL. (2012). Bone: the conundrum of glucocorticoid-induced osteoporosis. Nat Rev Endocrinol. 8(8): 451–452.

[75] Tjhia CK, Odvina CV, Rao DS, Stover SM, Wang X, Fyhrie DP. (2011). Mechanical property and tissue mineral density differences among severely suppressed bone turnover (SSBT) patients, osteoporotic patients, and normal subjects. Bone. 49(6): 1279–1289.

[76] Peel NF, Moore DJ, Barrington NA, Bax DE, Eastell R. (1995). Risk of vertebral fracture and relationship to bone mineral density in steroid treated rheumatoid arthritis. Ann Rheum Dis. 54(10): 801–806.

Section 4

Diet and Microbes in Lupus

Chapter 8

Diet and Microbes in the Pathogenesis of Lupus

Xin M. Luo, Michael R. Edwards,
Christopher M. Reilly, Qinghui Mu and
S. Ansar Ahmed

Additional information is available at the end of the chapter

http://dx.doi.org/10.5772/68110

Abstract

Systemic lupus erythematosus (SLE) is a complex autoimmune disorder with no known cure. It is characterized by severe and persistent inflammation that damages multiple organs. To date, treatment and prevention of disease flares have relied on long-term use of anti-inflammatory drugs where side effects are of particular concern. There is a need for better understanding of the disease and for better approaches in SLE treatment and management. In this chapter, we delineate the roles of diet and microbes in the pathogenesis of SLE.

Keywords: diet, microbiota, lupus, hygiene hypothesis, epigenetics

1. Introduction

Systemic lupus erythematosus (SLE) is an autoimmune disorder with complex genetic and environmental etiology. It is characterized by severe and persistent inflammation that leads to tissue damage in multiple organs. The cause is unclear, and there is currently no cure. Current standard of care treatments for SLE are primarily nonselective immunosuppressants, and not all patients respond to these regimens. Although current therapies can treat acute symptoms and reduce the risk of renal failure associated with SLE, side effects are a major cause of concern. Patients taking long-term immunosuppressants are prone to higher incidence of and more severe infections. There is an imperative need to develop new treatment strategies against SLE, for which a better understanding of disease pathogenesis is required. In this chapter, we delineate the roles of diet and microbes in the pathogenesis of SLE.

2. The hygiene hypothesis

Introduction. Environmental factors are known to impact lupus progression in both human and mouse. The role of environmental factors in the etiology of SLE is evidenced by the dramatic difference in disease incidence between West Africans and African-Americans, both derived from the same ethnic group but exposed to different environments. In addition, two remarkable cases of disease amelioration have been reported in SLE patients who had experienced multiple microbial infections. In lupus-prone mice, infections have also been demonstrated to attenuate lupus-like disease. The mechanisms behind these observations are unclear, but improvement in hygiene and absence of certain microbes may have contributed to the higher incidence and faster progression of lupus disease. In this subsection, we will describe the hygiene hypothesis and its relationship with the pathogenesis of SLE.

SLE and the hygiene hypothesis. Proposed by Strachan [1], the hygiene hypothesis initially states that the increased incidence of allergies stems from "declining family size, improvements in household amenities, and higher standards of personal cleanliness." Since then, the scope of the hypothesis has expanded to cover several autoimmune diseases, including type 1 diabetes (T1D), inflammatory bowel disease and multiple sclerosis. Many infectious agents have been described to be protective against autoimmunity [2, 3], whereas mouse models of these autoimmune diseases, such as NOD mice for T1D, are known to develop more progressive clinical signs in cleaner environments. In the case for SLE, it has been long recognized that lupus-prone mice exhibit different disease courses in different animal facilities, suggesting an important role for environmental factors in the etiology of SLE. In addition, the incidence of SLE increased at least threefold in the second half of the twentieth century [4, 5], which is strongly correlated with the increase in hygiene and the decrease of infections, particularly those of the gastrointestinal tract [6]. We therefore have recently extended the hygiene hypothesis to SLE [7].

Protective infectious agents against SLE. The increase in hygiene could reduce infections that are either pathogenic or protective in SLE. Known triggers of lupus development include parvovirus B-19 [8], rubella virus [9], Epstein-Barr virus and cytomegalovirus (CMV) [7, 10–15]. Infectious agents that have been shown to be protective against SLE, on the other hand, include *Helicobacter pylori*, hepatitis B virus (HBV), *Toxoplasma gondii*, malaria parasites such as *Plasmodium berghei* and *Plasmodium chabaudi* and more recently described, helminths. In a large cohort of African-Americans, *H. pylori* seronegativity was found to be associated with an increased risk and earlier onset of SLE [16, 17]. For HBV, only 2.5% of SLE patients were found to be positive for an HBV-specific antibody, suggesting prior infection, whereas in the general population, >10% of people are found positive for the same antibody [9, 18]. Besides human studies, it has been shown that the infection of *T. gondii* protects New Zealand Black (NZB)/New Zealand White (NZW) F1 hybrid (NZB/W F1) lupus-prone mice from developing SLE-like disease, with significantly decreased mortality, ameliorated lupus nephritis and reduced autoantibodies in the serum [19, 20]. Infections with malaria-causing parasites also protected NZB/W F1 mice from developing clinical signs of murine lupus [21–24]. In another classical mouse model of SLE, MRL/Mp-Fas^{lpr} (MRL/lpr), helminthic infection and administration of helminth (worm)-derived molecules have been recently shown to induce the regulatory functions of the immune system and attenuate SLE-like disease such as glomerulonephritis and development of anti-nuclear antibodies [25–27]. Similar results have also been obtained in NZB/W F1 mice, although with a different worm-derived compound [28]. Interestingly, all these protective infectious agents are highly prevalent in Africa where the incidence of SLE is low. Due to vaccinations and the increase in hygiene such as higher quality of drinking water, people in North America and Europe are much less likely to be infected by these agents. Conversely, SLE is of high prevalence in Western developed countries, especially for people of African descent.

It is most remarkable, however, that multiple infections led to complete amelioration of lupus disease in two female patients previously diagnosed with the most active form of SLE [20]. Both women were of childbearing age, where pregnancy was found to be a trigger of lupus flares. In addition, their disease was refractory to all available treatments. Due to drug-induced immunosuppression, they experienced multiple infections over several months that included CMV and *Staphylococcus aureus*, which unfortunately induced sepsis. One patient also experienced infections of *Pseudomonas aeruginosa* and *Pneumocystis carinii*, whereas the other experienced multiple *Escherichia coli* urinary tract infections. Both were treated with antivirals such as ganciclovir and antibiotics such as vancomycin and trimethoprim-sulfamethoxazole. Remarkably, the course of lupus disease changed dramatically in both women with improved autoantibody titers. They were reported to be symptom free after 3–5 years of follow-ups, and one patient even had a normal pregnancy afterwards. While the authors of the reports suggested that the infections had caused the amelioration of SLE symptoms, it is likely that the combination of infections and antiviral/antibacterial treatments had contributed to the change in disease course.

Mechanisms of protection. A couple of mechanisms could explain the protective effects of infectious agents against SLE. The first mechanism is competition. It is likely that the strong immune responses elicited by infectious agents can compete successfully for homeostatic signals (cytokines, growth factors, etc.) against the autoimmune response elicited by weaker autoantigens. The second mechanism is that regulatory cells stimulated by infectious agents can dampen autoimmune response. For example, type I interferons induced by some infectious agents can induce the generation of IL-10-producing regulatory T cells (Treg or Tr1 cells) [29, 30] and limit the production of IL-17 from T cells [31], both of which are mechanisms to suppress autoimmunity. Besides regulatory T cells, anti-inflammatory dendritic cells (DCs) that produce IL-10 and transforming growth factor β (TGF-β) and drive T helper (Th)-2 responses can be also induced by parasitic infections [3]. In addition, parasitic infections can promote IL-4 secretion from basophils and NKT cells, leading to a Th2-biased response to dampen Th1/Th17-induced autoimmunity [3]. Bacterial products, on the other hand, have been shown to directly induce IL-10-producing Treg cells [32]. Finally, toll-like receptors (TLR) appear to mediate the effects of protective infectious agents, which are TLR agonists, in preventing autoimmunity [6]. It is worth noting that these mechanistic studies were performed with regard to T1D.

Specifically for SLE, several studies have tried to pinpoint the mechanisms by which protective infectious agents prevent lupus-like disease in mice. In response to *T. gondii* infection, the levels of interferon (IFN)-γ and IL-10 decreased in NZB/W F1 mice, suggesting the repression of disease-facilitating Th1 and Th2 cytokines in the development of lupus-like nephritis [19]. In addition, alterations of the redox state in kidney and liver tissues may explain the protective effects of malarial infections against lupus nephritis [21]. A parasite-derived compound tuftsin-phosphorylcholine, on the other hand, was able to enhance the expression of TGF-β and IL-10 as well as the expansion of Treg cells in NZB/W F1 mice, while at the same time inhibiting the expression of IFN-γ and IL-17 [28]. This suggests a shift of the balance between Th1/Th17 and Treg toward a Treg-biased phenotype that may in turn attenuate lupus-like disease. Moreover, infection of *Schistosoma mansoni* skewed the Th1:Th2 balance to a Th2 phenotype in MRL/lpr mice, which significantly changed the pathophysiology of glomerulonephritis from diffuse proliferative lupus nephritis (more severe) to membranous lupus nephritis (less severe) [25]. Furthermore, it has been found that a parasitic worm product ES-62 targets MyD88-dependent effector functions of B cells (promoting regulatory B cells and inhibiting plasmablast differentiation) to suppress autoantibody production and proteinuria in MRL/lpr mice [26, 27]. Altogether, these studies suggest that infectious agents can protect against the development of SLE by inducing the regulatory functions of immune cells.

3. Diet and SLE

Introduction. Environmental factors beyond microbial infections contribute to the pathogenesis and severity of disease progression in mouse models, as well as lupus patients. Nutritional components including vitamins, caloric excess or restriction, polyunsaturated fatty acid composition, excess sodium intake and exogenous hormone containing compounds all influence the clinical signs and immune system cellular responses. Nutritional compounds such as vitamin D, omega-3 fatty acids and conjugated linoleic acid appear to have beneficial effects on some parameters of lupus, while high levels of vitamin E, omega-6 fatty acids, a modern "western diet," and high levels of circulating adipokines may exacerbate disease flares. Various commonly consumed phytoestrogens exert complex and differential effects, leading to regulation or exacerbation of SLE clinical signs. Modulating the immune system through dietary intervention to promote regulation of the immune response may form an adjunctive treatment to reduce signs of SLE both for maintenance as well as during disease flare-ups, while decreasing necessary dosages of systemic medications. In this section, we will discuss the role of diet in the pathogenesis of SLE.

Vitamin A. The three main isoforms of the ubiquitously expressed nuclear retinoic acid receptor (RAR), α, β and γ, heterodimerize with the retinoic X receptor (RXR) isoforms. Retinoic acid binding to these heterodimers leads to promotion of retinoic acid-responsive genes through retinoic acid response elements (RAREs). The RXR receptors are also associated with multiple nuclear receptors, including peroxisome proliferator-activated receptor (PPAR) and vitamin D receptor (VDR). Retinoic acid and 1,25-dihydroxyvitamin D3 (D3), the active hormonal metabolite of vitamin D, have been described to potentially antagonize each other's effects due to the similar binding patterns of RAR and VDR to RXR [33].

Retinoic acid has many roles in the development of both innate and cell-mediated immunity. Exposure of antigen presenting cells (APCs) to retinoic acid is critical for cell development and establishment of normal cellular function, leading to an increase in co-stimulatory molecules and induction of the expression of CD11b, a critical adhesion marker, on murine splenocytes and human monocytes [34, 35]. Retinoic acid appears to have differential effects on the induction of immune responses. 9-cis retinoic acid decreases the production of IL-12 in macrophages. However, when combined with lipopolysaccharide (LPS), it augmented the production of nitric oxide, leading to promotion of the Th2 phenotype through regulation of cytokine production by APCs [34, 36, 37].

The development and differentiation of B and T cells are also influenced by the exposure to retinoic acid. Administration of retinoic acid contributes to increased $CD19^+$ B cell numbers in the bone marrow and spleen, accelerated B cell maturation and increased expression of Pax-5, a transcription factor promoting early B cell development and expansion [33, 34]. Conversely, retinoic acid is reported by several groups to decrease mature B cell expansion by arresting B cells in the G0/G1 phase through increased expression of p27 (Kip1). This restricted proliferation may be necessary for the increased expression of CD38 leading to increased plasma cell numbers and production of IgG1 [34, 38–40]. Retinoic acid has also been reported to increase the proliferation of memory B cells when stimulated with the TLR9 ligand CpG and retinoic acid. Stimulation of B cells with both molecules led to a threefold increase in immunoglobulin secretion compared with cells stimulated with CpG alone [34].

Vitamin A deficiency has been associated with a decrease in $CD4^+$ T cells, a decrease in the $CD4^+$ to $CD8^+$ ratio, decreased splenic germinal center formation, decreased total splenocytes, as well as splenic and thymus organ mass [41–43]. Deficiency of vitamin A also contributed to an increase in a Th1-driven immune response, with increased IFN-γ and IL-12 and a decrease in IL-5 and IL-10 production [41]. Administration of retinoic acid contributed to an increase in CD4:CD8 ratio and the promotion of a Th2-driven immune response with an increase in IL-5 production, while repressing IFN-γ and the Th1 response [37, 44]. The administration of a single dose of all-*trans*-retinoic acid in a murine model of lupus nephritis reduced the disease severity and production of Th1-associated cytokines IL-2 and IFN-γ [45]. Another study in the same NZB/W F1 model of lupus reported prolonged survival with decreases in total IgG, IgG2a and anti-dsDNA autoantibodies in the serum [46]. A major contribution to the development of lupus nephritis is the deposition of immunoglobulins and complement proteins in the glomeruli. Multiple groups have reported the protective effect of retinoic acid on the development of glomerular disease, leading to decreased proteinuria and glomerular damage, while maintaining similar levels of IgG and C3 deposition within the glomeruli [47]. Another study reported that retinoic acid inhibits Th1-phenotype-related genes T-bet and IRF-1, leading to a decrease in Th1-related cytokines and altering the Th1/Th2 balance, skewing toward a type-2 response [48].

Retinoic acid administration to MRL/lpr mice contributes to the sustained function of natural T regulatory (Treg) cells and promotes the differentiation of inducible Treg cells in the peripheral tissues [36]. Enhanced differentiation of T cells to Treg cells was shown in the small intestine lamina propria, as well as upregulation of gut-homing receptors on Treg cells by the binding of retinoic acid [36, 49]. There is discrepancy as to whether DCs or macrophages are the predominant cell type to induce Treg cell differentiation in the small intestinal lamina propria, while DCs are known to contribute to Th17 cell differentiation. It has been shown that human SLE patients exhibit a defective induction of Treg cells through TGF-β induction and retinoic acid expansion [37]. This impaired induction led to increased numbers of Treg cells with defective regulatory function abilities, causing the inducible Treg cells to be ineffective at controlling the autoimmune inflammatory response. The studies described above clearly show that cells of both the innate and adaptive immune system are regulated by vitamin A/ retinoic acid. Therefore, it is conceivable that vitamin A and its metabolites may have an effect on patients suffering from SLE.

Vitamin D. Vitamin D3 and its metabolites have been extensively studied and have shown to influence multiple functions in the body, including the abilities to affect bone density and strength, and to modulate both the innate and adaptive immune branches. In this chapter, we will focus on the evidence of vitamin D's metabolites influence on the human immune system as it pertains to lupus. Vitamin D3 administration contributes to decreased pro-inflammatory cytokine production by human monocytes, along with decrease dendritic cell maturation, while increasing IL-10, impairing the differentiation of T cells into Th1 cells [50]. D3 is also able to decrease the expression of MHC class II, CD40, CD80 and CD86 co-stimulatory molecules, decreasing the ability of DCs to present antigens to T and B cells. The ability of D3 to activate human monocytes and macrophages in vitro led to increased cathelicidin and IL-1 production [48].

D3 decreases the expression of IL-2, IFN-γ and T cell proliferation in vitro, as well as decreasing $CD8^+$ cytotoxic activity. It is important in the regulation of many genes, including IL-2 and IFN-γ in T cells, through interaction with the vitamin D receptor-RXR heterodimer. Similar to retinoic acid, D3 inhibits the induction of the Th1-mediated immunity response in favor of the Th2 phenotype, through enhancing the production of IL-4 and decreasing IFN-γ. The Th17 cell response is also mitigated by vitamin D through the inhibition of IL-6 and IL-23 production, leading to the promotion of the Treg cell phenotype through expansion of Foxp3 [51, 52].

It has not yet been determined if D3 acts directly on B cells to decrease B cell proliferation and induction of apoptosis. D3 is also associated with decreased plasma cell differentiation and a subsequent decrease in IgG secretion. In one study, the authors showed that D3 has the ability to upregulate p27 mRNA; however, p18 and p21 were not similarly upregulated in human purified B cells from patients with SLE. The p27 gene is associated with inhibition of the cell cycle, leading to decreased proliferation in activated human B cells, especially memory B cells [53].

Mouse models of SLE have shown decreased proteinuria and prolonged survival when supplemented with D3. A commonly used therapy for human SLE patients is the administration of glucocorticoids to reduce inflammation and to broadly dampen the immune response [54]. Glucocorticoids have been shown to decrease the expression of the vitamin D receptor in multiple cell types. Conversely, D3 interferes with both glucocorticoid receptor and androgen receptor responsiveness through reduced receptor expression and impaired translocation to the nucleus due to alterations in phosphorylation status [55]. When administered as a medication, D3 can lead to adverse effects, including hypercalcemia and bone resorption [48].

Though in vitro evidence strongly supports an immune-regulatory role of vitamin D and its metabolites in the adaptive immune system, there are conflicting reports regarding vitamin D deficiency in SLE patients and the supportive role of vitamin D supplementation. The majority of studies describe decreased serum levels of D3 in patients with SLE compared to healthy patients, which correlated with increased disease activity. The current consensus is that vitamin D serum levels correlate inversely with disease activity, and vitamin D deficiency is associated with increased disease activity or severity [51, 56].

Vitamin E. Vitamin E is a potent antioxidant supporting the normal structure and function of cells by reducing damaging free radical reactive oxygen species (ROS). ROS have been implicated in tissue damage and an increase in pro-inflammatory cytokine production [57]. These factors support the development of autoimmune and degenerative disease severity. The preferentially absorbed form of vitamin E is α-tocopherol, which contributes to the normal function of the immune system in humans and mice. In one study, lowered antioxidant ability was found to precede the diagnosis of SLE, and oxidative damage was increased prior to diagnosis of SLE. This suggests that the decreased ability to control oxidative damage is a potential risk factor for development of SLE [58, 59].

Multiple studies in mouse models of SLE have shown that the dose of vitamin E had differential effects on the disease. Low-dose α-tocopherol increases the lifespan of NZB/W F1 mice while decreasing proteinuria, anti-dsDNA autoantibody IgG in the serum, IL-6 and IFN-γ production from splenocytes [60]. In the MRL/lpr mouse model, low-dose administration of vitamin E increases lifespan and IL-2 production. In contrast, high-dose vitamin E increases anti-DNA and cardiolipin IgM, as well as IL-4 and IL-10 from activated splenocytes. The authors conclude that the decreased survival in high-dose groups was due to the imbalance of Th1/Th2 cytokines, with Th2 cytokines leading to hyperactivation of the B cells in the MRL/lpr model [61]. Vitamin E also increases the pro-inflammatory chemokine MIP-1α in MRL/lpr mice, which activates granulocytes and promotes pro-inflammatory cytokine production [62]. A study comparing plasma antioxidant status between healthy patients and patients diagnosed with SLE showed that SLE patients have impaired plasma antioxidant status as well as a decreased antioxidant intake. The study was small and did not take into account dietary restrictions or food intolerance, limiting the ability to draw firm conclusions for a large set of SLE patients [58]. The above studies demonstrate that the dose of vitamin E is a critical determinant in amelioration or exacerbation of murine lupus. Response to vitamin E supplementation in human SLE patients needs to be thoroughly investigated to determine whether vitamin E supplementation is appropriate.

Omega 3:6 PUFA. Poly-unsaturated fatty acids (PUFAs) have been a popular topic of research in health due to their wide range of effects that can be exerted on the body. Omega-3 PUFAs generally have an anti-inflammatory role, lowering the severity of autoimmune disease and increasing survival in mouse models of SLE. In contrast, diets that are high in saturated fatty acids and omega-6 PUFAs lead to higher anti-dsDNA antibody, proteinuria and inflammatory cytokines in mice [63, 64]. Mouse survival rates were not measured in these studies.

Eicosapentaenoic acid (EPA) and docosahexaenoic acid (DHA) are the main bioactive constituents of omega-3 rich fish oil. SLE patients were shown to have decreased EPA in erythrocytes along with a decrease in the EPA to pro-inflammatory arachidonic acid ratio [65]. The evidence in human studies and clinical trials using omega-3 PUFAs in SLE patients is inconclusive at this time, with multiple studies showing no demonstrable effect on SLE disease activity index or other clinical scores and no effect of omega-3 fatty acids on glucocorticoid requirements when used as immunosuppressive medication.

In a mouse study using NZB/W F1 female mice, higher on concentrations of EPA and DHA led to increased lifespan, decreased glomerulonephritis, decreased anti-dsDNA antibodies, as well as a reduction in pro-inflammatory cytokines IL-1β, IL-6 and TNFα in splenocytes, relative to controls. The authors also demonstrated a reduction in nuclear factor-κB (NF-κB) and p65 nuclear translocation in mice fed higher concentrations of both EPA and DHA [66]. In studies using the MRL/lpr mouse model, fish oil altered pro-inflammatory chemokine production, leading to a decrease in RANTES and MCP-1 from splenocytes [62]. In NZB/W F1 mice, omega-6 PUFAs, conversely, led to an increase in IL-6 and TNFα production as well as prostaglandin E2 from macrophages, a decrease in TGF-β mRNA from splenocytes and lower anti-dsDNA IgG in the serum [67].

There is evidence that n-3 PUFAs remodel the lipid rafts in T cells, which can lead to a decrease in intracellular signaling through the T cell receptor, as well as binding to multiple PPARs. Omega-3 PUFAs bind to PPARα in T and B cells, whereas they bind to PPARγ in cells of myeloid lineage, leading to alterations in gene expression. The binding capacity to PPARs by n-3 and n-6 PUFAs is equal, suggesting that gene modulation between the different families is unlikely, though the possibility exists for differences in cellular metabolism of n-3 and n-6 PUFAs to allow for distinct PPAR activation [65]. In certain instances, the evidence is contradictory between ex vivo and in vivo studies, and cytokine levels have been shown to be opposite in mouse models compared to human data [65]. While there is inconclusive evidence for the anti-inflammatory effects of n-3 PUFAs in human clinical trials, it is still recommended by some that rheumatic patients supplement their diet with long-chain n-3 PUFA and gamma linoleic acid [65].

Conjugated linoleic acid. Conjugated linoleic acid (CLA) has been described to provide health benefits in humans and makes up a group of isomers of linoleic acid. These fatty acids occur naturally in dairy and beef. CLA is considered to have anti-carcinogenic, anti-atherosclerotic and immune-enhancing abilities, with respect to lymphocytic cytotoxic function, macrophage activation and lymphocyte proliferation [68]. The isomer of CLA that demonstrates the strongest anti-inflammatory effect is *cis*9, *trans*11-CLA, which accounts for up to 90% of the dietary CLAv [68].

Supplementation with CLA leads to a reduction in the loss of body mass during end-stage disease, along with an increase in survival after the onset of proteinuria in the NZB/W F1 mouse model [69, 70]. In a non-autoimmune mouse model and cell lines, CLA has a profound effect on macrophage functions. In BALB/c mice, CLA ameliorates LPS-induced body wasting and anorexia in vivo, decreases the production of nitric oxide from macrophages, and decreases the serum concentration of TNFα. Splenocytes from BALB/c mice fed the CLA supplement also have a lower level of IL-4 production and an increase in IL-2 production after stimulation with concanavalin A [71]. CLA also decreases macrophage adhesion as well as downregulating multiple atherogenic genes associated with leukocyte adhesion, while inducing the antagonist IL-1Rα in human umbilical cord vein endothelial cells and the RAW macrophage cell line [72].

CLA is able to exert immune-modulatory effects on dendritic cells and subsequent differentiation of T cells in mice. DCs produce multiple cytokines after activation and express MHC II on the cell surface to facilitate interactions with T cells and B cells. Exposure of DCs to CLA led to a decrease in IL-12 and an increase in IL-10 production, along with decreased migration to the lymph nodes [73]. CLA decreased the expression of MHC II and costimulatory molecules CD80 and CD86 on the surface of DCs, reducing the DC's ability to trigger T cell and B cells responses [74]. When exposed to LPS stimulation in mice fed a CLA rich diet, serum levels of IFN-γ, IL-1β and IL-12p40 were decreased [75]. CLA decreases the ability of DCs to induce the T helper cell differentiation into Th1 and Th17 cells, as well as directly suppressing the production of IL-17 and IL-2 by Th17 cells [74]. The mechanism for CLA influencing the DC response after activation with LPS was shown to be through suppression of both NF-κB and IRF3 downstream of TLR4 [75]. The immune-modulatory effects have been well described in mouse models, though data for the effects of CLA in human SLE patients are lacking at this time.

Western diet and obesity. Considerable attention has recently been given to the attributes of dietary components that make up the typical diet in the developed countries, termed the "western diet." These factors include high-fat, high-protein, high-sugar and high-salt, as well as consumption of a large portion of processed foods. These nutritional components promote obesity, metabolic syndrome and cardiovascular disease. In addition, a recent study has shown the role of the "western diet" in promotion of autoimmune disorders [76]. White adipose tissue is now considered to be a major endocrine organ, secreting more than 50 adipokines including leptin, adiponectin, resistin and visfatin, along with pro-inflammatory cytokines IL-6 and TNFα [76, 77]. Excess white adipose tissue drives a low-level steady state inflammation, which may contribute to various autoimmune and inflammatory-mediated diseases.

The connection between obesity and the development of SLE is complex, and contradictory information exists among studies. There was no correlation found in Danish women between obesity and the incidence of SLE after 11 years [77, 78]. This cohort study had multiple limitations, such as reliance on survey questionnaires regarding pre-pregnancy weights and diagnoses, potential socio-economic bias with women of lower socioeconomic status being underrepresented in the Danish National Birth Cohort, and the confounding factor of pregnancy and childbirth during the study, which do not allow for conclusions to be drawn regarding the link between obesity and SLE [78]. Childhood obesity rates correlated positively with incidence of childhood-onset SLE. The adipokine leptin has been extensively studied and exerts multiple effects on the body [79]. Leptin promotes satiety and stimulation of energy expenditure, by acting on the hypothalamic nuclei, as well as contributing to fertility, bone metabolism and having a profound effect on the immune system. Lack of leptin, due to starvation, testosterone or glucocorticoids, can lead to immunosuppression, while upregulation of leptin by inflammatory cytokines or female sex hormones, 17β-estradiol and progesterone, can lead to inflammation [79]. Leptin can induce the production of IL-6, IL-12 and TNFα pro-inflammatory cytokines from macrophages, while stimulating the proliferation of naïve T cells and promoting a Th1 immune response. Leptin inhibits the production of Th2 cytokines IL-4 and IL-10, along with inhibiting T regulatory cell proliferation [80]. The formation of a pro-inflammatory state through increased leptin levels may contribute to autoimmune disease development.

Leptin is commonly elevated in obese patients as well as SLE patients, which contributes to the survival of autoreactive T cells, and a decrease in the functional T regulatory cells, while promoting the proliferation of Th17 cells in a mouse model of SLE [81, 82]. Circulating serum leptin levels as well as leptin secretion have been shown to be higher in females compared to males, both in obese and non-obese subjects. The sex difference in leptin secretion may be a contributing factor in the development of female-predominant SLE. Leptin deficiency in murine models of SLE has led to decreased anti-dsDNA and a decrease in severity of SLE symptoms [83, 84]. The increased level of circulating leptin may also contribute to the exacerbation of cardiovascular damage in some SLE patients [85, 86]. Adiponectin deficiency was correlated with an increase in SLE disease severity [87, 88]; however, another study found increased levels of adiponectin in the serum and urine of human patient with lupus nephritis [89]. Little information is available regarding other adipokines and their involvement with SLE development.

Obesity is correlated with a predisposition to metabolic syndrome, with increased rates of hypertension, dyslipidemia and atherosclerosis, as well as subsequent cardiovascular disease. Atherosclerosis and cardiovascular disease are highly prevalent in patients with SLE, and a significant number of patient deaths occur due to cardiovascular disease, while obesity has been linked to worsening renal disease and cardiovascular disease in patients suffering from SLE [77]. High levels of inflammatory markers and elevated leptin concentrations found in SLE patients, and mice have been correlated with decreased cognitive function, increased renal damage and increased cardiovascular risks [90, 91].

Diets high in salt (sodium chloride) are found in multiple regions throughout the world, mainly in developed countries where processed foods and "fast food" are prevalent. Excess sodium intake has been attributed to cardiovascular disease and hypertension, as well as stroke, and is now being studied in the development of autoimmune diseases [76]. T cells in a hyperosmotic environment show an increase in p38/MAPK as well as transcription factor NFAT5, leading to an altered cellular response [92]. Sodium can be stored in the human body in various tissues, leading to hyper-osmotic environments in multiple tissues during high-dietary salt intake. Human and murine T cells were investigated under high salt conditions *in vivo* that led to the promotion of Th17 differentiation in vitro [93]. High salt intake has been associated with a decrease in glucocorticoid therapy response in a study of 260 Chinese SLE patients treated with prednisone and followed for 12 weeks [94]. Further studies need to be performed to determine the mechanism for hyperosmotic conditions to promote the highly pro-inflammatory Th17 cell differentiation.

http://dx.doi.org/10.5772/68110

Phytoestrogens. Endogenously produced estrogen contributes significantly to the development of SLE and disease progression. Estrogen is able to suppress IL-2, enhancing the effect of autoantigens. 17β-estradiol implants led to an increase in IFN-γ, nitric oxide and a range of cytokines and chemokines in murine splenocytes [95]. The estrogen receptors on cells comprise two subtypes, α and β. Estrogen receptor-α (ERα) mRNA was increased in the peripheral blood mononuclear cells of SLE patients, while estrogen receptor-β (ERβ) was decreased. ERα was shown to be predominantly pro-inflammatory in a mouse model of SLE, leading to increased proteinuria and decreased survival time when activated, while ERβ showed an immunosuppressive phenotype by decreased autoantibody anti-DNA IgG2 [96, 97].

Phytoestrogens are plant compounds that exert an estrogenic or an anti-estrogenic effect on the human body through interaction with both estrogen receptor α and β, with a preferential binding to ERβ [97]. Phytoestrogens can also block the binding of more potent estrogenic compounds to the ER and regulate target genes. Many types of phytoestrogens are found naturally, with soy-based phytoestrogens, isoflavones, present in many of the foods consumed in industrialized societies. Due to the ubiquity of phytoestrogens in normal diets, controlled human trials are lacking with regard to the specific effects of phytoestrogens on SLE disease development. Data from mouse experiments involving supplementation of isoflavones to MRL/lpr mice show a decrease in IFN-γ from splenocytes with a decrease in anti-dsDNA and cardiolipin levels in the serum, along with a reduction in proteinuria and renal damage through preferential binding of the ERβ [98]. Exclusion of dietary isoflavones through diets using casein as the protein source rather than soy led to amelioration of glomerulonephritis [99]. Alfalfa sprout extract supplementation to MRL/lpr mice produced similar results with decreased renal damage and increased survival, while decreasing IFN-γ and IL-4 production by splenocytes. Alfalfa sprout extract was also able to reduce TNFα, IL-6 and IL-1β pro-inflammatory cytokines in a mouse model of endotoxic shock [100]. Coumestrol, one phytoestrogen in alfalfa, was able to decrease anti-dsDNA IgG and decrease proteinuria in the NZB/W F1 mouse model [101]. However, these findings have not been observed in human SLE patients, where ingestion of alfalfa tablets, which contain all phytoestrogen components of the alfalfa plant, exacerbated disease severity [102].

Multiple phytoestrogens have been shown to upregulate VDR expression in various human cell lines. Genistein and glycitein upregulated VDR transcription and translation in colon cancer cells, while resveratrol and genistein also increased VDR expression in breast cancer cells [103, 104]. Along with receptor expression, genistein decreased CYP24, an enzyme responsible for metabolism of the vitamin D metabolite D3 [105]. Phytoestrogens are abundant in many diets throughout the world and are able to contribute to the modulation of the immune system through interaction with estrogen receptors, potentially ameliorating or exacerbating patients' clinical signs.

4. The role of gut microbiota

Introduction. The mammalian gut harbors trillions of microorganisms known as the microbiota. Increasing evidence in recent years suggests that host microbiota and immune system interact to maintain tissue homeostasis in healthy individuals. The importance of microbiota on the host is highlighted by altered immune responses in the absence of commensal bacteria. Higher susceptibility to infectious pathogens and in some cases, attenuated symptoms in autoimmune disorders, has been observed in mice raised under germ-free conditions. Indeed, perturbation of the host microbiota, especially that in the gut, has been shown to be associated with many autoimmune diseases, including SLE. Changes of gut microbiota in nephritic lupus mice versus healthy controls have recently been described, where a decrease of *Lactobacillaceae* and an increase of *Lachnospiraceae* were observed in lupus-prone mice. A cross-sectional study has also shown that a lower *Firmicutes* to *Bacteroidetes* ratio was present in the fecal microbiota of SLE patients with inactive disease, which is consistent with observations in other autoimmune diseases. In addition, oral antibiotics are known to trigger lupus flares, again suggesting a role for commensal bacteria in SLE. In this section, we will describe the existing data and a proposed role of gut microbiota in the pathogenesis of SLE.

Gut microbiota and SLE. Evidence is rapidly growing that mutualistic bacteria contribute to the development of a healthy functioning immune system, as well as the development of aberrant immune responses. The past 10 years have seen a rapid growth in the understanding of how the commensal microbiota is able to contribute to health and disease with the exploration of 16S rRNA sequencing along with the use of gnotobiotic animals. These newer methods of DNA sequencing have allowed researchers to investigate the effects of specific species or strains of organisms and how they interact with the immune system. Gnotobiotic animals are born into a sterile environment and develop under sterile conditions so that a specific group of bacteria, viruses, eukaryotes or parasites can be introduced to the animal, and the resulting effects can be studied without the interference of other organisms [106]. Intestinal microbial dysbiosis can lead to immune system effects at distant sites of the body [49, 107–112]. The systemic immune system is influenced by microbiota in the intestines, suggesting that microbiota at other sites of the body can also have a systemic effect on the host's immune system.

The host's genetic make-up is the primary factor in determining the composition of one's adult microbiota. Other contributing factors include mother's health in utero, the method of delivery during birth, if one is either breast fed or fed formula, the use of antibiotics during early childhood and types of foods consumed prior to, and during, weaning. The adult microbiota is not a static entity, however, and can be modified through many different environmental factors, and the composition will also change with age. Many of the previously discussed contributions to SLE are associated with alterations in the microbiota. Obese patients have an increased *Firmicutes* to *Bacterioidetes* ratio, with members of *Firmicutes* leading to increased energy harvest from dietary nutrients [113]. The "western diet" is associated with alterations in the gut microbiota as well. Children from a rural village in the West African country of Burkina Faso had increased microbial richness and greater *Prevotella* with decreased *Bacteroides* levels compared to European children. The microbiota of the Burkina Faso children also produced more short chain fatty acids than the intestinal microbiota of the European children [114]. These findings of agrarian societies with increased *Prevotella* and decreased *Bacteroides* have been supported in studies comparing rural South Americans and people from Bangladesh to people living in industrialized regions [115]. The source of dietary fat can impact microbiota composition as well, as mice fed diets with a fat source from either milk-fat, lard, safflower oil or a low-fat diet, all resulted in distinct phylogenetic profiles [116, 117].

Murine studies on how the microbiota affects the immune system have emerged recently. At the level of the intestinal lamina propria, bacteria compete with host defenses and establish homeostasis. T cells are kept in check between pro-inflammatory Th1, Th2 and Th17 cells as well as innate lymphoid cells, and the anti-inflammatory T regulatory cells [118–120]. Specific bacterial groups can elicit distinct immune responses, as evidenced by mice colonized with segmented filamentous bacteria developed elevated levels of Th17 cells in the lamina propria [121, 122]. Colonization of previously germ-free mice with clostridial strains from cluster IV and XIVa resulted in an expansion of the T regulatory cell population in the lamina propria and systemically [123]. Polysaccharide A derived from *Bacteroides fragilis* is able to induce IL-10 production in the lamina propria through binding to TLR2 on T regulatory cells, inhibiting the expansion of the local Th17 cell population [124]. Only a single study, reported in 1999, to date has explored the development of SLE in a germ-free mouse strain. That study used MRL/lpr mice and showed no difference in disease progression between conventionally raised mice and germ-free mice [125]. Due to the *Fas* mutation and the underlying cause of lupus disease in this strain of mice, the MRL/lpr strain may not be the best strain to understand the impact of gut microbiome in a germ-free setting on lupus. Few murine studies investigating the microbiota's role in SLE have been published to date. Regardless, gut microbiome in MRL/lpr mice has recently been shown to impact lupus. In the MRL/lpr mouse model of SLE, young female mice had lower numbers of *Lactobacilli* species and increased numbers of *Lachnospiraceae* density in the murine feces. The administration of retinoic acid restored the *Lactobacilli* density and correlated with reduced clinical signs and a reverse of multiple lupus-associated microbial functions. The increased density of *Lachnospiraceae* was also overrepresented in female lupus-prone mice along with butyrate producing *Clostridiaceae* species. There is potential that use of *Lactobacilli* containing probiotics and vitamin A may benefit lupus patients [49, 107].

There have been few human trials to determine the impact on intestinal microbiota specifically on SLE development. In 20 human SLE patients in remission compared to healthy controls, a decreased *Firmicutes* to *Bacterioidetes* ratio was found in fecal samples. This change in fecal microbiota is associated with an increase in oxidative phosphorylation and glycan utilization by the host microbiota [126, 127]. In contrast to the murine studies, *Lachnospiraceae* and *Clostridia* were associated with healthy patients, rather than lupus patients [126]. The intestinal microbiota is a complex conglomeration that can contribute to modulation of the local and systemic immune system. Current and future work will begin to target specific groups and mechanisms of microbial contribution to systemic autoimmune disease pathogenesis.

5. Bacterial metabolites and mechanisms of action

Introduction. Bacterial metabolites produced by the gut microbiota may have profound effects on immune function. Recently, several groups have found that short-chain fatty acids (SCFAs) produced by gut microbiota, especially butyrate produced by Clostridia, can promote the differentiation of regulatory T (Treg) cells in the colon, spleen and lymph nodes and suppress inflammation [128–131]. Treg deficiency leads to autoimmunity, while re-introduction of Treg cells can rescue animals from the disease. In human SLE, a pathogenic role of dysfunctional Treg cells has been suggested. In particular, the imbalance between Treg and Th17 cells and a bias toward IL 17-producing cells (both Th17 cells and double-negative T cells can produce IL-17 in SLE) are widely recognized for SLE. In the gut, the number and diversity of butyrate-producing bacteria are subject to factors related to age, disease and to diet. Butyrate and SCFAs are inhibitors of histone deacetylases (HDACs). HDAC inhibition can result in altering gene expression by making the chromatin more accessible to transcription factors by acetylating histone proteins at specific lysine residues and may also lead to post-translational modification of several transcription factors that reside both cytosolic and nuclear. Below, we have outlined the influence of SCFAs (predominately butyrate) on HDAC activity on the epithelia in the gut microbiota as it is likely to play an important role in regulation of the gut microbiota and lupus.

Role of epigenetics in immunity. Although genome-wide association studies have identified many genes that may play a role in the initiation or progression of SLE [132–134], these studies do not account for risk attributed to heritable factors [135] and have failed to identify a unifying switch. Epigenetics is the process in which alterations in gene expression and phenotype occur which are heritable but do not alter the DNA sequence [136]. There is increasing evidence that epigenetics plays a key role in SLE pathogenesis and epigenetically targeted therapies may be efficacious [137, 138]. In regard to epigenetics, interactions between DNA and core histone proteins are important in regulating the accessibility of transcription factors to bind promoter regions and thus regulate gene expression [139]. Histone acetyltransferases (HATs) and HDACs can alter the charge and subsequent binding affinity of core histone proteins to the chromatin through removal or addition of acetyl groups on lysine residues, respectively [140–142]. Recent investigations have revealed that HATs and HDACs are also capable of modifying lysine residues on numerous non-histone nuclear and cytosolic proteins [141, 143], which has driven some researchers to alternatively refer to the enzymes as lysine (K) acetyltransferases (KATs) and lysine deacetylases (KDACs).

HDAC enzymes. There are 18 mammalian HDACs, which remove acetyl groups from lysine residues in histones and other proteins to control multiple cellular functions including transcription, cell cycle kinetics, cell signaling and cellular transport processes [144]. HDACs are classified based on structure, homology to yeast HDACs and function into classes I–IV [145, 146]. Class I HDACs (HDAC-1, -2, -3 and -8) are nuclear exclusive enzymes found in a wide range of tissues and cells lines where they are known for histone modification and repression of transcription [147, 148]. Class II HDACs are further subdivided into class IIa (HDAC-4, -5, -7 and -9) and class IIb (HDAC-6 and -10) based on domain organization [149] and exhibit selective tissue expression, nucleocytoplasmic shuttling and function through recruitment of distinct cofactors [148]. Class III comprises the sirtuins, which act through a distinct NAD^+-dependent mechanism and are not considered "classical" HDACs [147]. HDAC11 is the sole member of class IV as phylogenetic analysis revealed very low similarity to HDACs in the other classes [150].

In addition to their initial relevance in cancer biology [151], HDAC enzymes are now increasingly being investigated as regulators of inflammation and immunity [147]. As reviewed by Shakespear et al., HDACs are documented to play a role in myeloid development, toll-like receptor (TLR) and interferon (IFN) signaling in innate immune cells, antigen presentation and development and function of B and T lymphocytes [147]. Subsequently, pharmacologic inhibition of HDACs has been evaluated as a possible treatment modality in a wide spectrum of diseases, including inflammatory and autoimmune diseases [152].

SCFAs. Intestinal bacteria provide the hosts with nutrients and confer resistance to infection. The delicate balance between pro- and anti-inflammatory mechanisms, essential for gut immune homeostasis, is affected by the composition of the commensal microbial community and has been reviewed by others [153]. Recent studies have shown that metabolism and immunology are intertwined and the field of immunometabolism has emerged which examines how gut metabolites influence immune cell function [154]. In the gut, carbohydrates resistant to breakdown in the stomach and small intestine are subject to colonic fermentation to result in the production of SCFAs, containing1–6 carbon atoms. Anaerobic bacteria generate the major SCFAs and include acetate, propionate and butyrate. The SCFA butyrate is produced by fermentation of dietary fiber by the intestinal microbiota and is the primary energy source of colonocytes [155]. Recently, Imhann and coworkers showed that patients with inflammatory bowel disease (IBD) had a decrease in the genus *Roseburia*. Furthermore, they noted that *Roseburia* spp. is acetate-to-butyrate converters suggesting that a lack of butyrate may contribute to IBD [156]. Furthermore, a reduction on butyrate producing *Roseburia* ssp. has been associated with chronic kidney disease progression [157]. On the other hand, butyrate has seen shown to aggravate dextran sulfate sodium induce colitis in an animal model [158]. In regard to HDAC inhibition, butyric acid has been reported to specifically inhibit the class I HDACs (1, 2, 3 and 8) [159].

T cells in gut immunity. Balanced mucosal immunity in the gut is critical for host homeostasis and defense. Naïve $CD4^+$ T cells when activated differentiate into T helper cell [Th1, Th2, Th17 or follicular helper (Tfh)] depending on cytokine exposure and B cell or antigen presenting cell influence. One specific subset of T cells (Treg cells) acts to suppress effect T cell function. The majority of Treg cells develop in the thymus (nTregs) and are selected for by strong or intermediate T cell receptor (TCR) signals while escaping negative selection [160]. Additionally, Treg cells can also be induced under certain circumstances from naïve T cells in the periphery (iTregs). This can happen systemically and has been shown to occur at interface with the environment in both whole animal and in in vitro assays [161]. Treg differentiation is strongly influenced by the presence of the anti-inflammatory cytokine transforming growth factor β (TGF-β). Furthermore, expression of the transcription factor Foxp3 is essential for Treg development and function and is regulated by genomic regulatory elements termed conserved noncoding DNA sequences (CNS). While CNS1 is unnecessary for nTreg differentiation, it has been reported to be crucial for iTreg generation in gut-associated lymphoid tissues (GALT) [162]. CNS2 is required for Foxp3 expression in the progeny of dividing Treg cells. CNS3 controls *de novo* Foxp3 expression and nTreg differentiation [163]. Studies have shown that Treg cells expressing transcription factor Foxp3 have a key role in limiting inflammatory responses in the intestine [164, 165].

Treg-Th17 balance. Th17 is a subset of T helper cells and serves to maintain the mucosal barrier and contribute to pathogen clearance at mucosal surfaces. However, they have also been implicated in autoimmune and inflammatory disorders as the loss of Th17 cells at mucosal surfaces has been shown to allow chronic inflammation and microbial translocation. In the gut, there exists a balance of Treg-Th17 cells as the signals that cause Th17s to differentiate actually inhibit Treg differentiation [166]. Since both Treg and Th17 cells are both pertinent to gut homeostasis and immune regulation, the balance of these T cells is critical for homeostasis [167]. Treg cells prevent systemic and tissue-specific autoimmunity and inflammatory lesions at mucosal interfaces [165]. Mice deficient in iTregs spontaneously developed pronounced Th2-type pathologies at mucosal sites including in the gastrointestinal tract and lungs and shows hallmarks of allergic inflammation and asthma [168]. Studies have shown that in the gut, iTreg cells are the prominent phenotype and are rapidly induced following naïve T cell activation which is dependent on Notch2-singling and may be somewhat independent of TGF-β [165]. This suggests that whereas nTreg cells generated in the thymus appear sufficient for control of systemic and tissue-specific autoimmunity, extrathymic differentiation of iTregs affects the commensal microbiota composition and serves a distinct, essential function in maintaining the inflammatory response at mucosal interfaces. Furthermore, when the animals were given the SCFA (butyrate), Treg cell differentiation in the gut increased and this was dependent on CNS1 expression [129]. In addition to butyrate, de novo iTreg generation in the periphery was potentiated by propionate, another SCFA of microbial origin capable of HDAC inhibition, but not acetate, which lacks this HDAC-inhibitory activity, suggesting that bacterial metabolites mediate communication between the commensal microbiota and the immune system. Other studies have also reported that a butyrate-mediated increase in the Treg cell subset in vivo was due to increased extrathymic generation of Treg cells and not due to their increased nTreg cells [169]. In addition to butyrate inducing a Treg phenotype, butyrate has also been shown to increases macrophage phagocytosis and killing of bacteria. When Treg cells were cultured with stimulated macrophages exposed to IL-4 and butyrate, less inflammatory cytokines were produced compared to macrophages treated with IL-4 indicating that microbial-derived butyrate decreases inflammatory mediator production in the gut [170]. In other studies using the antibiotic vancomycin, which targets Gram-positive bacteria, the level of iTregs was reduced. This could be due to the decrease in *Roseburia* spp. that is the butyrate-producing, Gram-positive anaerobic bacteria that inhabit the human colon. However, when specific pathogen-free mice were treated with a combination of vancomycin and SCFAs, the reduction in iTregs was completely restored suggesting that SCFAs play a role in iTreg homeostasis [128].

HDAC and Treg-Th17 balance in lupus. HDAC inhibition has been shown to decrease disease in lupus-prone MRL/lpr and NZB/W F1 mice [171–174]. Mechanisms by which HDAC inhibition decreases SLE disease have previously been reviewed by Reilly and others [142, 175]. HDAC inhibition may act in several ways including correction the hypoacetylation states of histones H3 and H4 [176], increased $CD4^{+}CD25^{+}Foxp3^{+}$ Treg cells [172, 174], reduced Th1- and Th17-inducing cytokines (IL-12 and IL-23) as well as Th1-attracting chemokines [142], and inhibition of germline and post-switch immunoglobulin transcripts in splenic B cells [177]. More importantly in SLE, decreased renal disease (glomerulonephritis and proteinuria) has been consistently reported in studies investigating the use of HDAC inhibitors to treat lupus in various mouse models [171–174]. Pan and selective HDAC inhibitors are being evaluated in the clinic for inflammatory diseases with some mixed results and adverse effects such as fatigue, nausea, vomiting, diarrhea, thrombocytopenia, neutropenia and cardiac irregularities [178]. Investigations of specific functions for each HDAC isoform in knockout mice have revealed that elimination of class I and class IIa HDACs result in embryonic lethal phenotypes or fatal cardiac, vascular, musculoskeletal or neural crest defects, and specific HDAC isoform activity is required for normal cells development [178, 179]. The observed butyrate-mediated increase in the Treg cell subsets in vivo due to increased extrathymic generation of Treg cells and not due to their increased thymic output would support a role of HDACi in gut homeostasis [169]. In studies involving lupus patients, while Treg or Th17 cells alone were not correlated with SLE development, the ratio of Treg to Th17 cells in active SLE patients was significantly lower than that in inactive SLE patients and healthy controls. Moreover, corticosteroid treatment increased the ratio of Treg to Th17 cells in active SLE patients. Indeed, the Treg/Th17 cell ratio is inversely correlated with the severity of active SLE, indicating that in active SLE, there appears to exist an imbalance between Treg and Th17 cells [180]. Inducible Tregs cells are dependent on the expression of the transcription factor Foxp3 which may be transiently expressed allowing for plasticity of the Tregs/Th17 phenotype [181]. Interestingly, when Foxp3 is acetylated, the transcription factor becomes more stable and has greater propensity to bind DNA yielding a more stable and effective Treg population [182]. In addition to the regulation of Treg differentiation, butyrate has also been shown to increase the tri-methylation of lysine 27 on histone 3 (H3K27me3) in the promoter of nuclear factor-κB1 (NF-κB1) in colon tissue resulting in repression of inflammation [183]. In our lupus mouse studies, we found a marked depletion of lactobacilli in our lupus animals and increases in *Lachnospiraceae* compared to age-matched health controls. Interestingly, we also found that *Lachnospiraceae*, butyrate-producing genera, was more abundant in the gut of lupus-prone mice at specific time points during lupus progression [49]. Whether this was causative or in response to disease pathogenesis is an active area of investigation in our laboratory. Nonetheless, our results and others demonstrate the dynamics of gut microbiota as that bacterial production of SCFAs and butyrate may play a role in the initiation and progression of inflammation and autoimmunity.

Author details

Xin M. Luo*, Michael R. Edwards, Christopher M. Reilly, Qinghui Mu and S. Ansar Ahmed

*Address all correspondence to: xinluo@vt.edu

Department of Biomedical Sciences and Pathobiology, College of Veterinary Medicine, Virginia Polytechnic Institute and State University, Blacksburg, VA, USA

References

[1] Strachan DP. Hay fever, hygiene, and household size. BMJ. 1989;299(6710):1259–60.

[2] Cooke A. Infection and autoimmunity. Blood Cells Mol Dis. 2009;42(2):105–7.

[3] Zaccone P, Cooke A. Infectious triggers protect from autoimmunity. Semin Immunol. 2011;23(2):122–9.

[4] Uramoto KM, Michet CJ, Jr., Thumboo J, Sunku J, O'Fallon WM, Gabriel SE. Trends in the incidence and mortality of systemic lupus erythematosus, 1950–1992. Arthritis Rheum. 1999;42(1):46–50.

[5] Danchenko N, Satia JA, Anthony MS. Epidemiology of systemic lupus erythematosus: a comparison of worldwide disease burden. Lupus. 2006;15(5):308–18.

[6] Bach JF. Infections and autoimmune diseases. J Autoimmun. 2005;25(Suppl):74–80.

[7] Mu Q, Zhang H, Luo XM. SLE: another autoimmune disorder influenced by microbes and diet? Front Immunol. 2015;6:608.

[8] Severin MC, Levy Y, Shoenfeld Y. Systemic lupus erythematosus and parvovirus B-19: casual coincidence or causative culprit? Clin Rev Allergy Immunol. 2003;25(1):41–8.

[9] Kivity S, Agmon-Levin N, Blank M, Shoenfeld Y. Infections and autoimmunity—friends or foes? Trends Immunol. 2009;30(8):409–14.

[10] Hayashi T, Lee S, Ogasawara H, Sekigawa I, Iida N, Tomino Y, et al. Exacerbation of systemic lupus erythematosus related to cytomegalovirus infection. Lupus. 1998;7(8):561–4.

[11] James JA, Kaufman KM, Farris AD, Taylor-Albert E, Lehman TJ, Harley JB. An increased prevalence of Epstein-Barr virus infection in young patients suggests a possible etiology for systemic lupus erythematosus. J Clin Investig. 1997;100(12):3019–26.

[12] Nawata M, Seta N, Yamada M, Sekigawa I, Lida N, Hashimoto H. Possible triggering effect of cytomegalovirus infection on systemic lupus erythematosus. Scand J Rheumatol. 2001;30(6):360–2.

[13] Nelson P, Rylance P, Roden D, Trela M, Tugnet N. Viruses as potential pathogenic agents in systemic lupus erythematosus. Lupus. 2014;23(6):596–605.

[14] Rasmussen NS, Draborg AH, Nielsen CT, Jacobsen S, Houen G. Antibodies to early EBV, CMV, and HHV6 antigens in systemic lupus erythematosus patients. Scand J Rheumatol. 2015;44(2):143–9.

[15] Sundar K, Jacques S, Gottlieb P, Villars R, Benito ME, Taylor DK, et al. Expression of the Epstein-Barr virus nuclear antigen-1 (EBNA-1) in the mouse can elicit the production of anti-dsDNA and anti-Sm antibodies. J Autoimmun. 2004;23(2):127–40.

[16] Esposito S, Bosis S, Semino M, Rigante D. Infections and systemic lupus erythematosus. Eur J Clin Microbiol Infect Dis. 2014;33(9):1467–75.

[17] Sawalha AH, Schmid WR, Binder SR, Bacino DK, Harley JB. Association between systemic lupus erythematosus and Helicobacter pylori seronegativity. J Rheumatol. 2004;31(8):1546–50.

[18] Ram M, Anaya JM, Barzilai O, Izhaky D, Porat Katz BS, Blank M, et al. The putative protective role of hepatitis B virus (HBV) infection from autoimmune disorders. Autoimmun Rev. 2008;7(8):621–5.

[19] Chen M, Aosai F, Norose K, Mun HS, Ishikura H, Hirose S, et al. *Toxoplasma gondii* infection inhibits the development of lupus-like syndrome in autoimmune (New Zealand Black × New Zealand White) F1 mice. Int Immunol. 2004;16(7):937–46.

[20] Praprotnik S, Sodin-Semrl S, Tomsic M, Shoenfeld Y. The curiously suspicious: infectious disease may ameliorate an ongoing autoimmune destruction in systemic lupus erythematosus patients. J Autoimmun. 2008;30(1–2):37–41.

[21] Al-Quraishy S, Abdel-Maksoud MA, El-Amir A, Abdel-Ghaffar FA, Badr G. Malarial infection of female BWF1 lupus mice alters the redox state in kidney and liver tissues and confers protection against lupus nephritis. Oxid Med Cell Longev. 2013; 2013:156562.

[22] Greenwood BM, Herrick EM, Voller A. Suppression of autoimmune disease in NZB and (NZB x NZW) F1 hybrid mice by infection with malaria. Nature. 1970;226(5242):266–7.

[23] Sato MN, Minoprio P, Avrameas S, Ternynck T. Changes in the cytokine profile of lupus-prone mice (NZB/NZW)F1 induced by *Plasmodium chabaudi* and their implications in the reversal of clinical symptoms. Clin Exp Immunol. 2000;119(2):333–9.

[24] Butcher G. Autoimmunity and malaria. Trends Parasitol. 2008;24(7):291–2.

[25] Miyake K, Adachi K, Watanabe M, Sasatomi Y, Ogahara S, Abe Y, et al. Parasites alter the pathological phenotype of lupus nephritis. Autoimmunity. 2014;47(8):538–47.

[26] Rodgers DT, McGrath MA, Pineda MA, Al-Riyami L, Rzepecka J, Lumb F, et al. The parasitic worm product ES-62 targets myeloid differentiation factor 88-dependent effector mechanisms to suppress antinuclear antibody production and proteinuria in MRL/lpr mice. Arthritis Rheumatol. 2015;67(4):1023–35.

[27] Rodgers DT, Pineda MA, Suckling CJ, Harnett W, Harnett MM. Drug-like analogues of the parasitic worm-derived immunomodulator ES-62 are therapeutic in the MRL/Lpr model of systemic lupus erythematosus. Lupus. 2015;24(13):1437–42.

[28] Bashi T, Blank M, Ben-Ami Shor D, Fridkin M, Versini M, Gendelman O, et al. Successful modulation of murine lupus nephritis with tuftsin-phosphorylcholine. J Autoimmun. 2015;59:1–7.

[29] Levings MK, Sangregorio R, Galbiati F, Squadrone S, de Waal Malefyt R, Roncarolo MG. IFN-alpha and IL-10 induce the differentiation of human type 1 T regulatory cells. J Immunol. 2001;166(9):5530–9.

[30] Dikopoulos N, Bertoletti A, Kroger A, Hauser H, Schirmbeck R, Reimann J. Type I IFN negatively regulates CD8+ T cell responses through IL-10-producing CD4+ T regulatory 1 cells. J Immunol. 2005;174(1):99–109.

[31] Henry T, Kirimanjeswara GS, Ruby T, Jones JW, Peng K, Perret M, et al. Type I IFN signaling constrains IL-17A/F secretion by gammadelta T cells during bacterial infections. J Immunol. 2010;184(7):3755–67.

[32] Alyanakian MA, Grela F, Aumeunier A, Chiavaroli C, Gouarin C, Bardel E, et al. Transforming growth factor-beta and natural killer T-cells are involved in the protective effect of a bacterial extract on type 1 diabetes. Diabetes. 2006;55(1):179–85.

[33] Mora JR, Iwata M, von Andrian UH. Vitamin effects on the immune system: vitamins A and D take centre stage. Nat Rev Immunol. 2008;8(9):685–98.

[34] Ross AC, Chen Q, Ma Y. Augmentation of antibody responses by retinoic acid and costimulatory molecules. Semin Immunol. 2009;21(1):42–50.

[35] Ma Y, Ross AC. The anti-tetanus immune response of neonatal mice is augmented by retinoic acid combined with polyriboinosinic:polyribocytidylic acid. Proc Natl Acad Sci U S A. 2005;102(38):13556–61.

[36] Zhou X, Kong N, Wang J, Fan H, Zou H, Horwitz D, et al. Cutting edge: all-trans retinoic acid sustains the stability and function of natural regulatory T cells in an inflammatory milieu. J Immunol. 2010;185(5):2675–9.

[37] Sobel ES, Brusko TM, Butfiloski EJ, Hou W, Li S, Cuda CM, et al. Defective response of CD4(+) T cells to retinoic acid and TGFbeta in systemic lupus erythematosus. Arthritis Res Ther. 2011;13(3):R106.

[38] Ross AC, Chen Q, Ma Y. Vitamin A and retinoic acid in the regulation of B-cell development and antibody production. Vitamins Hormon. 2011;86:103–26.

[39] Duriancik DM, Lackey DE, Hoag KA. Vitamin A as a regulator of antigen presenting cells. J Nutr. 2010;140(8):1395–9.

[40] Long KZ, Santos JI, Rosado JL, Estrada-Garcia T, Haas M, Al Mamun A, et al. Vitamin A supplementation modifies the association between mucosal innate and adaptive immune responses and resolution of enteric pathogen infections. Am J Clin Nutr. 2011;93(3):578–85.

[41] Hall JA, Cannons JL, Grainger JR, Dos Santos LM, Hand TW, Naik S, et al. Essential role for retinoic acid in the promotion of CD4(+) T cell effector responses via retinoic acid receptor alpha. Immunity. 2011;34(3):435–47.

[42] Mucida D, Park Y, Kim G, Turovskaya O, Scott I, Kronenberg M, et al. Reciprocal TH17 and regulatory T cell differentiation mediated by retinoic acid. Science. 2007;317(5835):256–60.

[43] Ross AC. Vitamin A and retinoic acid in T cell-related immunity. Am J Clin Nutr. 2012;96(5):1166S–72S.

[44] Nozaki Y, Yamagata T, Sugiyama M, Ikoma S, Kinoshita K, Funauchi M. Anti-inflammatory effect of all-trans-retinoic acid in inflammatory arthritis. Clin Immunol. 2006;119(3):272–9.

[45] Kinoshita K, Yoo BS, Nozaki Y, Sugiyama M, Ikoma S, Ohno M, et al. Retinoic acid reduces autoimmune renal injury and increases survival in NZB/W F1 mice. J Immunol. 2003;170(11):5793–8.

[46] Nozaki Y, Yamagata T, Yoo BS, Sugiyama M, Ikoma S, Kinoshita K, et al. The beneficial effects of treatment with all-trans-retinoic acid plus corticosteroid on autoimmune nephritis in NZB/WF mice. Clin Exp Immunol. 2005;139(1):74–83.

[47] Pérez de Lema G L-CF, Molina A, Luckow B, Schmid H, de Wit C, Moreno-Manzano V, Banas B, Mampaso F, Schlöndorff D. Retinoic acid treatment protects MRL/lpr lupus mice from the development of glomerular disease. Kidney Int. 2004;66(3):1018–28.

[48] Hsieh CC, Lin BF. Dietary factors regulate cytokines in murine models of systemic lupus erythematosus. Autoimmun Rev. 2011;11(1):22–7.

[49] Zhang H LX, Sparks JB, Luo XM. Dynamics of gut microbiota in autoimmune lupus. Appl Environ Microbiol. 2014;80(24):7551–60.

[50] Almerighi C, Sinistro A, Cavazza A, Ciaprini C, Rocchi G, Bergamini A. 1 alpha,25-dihydroxyvitamin D3 inhibits CD40L-induced pro-inflammatory and immunomodulatory activity in human monocytes. Cytokine. 2009;45(3):190–7.

[51] Kriegel MA, Manson JE, Costenbader KH. Does vitamin D affect risk of developing autoimmune disease?: A systematic review. Semin Arthritis Rheum. 2011;40(6):512–31 e8.

[52] Proal AD, Albert PJ, Marshall TG. The human microbiome and autoimmunity. Curr Opin Rheumatol. 2013;25(2):234–40.

[53] Chen S, Sims GP, Chen XX, Gu YY, Chen S, Lipsky PE. Modulatory effects of 1,25-dihydroxyvitamin D3 on human B cell differentiation. J Immunol. 2007;179(3):1634–47.

[54] Lam NC, Ghetu MV, Bieniek ML. Systemic lupus erythematosus: primary care approach to diagnosis and management. Am Fam Phys. 2016;94(4):284–94.

[55] Kassi E, Nasiri-Ansari N, Spilioti E, Kalotychou V, Apostolou PE, Moutsatsou P, Papavassiliou AG. Vitamin D interferes with glucocorticoid responsiveness in human peripheral blood mononuclear target cells. Cell Mol Life Sci. 2016.

[56] Sahebari M NN, Salehi M. Correlation between serum 25(OH)D values and lupus disease activity: an original article and a systematic review with meta-analysis focusing on serum VitD confounders. Lupus. 2014;23(11):1164–77.

[57] Kurien BT, Scofield RH. Autoimmunity and oxidatively modified autoantigens. Autoimmun Rev. 2008;7(7):567–73.

[58] Bae SC, Kim SJ, Sung MK. Impaired antioxidant status and decreased dietary intake of antioxidants in patients with systemic lupus erythematosus. Rheumatol Int. 2002; 22(6):238–43.

[59] Shah D, Kiran R, Wanchu A, Bhatnagar A. Oxidative stress in systemic lupus erythematosus: relationship to Th1 cytokine and disease activity. ImmunolLett. 2010;129(1):7–12.

[60] Hsieh C-C, Lin B-F. The effects of vitamin E supplementation on autoimmune-prone New Zealand black × New Zealand white F1 mice fed an oxidised oil diet. Br J Nutr. 2007;93(05):655.

[61] Hsieh CC, Lin BF. Opposite effects of low and high dose supplementation of vitamin E on survival of MRL/lpr mice. Nutrition. 2005;21(9):940–8.

[62] Venkatraman J MK. Effects of dietary omega3 and omega6 lipids and vitamin E on chemokine levels in autoimmune-prone MRLMpJ-lprlpr mice. J Nutr Biochem. 2002;13(8):479.

[63] Fernandes G. Dietary lipids and risk of autoimmune disease. Clin Immunol Immunopathol. 1994;72(2):193–7.

[64] Lin BF, Jeng SJ, Chiang BL, Huang CC. Dietary fat affects lipids and anti-cardiolipin antibody levels in autoimmune-prone NZB/W F1 mice. Br J Nutr. 1997;77(4):657–69.

[65] Fritsche K. Fatty acids as modulators of the immune response. Ann Rev Nutr. 2006;26: 45–73.

[66] Reifen R BM, Afek A, Kopilowiz Y, Sklan D, Gershwin ME, German B, Yoshida S, Shoenfeld Y. Dietary polyunsaturated fatty acids decrease anti-dsDNA and anti-cardiolipin antibodies production in idiotype induced mouse model of systemic lupus erythematosus. Lupus. 1998;7(3):192–7.

[67] Chandrasekar B TD, Venkatraman JT, Fernandes G. Dietary omega-3 lipids delay the onset and progression of autoimmune lupus nephritis by inhibiting transforming growth factor beta mRNA and protein expression. J Autoimmunol. 1995;8(3):381–93.

[68] Reynolds CM, Roche HM. Conjugated linoleic acid and inflammatory cell signalling. Prostaglandins Leukot Essent Fatty Acids. 2010;82(4–6):199–204.

[69] Halade GV, Williams PJ, Veigas JM, Barnes JL, Fernandes G. Concentrated fish oil (Lovaza(R)) extends lifespan and attenuates kidney disease in lupus-prone short-lived (NZB×NZW)F1 mice. Exp Biol Med. 2013;238(6):610–22.

[70] Yang M PM, Cook ME. Dietary conjugated linoleic acid protects against end stage disease of systemic lupus erythematosus in the NZB/W F1 mouse. Immunopharmacol Immunotoxicol. 2000;22(3):433–49.

[71] Yang M CM. Dietary conjugated linoleic acid decreased cachexia, macrophage tumor necrosis factor-alpha production, and modifies splenocyte cytokines production. Exp Biol Med. 2003;228(1):51–8.

[72] Lee Y, Vanden Heuvel JP. Inhibition of macrophage adhesion activity by 9trans,11trans-conjugated linoleic acid. J Nutr Biochem. 2010;21(6):490–7.

[73] Dowling JK, McCoy CE, Doyle SL, BenLarbi N, Canavan M, O'Neill LA, et al. Conjugated linoleic acid suppresses IRF3 activation via modulation of CD14. J Nutr Biochem. 2013;24(5):920–8.

[74] Draper E, DeCourcey J, Higgins SC, Canavan M, McEvoy F, Lynch M, et al. Conjugated linoleic acid suppresses dendritic cell activation and subsequent Th17 responses. J Nutr Biochem. 2014;25(7):741–9.

[75] Yu Y CP, Vanden Heuvel JP. Conjugated linoleic acid decreases production of pro-inflammatory products in macrophages: evidence for a PPAR gamma-dependent mechanism. Biochim Biophys Acta. 2002;1581(3):89–99.

[76] Manzel A, Muller DN, Hafler DA, Erdman SE, Linker RA, Kleinewietfeld M. Role of "Western diet" in inflammatory autoimmune diseases. Curr Allergy Asthma Rep. 2014;14(1):404.

[77] Versini M, Jeandel PY, Rosenthal E, Shoenfeld Y. Obesity in autoimmune diseases: not a passive bystander. Autoimmun Rev. 2014;13(9):981–1000.

[78] Harpsoe MC, Basit S, Andersson M, Nielsen NM, Frisch M, Wohlfahrt J, et al. Body mass index and risk of autoimmune diseases: a study within the Danish National Birth Cohort. Int J Epidemiol. 2014;43(3):843–55.

[79] Sinicato NA, Postal M, Peres FA, Pelicari Kde O, Marini R, dos Santos Ade O, et al. Obesity and cytokines in childhood-onset systemic lupus erythematosus. J Immunol Res. 2014;2014:162047.

[80] Amarilyo G, Iikuni N, Shi FD, Liu A, Matarese G, La Cava A. Leptin promotes lupus T-cell autoimmunity. Clin Immunol. 2013;149(3):530–3.

[81] Yu Y, Liu Y, Shi FD, Zou H, Matarese G, La Cava A. Cutting edge: Leptin-induced RORgammat expression in CD4+ T cells promotes Th17 responses in systemic lupus erythematosus. J Immunol. 2013;190(7):3054–8.

[82] Lim H, Kim YU, Sun H, Lee JH, Reynolds JM, Hanabuchi S, et al. Proatherogenic conditions promote autoimmune T helper 17 cell responses in vivo. Immunity. 2014; 40(1):153–65.

[83] Fujita Y, Fujii T, Mimori T, Sato T, Nakamura T, Iwao H, et al. Deficient leptin signaling ameliorates systemic lupus erythematosus lesions in MRL/Mp-Fas lpr mice. J Immunol. 2014;192(3):979–84.

[84] Parker J, Menn-Josephy H, Laskow B, Takemura Y, Aprahamian T. Modulation of lupus phenotype by adiponectin deficiency in autoimmune mouse models. J Clin Immunol. 2011;31(2):167–73.

[85] Bagheri K EP, Naeimi S. Decreased serum level of soluble-leptin-receptor in patients with systemic lupus erythematosus. Iran Red Crescent Med J. 2012;14(9):587–93.

[86] McMahon M, Skaggs BJ, Sahakian L, Grossman J, FitzGerald J, Ragavendra N, et al. High plasma leptin levels confer increased risk of atherosclerosis in women with systemic lupus erythematosus, and are associated with inflammatory oxidised lipids. Ann Rheum Dis. 2011;70(9):1619–24.

[87] Vadacca M, Zardi EM, Margiotta D, Rigon A, Cacciapaglia F, Arcarese L, et al. Leptin, adiponectin and vascular stiffness parameters in women with systemic lupus erythematosus. Intern Emerg Med. 2013;8(8):705–12.

[88] Barbosa Vde S RJ, Antônio da Silva N. Possible role of adipokines in systemic lupus erythematosus and rheumatoid arthritis. Rev Bras Reumatol. 2012;52(2):278–87.

[89] Loghman M HA, Broumand B, Ataipour Y, Tohidi M, Marzbani C, Fakharran M. Association between urinary adiponectin level and renal involvement in systemic lupus erythematous. Int J Rheum Dis. 2016;19(7):678–84.

[90] Gilbert EL, Ryan MJ. High dietary fat promotes visceral obesity and impaired endothelial function in female mice with systemic lupus erythematosus. Gend Med. 2011;8(2):150–5.

[91] Ryan MJ. The pathophysiology of hypertension in systemic lupus erythematosus. Am J Physiol Regul Integr Comp Physiol. 2009;296(4):R1258–67.

[92] Kleinewietfeld M, Manzel A, Titze J, Kvakan H, Yosef N, Linker RA, et al. Sodium chloride drives autoimmune disease by the induction of pathogenic TH17 cells. Nature. 2013;496(7446):518–22.

[93] Wu C, Yosef N, Thalhamer T, Zhu C, Xiao S, Kishi Y, et al. Induction of pathogenic TH17 cells by inducible salt-sensing kinase SGK1. Nature. 2013;496(7446):513–7.

[94] Zou YF, Xu JH, Tao JH, Xu SQ, Liu S, Chen SY, et al. Impact of environmental factors on efficacy of glucocorticoids in Chinese population with systemic lupus erythematosus. Inflammation. 2013;36(6):1424–30.

[95] Khan D, Dai R, Karpuzoglu E, Ahmed SA. Estrogen increases, whereas IL-27 and IFN-gamma decrease, splenocyte IL-17 production in WT mice. Eur J Immunol. 2010;40(9): 2549–56.

[96] Menon R WS, Thomas LN, Allred CD, Dabney A, Azcarate-Peril MA, Sturino JM. Diet complexity and estrogen receptor β status affect the composition of the murine intestinal microbiota. Appl Environ Microbiol. 2013;79(18):5763–73.

[97] Morito K AT, Hirose T, Kinjo J, Hasegawa J, Ogawa S, Inoue S, Muramatsu M, Masamune Y. Interaction of phytoestrogens with estrogen receptors alpha and beta (II). Biol Pharm Bull. 2002;25(1):48–52.

[98] Hong Y WT, Huang C, Cheng W, Lin B. Soy isoflavones supplementation alleviates disease severity in autoimmune-prone MRL-lpr/lpr mice. Lupus. 2008;17(9):814–21.

[99] Zhao JH, Sun SJ, Horiguchi H, Arao Y, Kanamori N, Kikuchi A, et al. A soy diet accelerates renal damage in autoimmune MRL/Mp-lpr/lpr mice. Int Immunopharmacol. 2005;5(11):1601–10.

[100] Hong YH HC, Wang SC, Lin BF. The ethyl acetate extract of alfalfa sprout ameliorates disease severity of autoimmune-prone MRL-lpr/lpr mice. Lupus. 2009;18(3):206–15.

[101] Schoenroth LJ, Hart DA, Pollard KM, Fritzler MJ. The effect of the phytoestrogen coumestrol on the NZB/W F1 murine model of systemic lupus. J Autoimmun. 2004;23(4):323–32.

[102] Akaogi J, Barker T, Kuroda Y, Nacionales DC, Yamasaki Y, Stevens BR, et al. Role of non-protein amino acid L-canavanine in autoimmunity. Autoimmun Rev. 2006;5(6):429–35.

[103] Gilad LA, Tirosh O, Schwartz B. Phytoestrogens regulate transcription and translation of vitamin D receptor in colon cancer cells. J Endocrinol. 2006;191(2):387–98.

[104] Wietzke JA, Welsh J. Phytoestrogen regulation of a Vitamin D3 receptor promoter and 1,25-dihydroxyvitamin D3 actions in human breast cancer cells. J Steroid Biochem Mol Biol. 2003;84(2–3):149–57.

[105] Lechner D, Cross HS. Phytoestrogens and 17beta-estradiol influence vitamin D metabolism and receptor expression-relevance for colon cancer prevention. Recent Results Cancer Res. 2003;164:379–91.

[106] Vieira SM PO, Kriegel MA. Diet, microbiota and autoimmune diseases. Lupus. 2014;23(6):518–26.

[107] Zhang H, Sparks JB, Karyala SV, Settlage R, Luo XM. Host adaptive immunity alters gut microbiota. ISME J. 2015;9(3):770–81.

[108] Kwon HK, Lee CG, So JS, Chae CS, Hwang JS, Sahoo A, et al. Generation of regulatory dendritic cells and CD4+Foxp3+ T cells by probiotics administration suppresses immune disorders. Proc Natl Acad Sci U S A. 2010;107(5):2159–64.

[109] Calcinaro F, Dionisi S, Marinaro M, Candeloro P, Bonato V, Marzotti S, et al. Oral probiotic administration induces interleukin-10 production and prevents spontaneous autoimmune diabetes in the non-obese diabetic mouse. Diabetologia. 2005;48(8):1565–75.

[110] Kunisawa J, Kiyono H. Peaceful mutualism in the gut: revealing key commensal bacteria for the creation and maintenance of immunological homeostasis. Cell Host Microbe. 2011;9(2):83–4.

[111] Jarchum I, Pamer EG. Regulation of innate and adaptive immunity by the commensal microbiota. Curr Opin Immunol. 2011;23(3):353–60.

[112] Brusca SB, Abramson SB, Scher JU. Microbiome and mucosal inflammation as extra-articular triggers for rheumatoid arthritis and autoimmunity. Curr Opin Rheumatol. 2014;26(1):101–7.

[113] Turnbaugh PJ, Ley RE, Mahowald MA, Magrini V, Mardis ER, Gordon JI. An obesity-associated gut microbiome with increased capacity for energy harvest. Nature. 2006;444(7122):1027–31.

[114] De Filippo C, Cavalieri D, Di Paola M, Ramazzotti M, Poullet JB, Massart S, et al. Impact of diet in shaping gut microbiota revealed by a comparative study in children from Europe and rural Africa. Proc Natl Acad Sci U S A. 2010;107(33):14691–6.

[115] Albenberg LG, Wu GD. Diet and the intestinal microbiome: associations, functions, and implications for health and disease. Gastroenterology. 2014;146(6):1564–72.

[116] Huang EY, Leone VA, Devkota S, Wang Y, Brady MJ, Chang EB. Composition of dietary fat source shapes gut microbiota architecture and alters host inflammatory mediators in mouse adipose tissue. J Parenter Enter Nutr. 2013;37(6):746–54.

[117] Hildebrandt MA, Hoffmann C, Sherrill-Mix SA, Keilbaugh SA, Hamady M, Chen YY, et al. High-fat diet determines the composition of the murine gut microbiome independently of obesity. Gastroenterology. 2009;137(5):1716–24 e1–2.

[118] Tlaskalova-Hogenova H, Stepankova R, Hudcovic T, Tuckova L, Cukrowska B, Lodinova-Zadnikova R, et al. Commensal bacteria (normal microflora), mucosal immunity and chronic inflammatory and autoimmune diseases. Immunol Lett. 2004;93(2–3):97–108.

[119] Owyang C, Wu GD. The gut microbiome in health and disease. Gastroenterology. 2014;146(6):1433–6.

[120] Cerf-Bensussan N, Gaboriau-Routhiau V. The immune system and the gut microbiota: friends or foes? Nat Rev Immunol. 2010;10(10):735–44.

[121] Ivanov, II, Atarashi K, Manel N, Brodie EL, Shima T, Karaoz U, et al. Induction of intestinal Th17 cells by segmented filamentous bacteria. Cell. 2009;139(3):485–98.

[122] Wu HJ, Ivanov, II, Darce J, Hattori K, Shima T, Umesaki Y, et al. Gut-residing segmented filamentous bacteria drive autoimmune arthritis via T helper 17 cells. Immunity. 2010;32(6):815–27.

[123] Atarashi K, Tanoue T, Oshima K, Suda W, Nagano Y, Nishikawa H, et al. Treg induction by a rationally selected mixture of Clostridia strains from the human microbiota. Nature. 2013;500(7461):232–6.

[124] Ochoa-Reparaz J, Mielcarz DW, Wang Y, Begum-Haque S, Dasgupta S, Kasper DL, et al. A polysaccharide from the human commensal *Bacteroides fragilis* protects against CNS demyelinating disease. Mucosal Immunol. 2010;3(5):487–95.

[125] Maldonado MA KV, MacDonald GC, Chen F, Reap EA, Balish E, Farkas WR, Jennette JC, Madaio MP, Kotzin BL, Cohen PL, Eisenberg RA. The role of environmental antigens in the spontaneous development of autoimmunity in MRL-lpr mice. J Immunol. 1999;162(11):6322–30.

[126] Hevia A, Milani C, Lopez P, Cuervo A, Arboleya S, Duranti S, et al. Intestinal dysbiosis associated with systemic lupus erythematosus. mBio. 2014;5(5):e01548–14.

[127] de Araujo Navas EA, Sato EI, Pereira DF, Back-Brito GN, Ishikawa JA, Jorge AO, et al. Oral microbial colonization in patients with systemic lupus erythematous: correlation with treatment and disease activity. Lupus. 2012;21(9):969–77.

[128] Smith PM, Howitt MR, Panikov N, Michaud M, Gallini CA, Bohlooly YM, et al. The microbial metabolites, short-chain fatty acids, regulate colonic Treg cell homeostasis. Science. 2013;341(6145):569–73.

[129] Arpaia N, Campbell C, Fan X, Dikiy S, van der Veeken J, deRoos P, et al. Metabolites produced by commensal bacteria promote peripheral regulatory T-cell generation. Nature. 2013;504(7480):451–5.

[130] Furusawa Y, Obata Y, Fukuda S, Endo TA, Nakato G, Takahashi D, et al. Commensal microbe-derived butyrate induces the differentiation of colonic regulatory T cells. Nature. 2013;504(7480):446–50.

[131] Singh V, Kumar A, Raheja G, Anbazhagan AN, Priyamvada S, Saksena S, et al. *Lactobacillus acidophilus* attenuates downregulation of DRA function and expression in inflammatory models. Am J Physiol Gastrointest Liver Physiol. 2014;307(6):G623–31.

[132] Armstrong DL, Zidovetzki R, Alarcon-Riquelme ME, Tsao BP, Criswell LA, Kimberly RP, et al. GWAS identifies novel SLE susceptibility genes and explains the association of the HLA region. Genes Immun. 2014;15(6):347–54.

[133] Cui Y, Sheng Y, Zhang X. Genetic susceptibility to SLE: recent progress from GWAS. J Autoimmun. 2013;41:25–33.

[134] Graham RR, Hom G, Ortmann W, Behrens TW. Review of recent genome-wide association scans in lupus. J Intern Med. 2009;265(6):680–8.

[135] Rullo OJ, Tsao BP. Recent insights into the genetic basis of systemic lupus erythematosus. Ann Rheum Dis. 2013;72(Suppl 2):ii56–61.

[136] Choi JK. Systems biology and epigenetic gene regulation. IET Syst Biol. 2010;4(5):289.

[137] Guo Y, Sawalha AH, Lu Q. Epigenetics in the treatment of systemic lupus erythematosus: potential clinical application. Clin Immunol. 2014;155(1):79–90.

[138] Hedrich CM, Tsokos GC. Epigenetic mechanisms in systemic lupus erythematosus and other autoimmune diseases. Trends Mol Med. 2011;17(12):714–24.

[139] DesJarlais R, Tummino PJ. Role of histone-modifying enzymes and their complexes in regulation of chromatin biology. Biochemistry. 2016;55(11):1584–99.

[140] Hong L, Schroth GP, Matthews HR, Yau P, Bradbury EM. Studies of the DNA binding properties of histone H4 amino terminus. Thermal denaturation studies reveal that acetylation markedly reduces the binding constant of the H4 "tail" to DNA. J Biol Chem. 1993;268(1):305–14.

[141] Xu WS, Parmigiani RB, Marks PA. Histone deacetylase inhibitors: molecular mechanisms of action. Oncogene. 2007;26(37):5541–52.

[142] Reilly CM, Regna N, Mishra N. HDAC inhibition in lupus models. Mol Med. 2011;17(5–6): 417–25.

[143] Choudhary C, Kumar C, Gnad F, Nielsen ML, Rehman M, Walther TC, et al. Lysine acetylation targets protein complexes and co-regulates major cellular functions. Science. 2009;325(5942):834–40.

[144] Li G, Jiang H, Chang M, Xie H, Hu L. HDAC6 alpha-tubulin deacetylase: a potential therapeutic target in neurodegenerative diseases. J Neurol Sci. 2011;304(1–2):1–8.

[145] YangY,RaoR,ShenJ,TangY,FiskusW,NechtmanJ,etal.Roleofacetylationandextracellular location of heat shock protein 90alpha in tumor cell invasion. Cancer Res. 2008;68(12): 4833–42.

[146] de Ruijter AJ, van Gennip AH, Caron HN, Kemp S, van Kuilenburg AB. Histone deacetylases (HDACs): characterization of the classical HDAC family. Biochem J. 2003;370(Pt 3):737–49.

[147] Shakespear MR, Halili MA, Irvine KM, Fairlie DP, Sweet MJ. Histone deacetylases as regulators of inflammation and immunity. Trends Immunol. 2011;32(7):335–43.

[148] Verdin E, Dequiedt F, Kasler HG. Class II histone deacetylases: versatile regulators. Trends Genet. 2003;19(5):286–93.

[149] Martin M, Kettmann R, Dequiedt F. Class IIa histone deacetylases: regulating the regulators. Oncogene. 2007;26(37):5450–67.

[150] Yang XJ, Seto E. The Rpd3/Hda1 family of lysine deacetylases: from bacteria and yeast to mice and men. Nat Rev Mol Cell Biol. 2008;9(3):206–18.

[151] Marks PA, Rifkind RA, Richon VM, Breslow R. Inhibitors of histone deacetylase are potentially effective anticancer agents. Clin Cancer Res. 2001;7(4):759–60.

[152] Dinarello CA, Fossati G, Mascagni P. Histone deacetylase inhibitors for treating a spectrum of diseases not related to cancer. Mol Med. 2011;17(5–6):333–52.

[153] Nagpal R, Kumar M, Yadav AK, Hemalatha R, Yadav H, Marotta F, et al. Gut microbiota in health and disease: an overview focused on metabolic inflammation. Benef Microbes. 2016;7(2):181–94.

[154] Rathmell JC. Metabolism and autophagy in the immune system: immunometabolism comes of age. Immunol Rev. 2012;249(1):5–13.

[155] Scott KP, Gratz SW, Sheridan PO, Flint HJ, Duncan SH. The influence of diet on the gut microbiota. Pharmacol Res. 2013;69(1):52–60.

[156] Imhann F, Vich Vila A, Bonder MJ, Fu J, Gevers D, Visschedijk MC, et al. Interplay of host genetics and gut microbiota underlying the onset and clinical presentation of inflammatory bowel disease. Gut. 2016–312135.

[157] Jiang S, Xie S, Lv D, Zhang Y, Deng J, Zeng L, et al. A reduction in the butyrate producing species *Roseburia* spp. and *Faecalibacterium prausnitzii* is associated with chronic kidney disease progression. Antonie Van Leeuwenhoek. 2016;109(10):1389–96.

[158] Zhang Q, Wu Y, Wang J, Wu G, Long W, Xue Z, et al. Accelerated dysbiosis of gut microbiota during aggravation of DSS-induced colitis by a butyrate-producing bacterium. Sci Rep. 2016;6:27572.

[159] Newman JC, Verdin E. Beta-hydroxybutyrate: much more than a metabolite. Diabetes Res Clin Pract. 2014;106(2):173–81.

[160] Kieback E, Hilgenberg E, Stervbo U, Lampropoulou V, Shen P, Bunse M, et al. Thymus-derived regulatory T cells are positively selected on natural self-antigen through cognate interactions of high functional avidity. Immunity. 2016;44(5):1114–26.

[161] Chang WS, Chiu NC, Chi H, Li WC, Huang FY. Comparison of the characteristics of culture-negative versus culture-positive septic arthritis in children. J Microbiol Immunol Infect. 2005;38(3):189–93.

[162] Zheng Y, Josefowicz S, Chaudhry A, Peng XP, Forbush K, Rudensky AY. Role of conserved non-coding DNA elements in the Foxp3 gene in regulatory T-cell fate. Nature. 2010;463(7282):808–12.

[163] Feng Y, van der Veeken J, Shugay M, Putintseva EV, Osmanbeyoglu HU, Dikiy S, et al. A mechanism for expansion of regulatory T-cell repertoire and its role in self-tolerance. Nature. 2015;528(7580):132–6.

[164] Aoki K, Sato N, Yamaguchi A, Kaminuma O, Hosozawa T, Miyatake S. Regulation of DNA demethylation during maturation of CD4+ naive T cells by the conserved non-coding sequence 1. J Immunol. 2009;182(12):7698–707.

[165] Nutsch K, Chai JN, Ai TL, Russler-Germain E, Feehley T, Nagler CR, et al. Rapid and efficient generation of regulatory T cells to commensal antigens in the periphery. Cell Rep. 2016;17(1):206–20.

[166] Hartigan-O'Connor DJ, Hirao LA, McCune JM, Dandekar S. Th17 cells and regulatory T cells in elite control over HIV and SIV. Curr Opin HIV AIDS. 2011;6(3):221–7.

[167] Shen X, Du J, Guan W, Zhao Y. The balance of intestinal Foxp3+ regulatory T cells and Th17 cells and its biological significance. Expert Rev Clin Immunol. 2014;10(3):353–62.

[168] Nagata DE, Ting HA, Cavassani KA, Schaller MA, Mukherjee S, Ptaschinski C, et al. Epigenetic control of Foxp3 by SMYD3 H3K4 histone methyltransferase controls iTreg development and regulates pathogenic T-cell responses during pulmonary viral infection. Mucosal Immunol. 2015;8(5):1131–43.

[169] Josefowicz SZ, Niec RE, Kim HY, Treuting P, Chinen T, Zheng Y, et al. Extrathymically generated regulatory T cells control mucosal TH2 inflammation. Nature. 2012;482(7385):395–9.

[170] Fernando MR, Saxena A, Reyes JL, McKay DM. Butyrate enhances antibacterial effects while suppressing other features of alternative activation in IL-4-induced macrophages. Am J Physiol Gastrointest Liver Physiol. 2016;310(10):G822–31.

[171] Mishra N, Reilly CM, Brown DR, Ruiz P, Gilkeson GS. Histone deacetylase inhibitors modulate renal disease in the MRL-lpr/lpr mouse. J Clin Invest. 2003;111(4):539–52.

[172] Regna NL, Chafin CB, Hammond SE, Puthiyaveetil AG, Caudell DL, Reilly CM. Class I and II histone deacetylase inhibition by ITF2357 reduces SLE pathogenesis in vivo. Clin Immunol. 2014;151(1):29–42.

[173] Reilly CM, Mishra N, Miller JM, Joshi D, Ruiz P, Richon VM, et al. Modulation of renal disease in MRL/lpr mice by suberoylanilide hydroxamic acid. J Immunol. 2004;173(6):4171–8.

[174] Reilly CM, Thomas M, Gogal R, Jr., Olgun S, Santo A, Sodhi R, et al. The histone deacetylase inhibitor trichostatin A upregulates regulatory T cells and modulates autoimmunity in NZB/W F1 mice. J Autoimmun. 2008;31(2):123–30.

[175] Cantley MD, Haynes DR. Epigenetic regulation of inflammation: progressing from broad acting histone deacetylase (HDAC) inhibitors to targeting specific HDACs. Inflammopharmacology. 2013;21(4):301–7.

[176] Garcia BA, Busby SA, Shabanowitz J, Hunt DF, Mishra N. Resetting the epigenetic histone code in the MRL-lpr/lpr mouse model of lupus by histone deacetylase inhibition. J Proteome Res. 2005;4(6):2032–42.

[177] Lu ZP, Ju ZL, Shi GY, Zhang JW, Sun J. Histone deacetylase inhibitor Trichostatin A reduces anti-DNA autoantibody production and represses IgH gene transcription. Biochem Biophys Res Commun. 2005;330(1):204–9.

[178] Balasubramanian S, Verner E, Buggy JJ. Isoform-specific histone deacetylase inhibitors: the next step? Cancer Lett. 2009;280(2):211–21.

[179] Witt O, Lindemann R. HDAC inhibitors: magic bullets, dirty drugs or just another targeted therapy. Cancer Lett. 2009;280(2):123–4.

[180] Ma J, Yu J, Tao X, Cai L, Wang J, Zheng SG. The imbalance between regulatory and IL-17-secreting CD4+ T cells in lupus patients. Clin Rheumatol. 2010;29(11):1251–8.

[181] Schmidt A, Elias S, Joshi RN, Tegner J. In vitro differentiation of human CD4+FOXP3+ induced regulatory T cells (iTregs) from naive CD4+ T cells using a TGF-beta-containing protocol. J Vis Exp. 2016;(118).

[182] Tao R, de Zoeten EF, Ozkaynak E, Chen C, Wang L, Porrett PM, et al. Deacetylase inhibition promotes the generation and function of regulatory T cells. Nat Med. 2007;13(11):1299–307.

[183] Liu Y, Upadhyaya B, Fardin-Kia AR, Juenemann RM, Dey M. Dietary resistant starch type 4-derived butyrate attenuates nuclear factor-kappa-B1 through modulation of histone H3 trimethylation at lysine 27. Food Funct. 2016;7(9):3772–81.